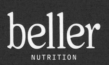

Spice Rack

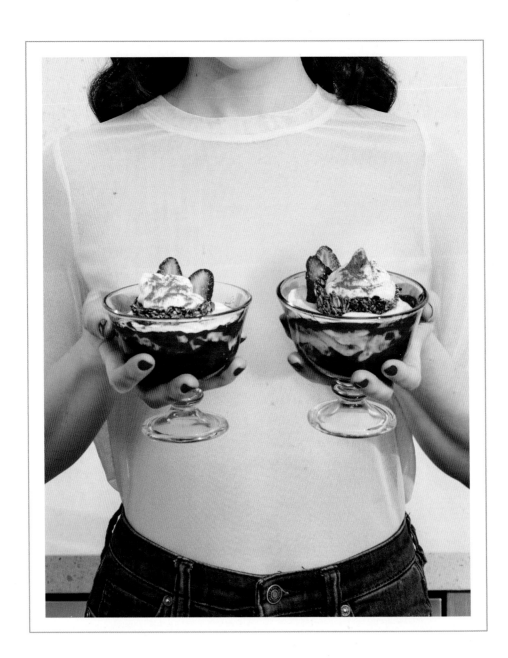

Spice Rack

A *Spicy* Action Plan with Recipes to Reduce
Breast Cancer Risk & Manage Your Weight

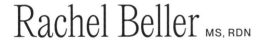

Rachel Beller MS, RDN

YOU
LIVE
RIGHT
PUBLISHERS

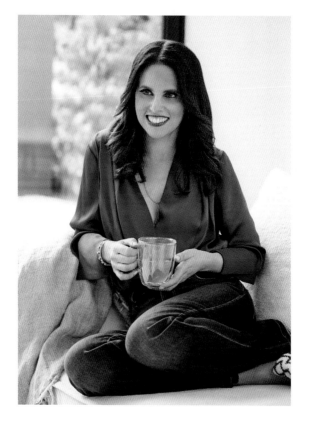

TO MY PARENTS
THE LOVING FORCES OF MY LIFE

TO MY FOUR KIDS
FOR BEING AMAZING & MAKING ME LAUGH DAILY

TO MY HUSBAND
WHO IS MY BEST FRIEND

TO ALL THE THRIVERS & THOSE
TOUCHED BY CANCER
YOU ARE NOT ALONE—
WE'RE IN THIS FIGHT TOGETHER!

Table of Contents

Foreword

When it comes to breast cancer there are two certainties; the first is that every woman who reaches reproductive age faces a risk of breast cancer. The second is that the risk of breast cancer, regardless of what the level of risk is, can be reduced through nutrition and exercise. As a cancer geneticist my practice is focused on how to identify, individualize, and reduce risk for all cancers. Breast cancer is one of the most responsive to diet and lifestyle changes.

Among the known risks for breast cancer, several are unchangeable: age, family history, and genetics. However, I often say, **"Genetics is the switch, but environment turns it on."** For example, Japanese women living in Japan and eating a traditional diet have one of the world's lowest risks for breast cancer. But within one generation of moving to the United States and adopting a Western diet, their risk approaches that of any other woman in the U.S. The foods you choose and the way you eat can be the first step in a life-changing process.

When thinking about breast cancer, genetics plays an increasingly important role in identifying those at high risk. But we know women can carry an ultra-high risk like a BRCA mutation and never get cancer, or conversely be 40 years young with no family history and develop breast cancer. The modifiers of this risk for any one person are complex, but this is where lifestyle, particularly nutrition, exposure, and exercise, have a huge impact. Since this is a cookbook, perhaps the correct analogy for me to use is the following: **"Genetics is the oven, but environment sets the temperature AND can even turn the oven on and off!"**

Rachel Beller, registered dietitian nutritionist, has focused her career on using nutritional science to improve health and wellness and reduce the risk of cancer. She has written a score of cookbooks and *SpiceRack* may be her most important work thus far. It combines a meticulously researched review of literature on nutraceutics (the medicinal property of spices and herbs) with easy-to-follow guidance on how to utilize herbs and spices. The book provides a transformative nutritional framework to reduce inflammation and cancer risk with elegant and delicious recipes.

Her recommendations are easily digested (pun intended!) and written in a warm and empowering style. Readers of *SpiceRack* will come away feeling like they have had hours of a private consultation with an expert dietitian and will have a resource to bookmark pages and return to them whenever needed. In addition, the recipes are simple, flavorful, and achieveable by novice and culinary experts alike.

This book addresses and answers all of the questions I face in my high-risk prevention program including "What can I do to reduce my risk for breast cancer?" "Do soy, dairy, and sugar cause cancer?" And of course "What is the ideal diet for cancer risk reduction and weight loss?" *SpiceRack* breaks down each component of risk and then provides practical, attainable actions to optimize diet for weight management and cancer prevention. For example, level up your anti-cancer nutrition by stirring flaxseed and Ceylon cinnamon into your oatmeal, and adding broccoli sprouts to your salads and smoothies! *SpiceRack* goes beyond any other health or cookbook with a step-by-step guide for goal setting and truly sustainable success based on Rachel Beller's many years as a renowned expert dietitian.

This is a book that will change lives!

—Ora Karp Gordon, MD, MS, FACMG

Medical Director, Providence Clinical Genetics & Genomics Program
Professor of Genetics, St John Cancer Institute
Health Sciences Clinical Professor, UCLA Geffen School of Medicine

Introduction

It all began with a mission:

"To change the way people think about what they choose to put into their bodies, to provide them with a simple action plan for weight management and cancer risk reduction, and to help them feel their amazing best."

How did I get here? In my mid-20s I lost my father to cancer. It was an incredibly challenging time, and I vividly remember how desperate my family was to find credible information about nutrition and cancer. The disappointment and pain from that period in my life ignited a deep sense of passion within me to pursue a career in nutritional oncology and research.

On another personal note, I struggled with my weight in my teens—I wasn't always comfortable wearing the same clothes as my peers and was self-conscious when I went out. I started to experiment with nutrition and by my late teens I noticed that the foods I ate made a big difference in how I felt in my body. In graduate school, I learned the science of nutrition and discovered how to nourish myself in a way that kept the weight off—with a method that was healthy, sustainable, and enjoyable.

I then discovered that research shows there's an undeniable connection between weight management and cancer risk reduction. A light bulb went off. I could take my personal pain from my father's battle with cancer and my weight loss journey and turn it into possibilities for others. I could use my passion and nutritional training to empower those who may be going through similar things: individuals who want to manage their weight to optimize their health, those touched by cancer who are looking to support thrivership, and families searching for evidence-based guidance for their loved one.

After I became a dietitian, I worked in front-line breast cancer research for 10 years before opening my own practice in Beverly Hills where I'm able to combine my effective approach for weight management with my passion for cancer risk reduction. I know that navigating food choices when it comes to breast cancer can be overwhelming and confusing. So I created an action plan that applies my years of research and practice into an all-in-one and easy-to-follow method. Over time I have been able to expand my message via community outreach programs, giving lectures to doctors and medical staff, sitting on medical advisory boards, and educating the world via media outlets.

But there was a gap that I kept seeing on bookshelves when it came to nutrition and breast cancer books. On one hand, there were dry textbook-like volumes that didn't show you how to eat; on the other hand there were anti-cancer cookbooks that didn't include the science or provide guidance for day-to-day eating outside of recipe guidelines.

There wasn't anything that explained the research of breast cancer and nutrition (and there's a lot!) in an approachable manner and translated that to day-to-day life. So I was inspired to write *SpiceRack*.

I know that it is essential to understand the WHY behind the method–it creates motivation to follow through, for life. So the first section of this book distills what research has revealed about breast cancer nutrition in an accessible, action-oriented way. The recipes in the second section are SO easy and SO tasty–it makes the method do-able with flexibility and sustainability. It's not about rules. It's about understanding nutrition principles that will forever change the way you think and feel about your food choices.

I know from experience that boring diets get dropped, fast. But this isn't a diet—it's a lifestyle. And it's not boring—it's Power Spiced up and I guarantee it'll keep things flavorful.

Spices are the easiest, most powerful way to completely transform the nutritional value of your meal with literally just a pinch! There have been thousands of studies revealing potent anti-inflammatory, antioxidant, and potential anti-cancer properties of spices. I've spent hundreds of hours sifting through the evidence and

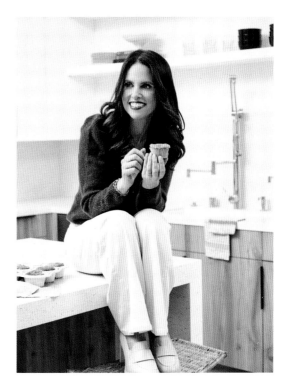

have picked out my top picks for breast cancer risk reduction–consistently spicing can have a cumulative benefit and may help protect your rack against cancer.

If you're ready to feel EMPOWERED and forever change how you think about what you choose to put in your body while optimizing your health, I'm here for you.

I wish that I could be right there with you in your kitchen, explaining the science and cooking a delicious (and spicy!) meal with you! Through *SpiceRack*, I hope that I can come close–think of me as holding your hand through this nutrition journey so that you can have clarity and confidence about what you're choosing to put into your body. For now, and for life.

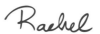

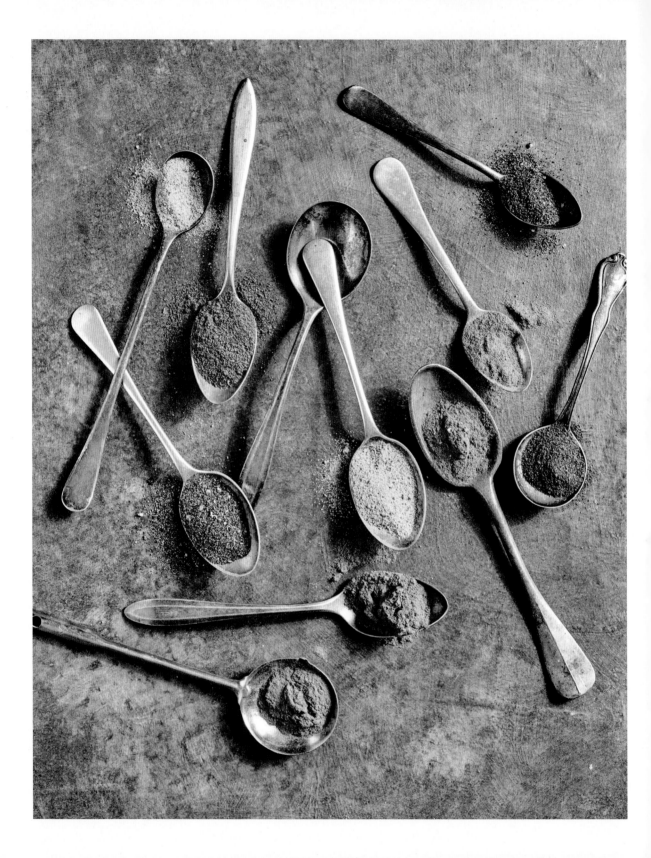

Discover the Power of Spicing

DAILY POWER—AND FLAVOR—IN JUST A PINCH
WHY POWER SPICE?

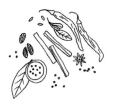

Power Spicing is about elevating your food beyond the basics. Spices are incredibly powerful when it comes to potential anti-cancer, antioxidant, and anti-inflammatory properties–that is why Power Spicing is central to my strategic nutrition plan. By adding spices to your daily routine, you can transform any meal or snack into a supercharged (and delicious) nutritional opportunity. I've incorporated my top spices for breast cancer risk reduction into the recipes in section 2 of this book. Your job is to keep spicing and reap the cumulative benefits over time.

Discover the Power of Spicing

DAILY POWER—AND FLAVOR—IN JUST A PINCH
WHY POWER SPICE?

I love spices—*naturally*—and think everyone should use them.

Not only do spices take healthy dishes from bland to in-demand (oatmeal? no problem! steamed broc? bring it on!), but my years of research have revealed that spices also add "daily power" in the form of nutritional value and potent cancer protective properties...the spice rack that you have in your kitchen is actually a useful tool for breast cancer risk reduction!

SpiceRack is an actionable plan for breast cancer risk reduction and more, and Power Spicing is the secret sauce that elevates the method beyond the basics. This chapter unlocks the power of spices and reveals how just a pinch can dramatically double—*or even triple*—the nutritional value and cancer-fighting potential of your meals. It explains WHY I've titled this book "*SpiceRack*"—there is immense value in using spices liberally and consistently to level up your nutrition. Power Spicing is an absolutely essential concept of *SpiceRack*.

For thousands of years, cultures around the world have prized spices not only for their culinary prowess, but also for their medicinal powers. Our ancestors were onto something—a convincing and growing body of modern research is uncovering a wealth of health benefits conveyed by spices.

In 2013, I read an article by the American Institute for Cancer Research that described how just a pinch of spices could deliver a significant amount of anti-inflammatory, cancer-protective benefits. That piqued my interest, and I dove into the scientific literature to find out more. And there was much, much more: in just the past five years, more than 1,900 studies have been conducted on turmeric, 1,600 on cayenne, 1,400 on garlic, 800 on cloves, 750 on cinnamon...the list goes on and on!

Spices and herbs are *the most* concentrated source of antioxidants and phytochemicals—yes, even more than berries, tea, and dark chocolate, and are far more powerful and sustainable than vitamin and supplement pills Americans pour millions of dollars into every year.

Then there's my favorite discovery, which I dubbed "Spice Synergy." When used in combination, certain spices can boost each other's nutritional effects. Think of these combos as the ultimate power couples (and trios, and more). For example, a compound in parsley called quercetin can actually help your body better absorb turmeric's anti-inflammatory nutrient called curcumin...so using parsley and turmeric together yields a more powerful effect. I'll teach you which spices to combine and how to create optimal blends for breast cancer risk reduction.

All of this research and experimenting with spice combos forever changed the way I think about spices. I've found that they are such a simple way to truly transform the nutritional profile of your diet...and I'll explain why. Plus it's an easy habit to sustain—incorporate Power Spicing into your daily routine and you'll have cumulative benefits, for life!

5 Irresistible Reasons to Spice Up Your Life

Don't just take my word for it. Let's dive into what literally hundreds of scientific studies have revealed about the power of spices! Aside from tasting great, here are my TOP reasons why Spicing is essential for optimal breast cancer risk reduction.

 SPICES HAVE MAJOR ANTI-CANCER PROPERTIES

Think of spices as jacks of all trades—they may fight cancer via a multitude of cellular mechanisms. Scientific studies show that dozens of compounds in spices may inhibit cancer cell growth, prevent cancer cell proliferation, block tumor spread (metastasis), and even kill malignant cells. Other compounds may bolster your immune system so that it can effectively work to fight tumor cells. Still other compounds may block the growth of blood vessels to tumor sites, cutting off cancer's access to nutrients and fuel. And as we'll learn in a few pages, spices are incredibly concentrated in antioxidant and anti-inflammatory compounds, which may help keep regular cells from transforming into cancerous ones.

There are hundreds of studies on spices and their anti-cancer effects (there's evidence for breast, colon, gastric, lung, prostate, skin cancer...and more), but let's just focus in on some of the star spices for breast cancer:

- **Parsley's** star player is apigenin, a flavonoid that may exert anti-estrogenic activities. Apigenin also has been shown to prevent

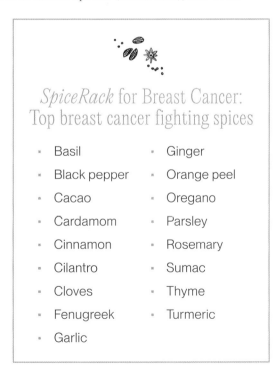

SpiceRack for Breast Cancer:
Top breast cancer fighting spices

· Basil	· Ginger
· Black pepper	· Orange peel
· Cacao	· Oregano
· Cardamom	· Parsley
· Cinnamon	· Rosemary
· Cilantro	· Sumac
· Cloves	· Thyme
· Fenugreek	· Turmeric
· Garlic	

the proliferation of breast cancer tumor cells and inhibit a cancer cell's ability to take in fuel.

- **Turmeric** contains curcumin, an intensely powerful anti-inflammatory and anti-cancer compound. It's been shown that curcumin may inhibit the expression of a gene that may lead to breast cancer, which may reduce risk. Research also indicates it may halt metastasis, block cancer cell growth, and kill tumor cells.

- **Orange peel's** fragrant oils contain the compounds hesperidin and D-limonene. Both of these have been shown to fight breast cancer cells—hesperidin may reduce tumor cell proliferation and damage cancer cell DNA, and D-limonene may boost the actions of enzymes that break down carcinogens. And I bet you didn't know: orange peels are a more concentrated source of antioxidants than the pulp!

- **Cacao**—yes, the source of chocolate—is absolutely packed with polyphenols (namely epicatechin and catechin), which have major anti-cancer effects. Lab studies show these polyphenols may inhibit cancer cell growth and spread, and may even cause cancer cell death. They may also boost your body's natural antioxidant enzymes, thus protecting your own cells against cellular damage that could contribute to cancer risk.

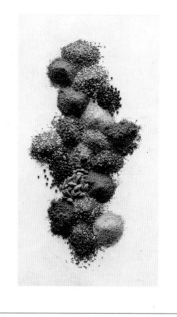

Scientific studies show that dozens of compounds in spices may inhibit cancer cell growth.

- **Rosemary's** leaves contain an essential oil rich in three acids (carnosic, rosmarinic, and ursolic acid) that work together on a cellular level to magnify their antioxidant and anti-inflammatory effects. These acids have been shown to inhibit DNA damage that may lead to cancerous cells, and may inhibit the spread of breast cancer tumor cells. Rosemary extract may also modify estrogen metabolism and decrease the viability of HER2+ breast cancer tumor cells.

- **Cardamom's** phytochemicals may activate the activity of our immune system's natural "tumor killing" cells, making it an all-star cancer fighter. Specifically, the compounds cineole and limonene have been shown to slow and possibly reverse breast cancer development.

- **Sumac** is rich in multiple antioxidant phytochemicals and also may help improve the action of our body's natural antioxidant enzymes. Altogether its antioxidant properties are especially powerful in protecting DNA from damage, which may help reduce cancer risk. Research has found it to potentially decrease the ability of breast cancer cells to grow and metastasize.

Those are just a few examples of the proposed anti-cancer cellular mechanisms of spices—the emerging research is exciting. While many of these studies are still at the cellular and laboratory level, scientists have started to investigate the use of spice phytochemicals in cancer treatment in clinical trials. These studies take time...but while we're awaiting the results, let's keep Spicing Up all our meals (and snacks) for optimal health and flavor.

 SPICES ARE THE #1 SOURCES OF ANTIOXIDANT AND ANTI-INFLAMMATORY COMPOUNDS

Maybe you've heard everything you need to know about antioxidants, but if not, let me tell you why they should be as big a fixture of your diet as protein and fiber.

Antioxidants are compounds that repair your body on a cellular level. They do so by neutralizing unstable molecules called free radicals, which are chemicals that damage cells and potentially contribute to cancer development. Therefore, antioxidants help protect your body by preventing undue damage to cellular structures including DNA. They preserve your cellular function and ultimately may help reduce risk of cancer development.

Your body makes a small amount of natural antioxidants, but it largely relies on dietary sources. And while it may be tempting to want to take antioxidant supplements, scientific studies have consistently found that antioxidant supplements have not been beneficial in cancer prevention. Instead, major research organizations like the American Cancer Society

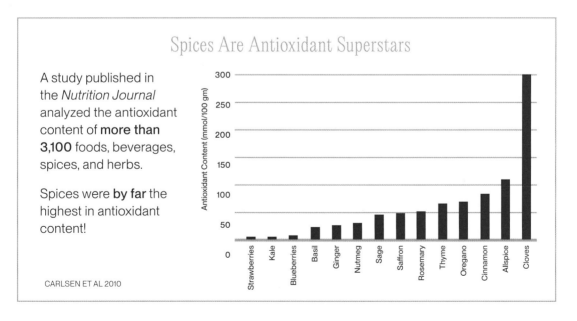

Spices Are Antioxidant Superstars

A study published in the *Nutrition Journal* analyzed the antioxidant content of **more than 3,100** foods, beverages, spices, and herbs.

Spices were **by far** the highest in antioxidant content!

CARLSEN ET AL 2010

and the American Institute of Cancer Research urge people to get their antioxidant fix from whole plant foods.

Now, once upon a time everyone thought blueberries were the best source of antioxidants. But today we know that spices outshine produce *by far*. A 2010 study by Harvard and the University of Oslo tested over 3,100 foods, and they made some eye-opening discoveries. For example, just a mere teaspoon of ground cloves has around 50% more antioxidant content than a half cup of blueberries. And if you add just a few pinches of cinnamon and nutmeg, you more than double your antioxidant dose.

Just a Pinch makes a big Punch! Let's dig into some science to explain. One way scientists measure the antioxidant value of a food is by measuring its FRAP value (ferric-reducing ability of plasma). These measurements allow us to roughly calculate how spices transform a meal. The higher the FRAP value, the better. Here's a real-life example:

A bowl of oatmeal mixed with plant-based milk has an antioxidant value of approximately 136 calculated via FRAP assay. One teaspoon of

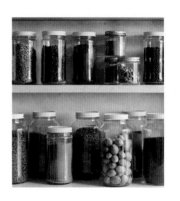

Spices contain phytochemicals that turn down pro-inflammatory cellular processes in the body, and turn up anti-inflammatory ones.

a spice mix made with Ceylon cinnamon, cacao, and turmeric has an antioxidant value of 1,156. When you add the spice mix to the oats, the total antioxidant value jumps to 1,292— a 9.5 times increase!

I can't emphasize enough how easy it is to radically boost the antioxidant content with just a few pinches of spices. Spices are REALLY that powerful...and the transformation is REALLY that easy. Not to mention the flavor upgrade you'll get as well!

Now let's move on to inflammation. Inflammation in itself isn't bad...it's your body's natural response to injury and illness. The swelling, heat, and redness that comes as a result of a cut or bacterial infection helps your body heal. Inflammation becomes a problem when it is long term, otherwise known as chronic. Chronic inflammation has been linked to some cancers, rheumatoid arthritis, heart disease, Alzheimer's disease, and more. Studies have shown that high levels of inflammation (measured via cellular inflammatory markers like tumor necrosis factor alpha, interleukin-6, and C reactive protein) play a role in the development of breast cancer.

So what is one thing you can do? Bring on the spices, of course! Research consistently shows that spices contain phytochemicals that turn down pro-inflammatory cellular processes in the body, and turn up anti-inflammatory ones.

One of my favorite studies comes from scientists at the University of Florida and Penn State. They wanted to see if eating spices can actually reduce the inflammatory markers in your blood. The researchers had participants in the intervention group eat about a half teaspoon of spices or herbs for a week (ginger, rosemary, turmeric, and cloves); participants in the control group did not eat the spices. Then they drew some blood samples and dripped them onto human white blood cells in a petri dish that had been exposed to inflammation.

The scientists found that the blood from participants who ate the spices resulted in significantly lower levels of a chemical called TNF-alpha, which means that the blood lowered inflammation levels. They also found there were less DNA strand breaks, indicating that the spices conveyed more antioxidant activity. These are amazing results! With just ½ teaspoon of spice intake per day over the course of seven days, there was a measurable change in the antioxidant and anti-inflammatory activity. Now, imagine if you were Spicing for years!

 SPICES MAY HELP WITH WEIGHT MANAGEMENT

As you'll read in the following chapter, weight management is essential for breast cancer risk reduction. Of course, weight loss is dependent on a nutritious diet and active lifestyle—you can't expect to drop a dress size simply by Spicing while still eating donuts and burgers all day (if only it were that easy!). But spices *do* offer a little extra help when the going's tough. I like to think of them as "sprinkles of support."

Let's look at cayenne, for example. Its major compound is capsaicin, which has been shown to burn an additional 50 calories a day—plus it may help reduce your appetite. While this sounds like a small boost, it can really add up over time. A 2014 study demonstrated that just a half teaspoon of cumin may lead to greater weight loss. And other spices such as fenugreek, ginger, nutmeg, and orange peel have been shown to regulate digestion and reduce feelings of hunger by activating hormones that make you feel full.

 SPICES NOURISH YOUR GUT MICROBIOME

Spices have antibacterial effects against disease-causing microorganisms—some herb extracts even work as natural food preservatives—but they actually have positive effects on the all-important bacteria in our guts.

As you will read in the fiber chapter, we have trillions of bacteria that live within our digestive tract, collectively, called the gut microbiome. It's been shown that a healthy gut is key to reducing breast cancer risk—a healthy balance of bacteria results in proper toxin detoxification and estrogen metabolism. Fiber is key to maintaining a healthy gut microbiome, but what you may not know (but can likely guess!) is that spices can also affect our microbiome.

A key 2017 study published by scientists at UCLA's Center for Human Nutrition found that extracts of black pepper, cayenne, cinnamon, ginger, oregano, and rosemary promoted the growth of helpful bacteria from the families *Bifidobacterium* and *Lactobacillus*—the same types found in most commercial probiotics. In addition, the spices inhibited growth of nasty microbes from the *Fusobacterium, Clostridium,* and *Ruminococcus* groups—the ones found in unhealthy digestive tracts.

Although more research needs to be done, there is great potential for everyday spices and herbs to regulate the gut microbiome, all while making our dishes delicious.

⑤ SPICES HELP YOU EAT MORE WHOLESOME FOOD!

Speaking of delicious, who wouldn't get bored of steamed broccoli or plain oatmeal? The best eating pattern is the one you stick with, and from years of working with patients, I know that boring diets get dropped in no time.

Spices can amp up food without adding any calories. If you want to take those Brussels sprouts from zero to zapper, just add a few pinches of paprika, turmeric, pepper, and cayenne, plus a squeeze of lemon. For a savory-sweet twist, add cumin, cinnamon, paprika, and pepper. As for oatmeal, dress it for success by decking it out with some cinnamon and orange peel for a bright flavor, or cacao, turmeric, and ginger for a warmer note. The possibilities are endless—and exciting.

As with antioxidants, I do *not* recommend relying on supplements alone that consist of isolated compounds from spices such as curcumin from turmeric, or EGCG from matcha. Whole, real spices contain multiple phytochemicals—turmeric doesn't just contain curcumin; it also contains carotenoids, xanthophylls, and eugenol, which all have their own benefits. Don't miss out on these other nutrients with an isolated supplement. And you'd be neglecting Spice Synergy and the unique effects that spices have to augment the daily nutritional power of your foods. Plus, supplements may be contaminated with who-knows-what (the lack of regulation in the supplement industry is a story for another day!).

> Spices and herbs are the most concentrated source of antioxidants and phytochemicals—pinches of goodness add up to greatness.

Instead, I tell my patients to *get real* by eating a variety of natural, whole fruit and vegetables, and adding a wide range of spices and herbs. And they should do it consistently—over time, pinches of goodness add up to greatness!

Spice Synergy

While one spice is nice, don't stop there. Scientific studies have revealed that certain spice combinations may act together to boost each other's nutritional effects on a cellular level. Think of these as the ultimate power couples...or trios...or more!

There are 3 main categories of Spice Synergy:

Absorption Enhancers: Optimal absorption is key. Absorption enhancers are special spices that research has shown may boost each other's absorption, bioavailability, and utilization of the potent health-promoting compounds.

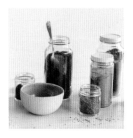

- **Cacao + matcha**

- **Cacao + turmeric**

- **Turmeric + parsley**

- **Black pepper + almost anything!**

  Black pepper is the ultimate sidekick. It works by enhancing our body's digestive and transportation enzymes by increasing blood flow to the gastrointestinal tract to help with nutrient absorption, and by slowing down the breakdown and elimination of certain healthy compounds. Researchers have found it may only take about ⅛ of a teaspoon of black pepper to yield these effects.

- **Black pepper + basil**

- **Black pepper + cayenne**

- **Black pepper + matcha**

- **Black pepper + paprika**

- **Black pepper + turmeric**—may enhance the effectiveness of curcumin, the anti-cancer compound in turmeric, by up to 2,000%!

- **Black pepper + almost any food:** it may enhance bioavailability of vitamins A, C, D, E, and B vitamins, selenium, magnesium, calcium, and iron!

Synergistic Action: Certain phytochemicals in spices and herbs have synergistic properties, meaning they may enhance each other's actions on a cellular level. This applies to antioxidant, anti-inflammatory, or disease-fighting effects!

- **Cacao + turmeric** = may work together to inhibit cancer cell growth

- **Cacao + cayenne** = may promote cancer cell death

- **Cayenne + matcha** = may have ten times greater inhibition of cancer cell growth

- **Ginger + cinnamon + matcha** = may regulate glucose levels to lower the risk of diabetes

- **Cumin + coriander** = increased antioxidant and antimicrobial properties

- **Garlic + fenugreek** = augmented antioxidant effect

- **Rosemary + turmeric** = may work together to have anti-cancer effects

- **Oregano + basil + thyme** = synergistic antimicrobial effect

- **Cumin + thyme** = boosted antimicrobial properties

- **Cardamom + turmeric** = may help prevent stomach ulcers

Double Dose: Some health-enhancing phytochemicals are found in multiple spices, so you can double up on the flavor and the benefits. Other compounds work toward the same health goal possibly via different chemical pathways. My motto: let's power up our meals from many angles!

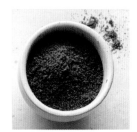

- **Ginger + cinnamon + cardamom + saffron** = may promote heart health

- **Basil + rosemary + thyme** = may also promote heart health

- **Garlic + onion** = may reduce the risk of cancer

- **Paprika + cayenne** = concentrated antioxidant and anti-inflammatory benefits

- **Turmeric + fenugreek** = may lower cholesterol levels

- **Garlic + turmeric** = may promote heart health

- **Saffron + turmeric + black pepper** = may decrease the risk of Alzheimer's disease

- **Garlic + ginger + cayenne** = may decrease cholesterol levels

Those are just some of the synergistic interactions that have been revealed so far in research studies—but there are potentially *so many more* that exist that we just haven't discovered yet. Spices really are better together!

Power Spicing Blends

Because of all the amazing benefits of spices, I've prescribed Spicing to my patients, lecture and television audiences, and masterclass participants for years. In 2017 I launched my own line of carefully crafted organic spice blends called Rachel Beller's Power Pantry as a cumulation of my research and experimentation with various spice combinations. My spice blends take advantage of Spice Synergy and prioritize spices that have been shown to potentially reduce cancer risk—and taste delicious together yet are universal for everyday use. I love being able to easily harness the power of spices as part of my Power Pantry, and it's been amazing to hear how people all over the globe have been able to use my spice blends to upgrade their nutrition. The blends are used in the recipes throughout this book—but of course, I've included substitutions.

Here's a quick overview of the Spice Synergy in my Power Pantry blends:

VEGITUDE POWER BLEND:

This is my specially formulated breast cancer protective blend— I chose each ingredient for its breast health benefits (and for the flavor, of course!).

- **Garlic and onion** have both been linked to lower breast cancer risk—they have been shown to have biologically active compounds that may potentially inhibit carcinogens, protect cell DNA, and suppress tumor cell proliferation.

- **Turmeric's** key nutrient, called curcumin, may block cancer cell growth, kill tumor cells, and halt metastasis.

- **Black pepper** may enhance the absorption of curcumin by up to 2,000%.

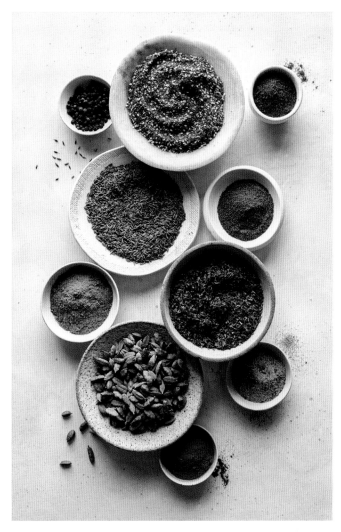

- **Parsley** is rich in apigenin, which is an antioxidant, that may have anti-estrogenic properties. It also contains quercetin, which may also improve curcumin absorption.

- All five of these spices also reduce inflammation.

EVERYTHING SAVORY BLEND:

Each spice in this all-purpose flavorful blend has research-supported cancer-fighting and anti-inflammatory effects...but the real magic of the blend lies in its all-star spice combos that work together to support your health.

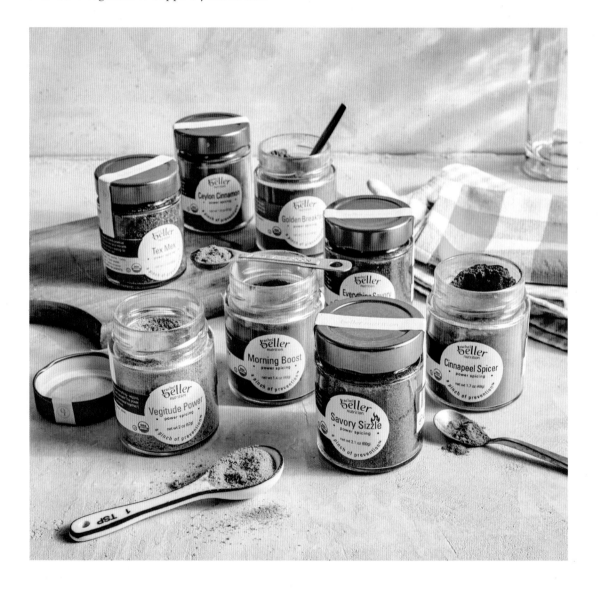

- **Cayenne** contains capsaicin, which may help burn fat. Additionally, cayenne has been shown to potentially kill tumor cells, stimulate digestion, and reduce inflammation.

- **Paprika** contains the antioxidants capsaicin, beta-carotene, and zeaxanthin, plus compounds such as capsanthin and capsorubin—exclusively found in paprika—which may reduce chronic inflammation.

- **Garlic's** main flavor-booster, allicin, has at least 33 active compounds, which have been shown to have potential anti-cancer properties.

- **Cumin** is rich in antioxidants and has potential weight loss benefits—which may help with risk reduction.

- **Paprika + Cayenne** provide a double dose of antioxidant and anti-inflammatory benefits from capsaicin.

- **Turmeric and Black Pepper** are a synergistic pair for cancer risk reduction as described above.

SAVORY SIZZLE BLEND:

This blend has the same ingredients as Everything Savory, but in different proportions to give a spicy kick...crank up the heat and nutritional power of your dish with this all-purpose flavor booster.

CINNAPEEL SPICER BLEND:

This is my go-to breakfast blend (but not limited to breakfast, of course) that delivers natural sweetness with a mild hint of citrus!

- **Ceylon Cinnamon** is "true" cinnamon—a lighter, sweeter version with 1,200 times less coumarin (a potential liver-toxic compound) than the standard grocery store cinnamon. It may regulate blood sugars, improve insulin sensitivity, and limit cancer cell growth.

- **Orange Peel** contains hesperidin and D-limonene, which may have antioxidant, anti-inflammatory, and anti-cancer effects. Bonus: it may also help suppress appetite and protect the liver from toxins.

- **Ginger** has 60+ phytonutrients, some of which may have anti-cancer effects (reduce cancer cell proliferation, alter gene expression, and decrease inflammation). Ginger may even help with weight loss by suppressing fat cell creation and helping you feel full after meals.

- All three spices may help with blood sugar control.

- All three spices have potential anti-cancer and anti-inflammatory effects.

GOLDEN BREAKFAST BLEND:

Everyone loves chocolate, but this blend takes it to the next level with a few key ingredients that spice up the sweetness! Each spice has major anti-inflammatory effects. In addition:

- **Cacao** is packed with polyphenols, which have been shown to potentially inhibit cancer cell growth and boost your body's natural antioxidant enzymes.

- **Cacao and turmeric** synergistically work together: the quercetin in cacao may enhance curcumin (in turmeric) absorption.

- **Ceylon cinnamon** has potential anti-cancer and blood sugar balancing properties.

MORNING BOOST BLEND:

This adds a warm, spicy-sweet depth (think apple pie!) to your breakfasts, smoothies, and snacks—along with an incredible boost of anti-inflammatory, antioxidant, and potential anti-cancer benefits.

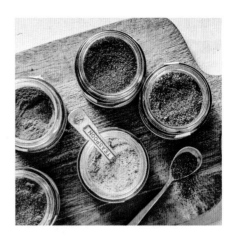

It's been shown that small amounts, from $1/8$ teaspoon to $1/2$ teaspoon, can exert significant actions on a cellular level to help reduce cancer risk, lower inflammation, and maintain cellular health.

- **Cloves** are ranked as the #1 food in terms of antioxidant content, and may have 3-15 times the antioxidant value compared to other spices and herbs.

- **Nutmeg** has major anti-inflammatory and possible anti-cancer properties.

- **Allspice's** major component, eugenol, has been shown to have potential anti-cancer, antioxidant, and anti-inflammatory activity.

- **Ginger** has over 60 powerful anti-inflammatory, antioxidant, and anti-cancer compounds.

- **Ceylon Cinnamon,** along with ginger, nutmeg, and allspice, may work to reduce blood sugar levels, which may in turn improve insulin sensitivity.

TEX MEX BLEND:

There's a lot of taco and chili spices out there, but this one kicks it up a notch with powerful antioxidant and anti-inflammatory spices. We've mentioned many of them above—paprika, cumin, garlic, onion, oregano, cloves, ancho chili, and a touch of Ceylon cinnamon. The result is a perfectly balanced, deep and savory blend that adds a not-too-spicy yet delicious flair (but without the added junk that's found in typical taco seasonings)!

Spice Up Your Day

Remember the concept of Antioxidant Meal Transformation we discussed a few pages ago? A spice blend will easily transform a simple dish into one that may help with cancer risk reduction in a multitude of ways. So here's some sage advice: adding pinches of spices a nd spice blends can have a cumulative effect over time! Even small amounts, from ⅛ to ½ teaspoon, can exert significant actions on a cellular level to help reduce cancer risk, lower inflammation, and maintain cellular health. Take every opportunity to Power Spice and savor the flavorful journey ahead—one pinch at a 'thyme'! Enjoy the power of spicing!

I'm talking about your:

- Beverages

- Breakfast

- Lunch

- Dinner

- Snacks

- Dessert

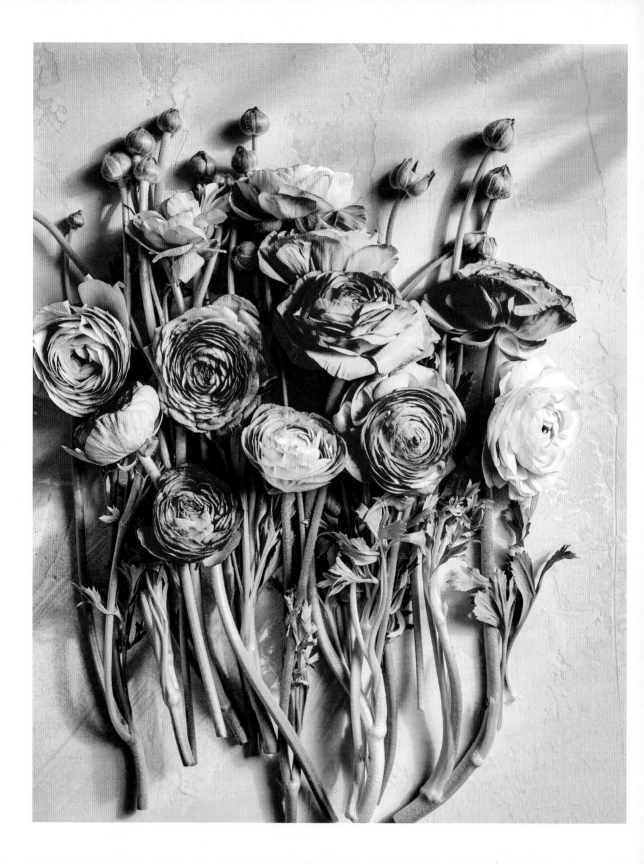

Consider the Weight Connection

Excess body fat is a strong driver of breast cancer risk. Research shows being overweight increases the hormones estrogen, insulin, and IGF-1, and these imbalances may be linked to the increased risk for cancer diagnosis, recurrence, and mortality. The good news is there are actionable steps you can take right now to help you lose excess weight in a healthy, sustainable way. I'll provide you with recipes and a clear nutrition plan rooted in science to help you reduce your risk of breast cancer and feel more confident and empowered about what you eat.

But before we dive into the recipes, let me first walk you through some of the foundational principles and explain the science behind the method.

Consider the Weight Connection

I spent the early part of my career working in cancer research, and over those years I came to realize the following: there's an undeniable connection between weight, estrogen, and cancer risk reduction. According to the World Health Organization, "overweight" and "obesity" are defined as abnormal or excessive fat accumulation that presents a risk to health. The number on the scale can increase if you increase muscle mass (which is a good thing!), so I want to be clear I am referencing increased body fat when discussing being overweight or gaining weight. Research has shown that excess body fat is a significant cancer risk factor, and losing the excess weight may be helpful. But losing weight isn't just about how we look and reducing clothing sizes; nor does it mean that you'll have to be on a boring, cardboard-food diet. And you're not powerless—the Beller Method is crafted to help with weight management and cancer risk reduction, for life! Before we dive into the Method, let's take a brief look at what the research says about weight status and breast cancer risk...

Being overweight increases the risk of diagnosis: Being overweight (defined in research as a BMI of 25-29.9 kg/m²) has been linked to higher risk of being diagnosed with postmenopausal breast cancer compared to maintaining a healthy mid-range weight (defined as a BMI of 18.5-25 kg/m²). How much higher? Studies show that women who are overweight after menopause have a *30-60%* increased risk of a breast cancer diagnosis! Though many of these studies are done with postmenopausal cases, it's never too early to be mindful about keeping weight in check and starting with a risk-reduction strategy.

Note: A small amount of research has shown that being overweight is associated with a lower risk of being diagnosed with *premenopausal* breast cancer. But this research is not significant enough to change my recommendation (or any major cancer organization's recommendations) to strive for a healthy balanced weight. Excessive weight gain should still be avoided for a myriad of reasons, breast health aside (think diabetes, inflammatory diseases, and heart disease prevention). Plus, many breast cancer diagnoses happen *after* menopause, and weight gain in early adulthood is likely to carry into your postmenopausal years. And I'll explain later that maintaining or losing weight throughout your whole adult life confers the lowest risk of breast cancer.

Weight gain, specifically through having excess body fat, may also increase breast cancer risk: Gaining weight over the course of your adult life also increases the risk of postmenopausal breast cancer. Over 87,000 women from the famous Nurse's Health Study were followed in an analysis that showed that women who gained 20 pounds after age 18 had a 15% higher risk of postmenopausal breast cancer compared to women who gained little or no weight. And a 55-pound gain was related to a 45% higher risk! Here's another way to demonstrate this point: A UK study published in the *British Medical Journal* reported that every 2 inch increase in waist circumference increased breast cancer risk by about 33%.

Excess weight is linked to a higher breast cancer mortality rate and risk of recurrence: The connection between high weight and breast cancer doesn't just exist for the initial diagnosis. A study published in the *Annals of Oncology* looked at 213,000 breast cancer survivors and found that mortality from breast cancer was 35% higher for obese women (obesity is defined as a BMI over 30 kg/m^2) than for women within the normal weight range. Another study discovered that for every 11 pounds a breast cancer patient gains, her mortality risk increases by 11%. We also have evidence that obesity is associated with a 35-40% higher rate of recurrence.

Why Does the Connection Exist?

Let's look at the science, not just at the numbers. On a molecular level, there are a few explanations why being overweight or obese has been linked to increased breast cancer risk, mortality, and recurrence rates. We'll focus on three important hormones: **estrogen, insulin, and insulin-like growth factor 1 (IGF-1).**

Estrogen is a hormone that helps develop breast tissue, regulate menstrual cycles, and more. But an excess amount of estrogen in the blood (and high lifetime exposure to estrogen) has been tied to breast cancer risk. This is because of:

- Its role in stimulating breast cell division

- Its action during critical times of breast growth and development

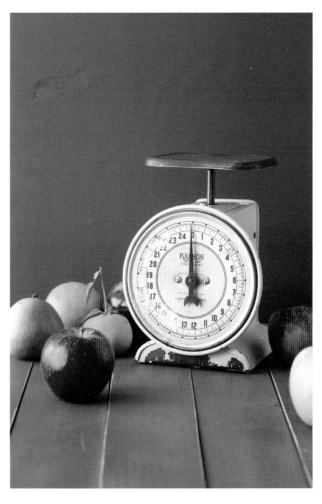

- Its effects on other hormones that stimulate breast cell division

- Its support of the growth of estrogen-responsive tumors (70% of breast cancers are estrogen-receptor positive)

After menopause, fat tissue becomes the main site of estrogen production. So having more fat tissue increases the amount of estrogen that's produced and is circulating in the blood. It's been shown that with increasing fat tissue, there is a significant increase in estrogen levels.

Another key hormone tied to weight and breast cancer is insulin. One of insulin's functions is to facilitate the transport of glucose (aka sugar) from your bloodstream, into your body's cells. Being overweight tends to be linked with high blood sugar levels, which requires higher insulin levels. When you have high insulin levels over time, your body becomes desensitized to the effects of insulin, and therefore needs to produce even *more* insulin to deal with the sugar rush. Insulin, in turn, activates a growth hormone called insulin-like growth factor 1 (IGF-1 for short). While regular levels of IGF-1 are essential for the development and function of many tissues in our body including mammary glands, it's been shown that excessive IGF-1 levels may actually stimulate breast tumor cell growth, proliferation, and migration. Research has suggested that elevated IGF-1 is linked to breast cancer risk, and may even be a causative factor. We discuss this in much more depth later, in the chapters on protein and sugar.

Other cellular mechanisms are being investigated, but scientists are beginning to understand that there are specific biochemical reasons why being overweight can increase your risk of breast cancer. Yes, there's much more to learn about weight and breast cancer. That's why scientists conduct research—and will never state that anything is "100 percent conclusive." But there's currently enough information and sound evidence for scientists and large organizations like the American Cancer Society, Susan G. Komen, and the American Institute

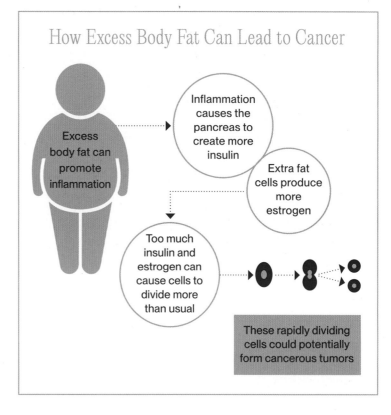

How Excess Body Fat Can Lead to Cancer

Excess body fat can promote inflammation

Inflammation causes the pancreas to create more insulin

Extra fat cells produce more estrogen

Too much insulin and estrogen can cause cells to divide more than usual

These rapidly dividing cells could potentially form cancerous tumors for Cancer Research to highlight the undeniable connection between excess body weight and breast cancer risk.

But What's the Good News?

You have the power to address this NOW, no matter what stage of life you're in.

Research has shown that losing weight and keeping the weight off—throughout your whole adult life—lowers your risk of breast cancer, likely by reducing estrogen, insulin, and IGF-1 levels. One large study found that women who lost between 4-11 pounds after menopause had more than 20% lower risk of breast cancer compared to women who didn't lose any weight at all. Another study following over 33,000 women enrolled in the Iowa Women's Health Study showed that the lowest risk groups were women who either maintained or lost weight when young, and again after menopause. And yet another study by the Epidemiology Research Program of the American Cancer Society showed that women who maintained at least a 10-pound weight loss had a lower breast cancer risk.

And it's not just breast cancer—being overweight or obese is linked to increased risk of 13 different cancers, including colon, rectal, esophagus, kidney, and pancreatic cancers, as well as cardiovascular disease and diabetes. Weight management is a long-term investment that's integral to your health as a whole.

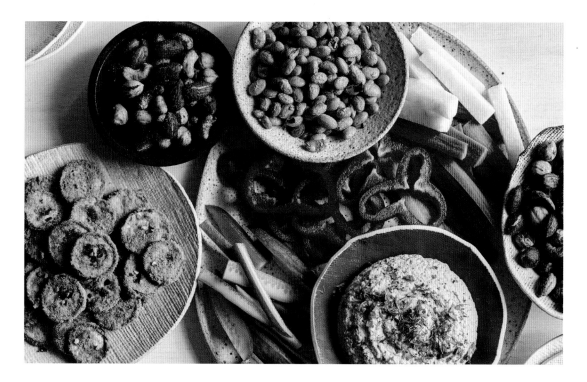

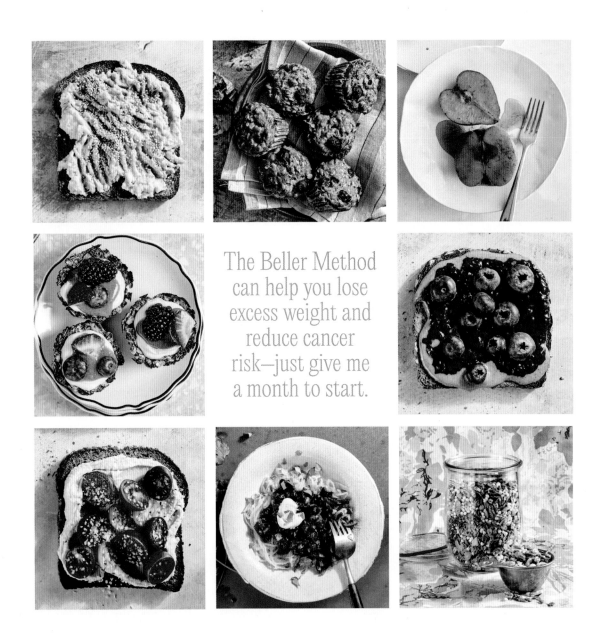

The Beller Method can help you lose excess weight and reduce cancer risk—just give me a month to start.

But it's easier said than done. That's where this book comes in.

The Beller Method can help you lose excess weight and reduce cancer risk—just give me a month to help you get started.

On average, most of my patients lose 6-10 pounds in 4-10 weeks, the healthy way. I help them develop and maintain a *sustainable nutrition plan*, and by consistently following the Beller Method those pounds go away and stay away. More importantly, I don't just shrink your portion sizes—any fad diet can do that. Instead, I've taken my years of experience within the breast cancer community and have applied scientific principles to create a simple method that promotes sustainable weight loss in a balanced way, and has you feeling empowered with what you choose to put into your body.

The Beller Method includes foods that work to maintain hormonal balance. It highlights certain foods that have been shown to be particularly beneficial for breast health, and may further reduce your risk through their antioxidant, anti-inflammatory, immunomodulatory, and anti-cancer properties. I did the hardcore research and detailed calculations to make sure your meals include all the essential fats, fiber, and other nutrients you need to protect your overall health—and in particular, promote breast cancer risk reduction. Remember, weight loss is a journey, and progress, not perfection, is key. I always tell my patients to remember that "it's what you do most of the time, not some of the time, that makes a difference when it comes to your long-term health." So let's get started!

> I always tell my patients to remember that "it's what you do most of the time, not some of the time, that makes a difference when it comes to your long-term health."

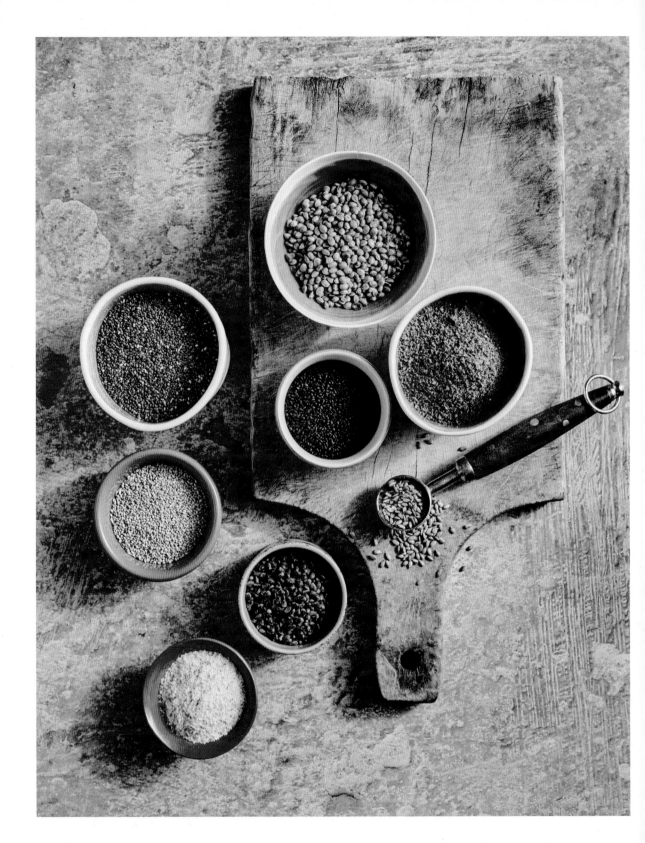

Fiber Up & Diversify

FOR HORMONAL BALANCE, IMMUNITY, GUT HEALTH, AND MORE

Fiber is absolutely key for breast cancer risk reduction—not only does it support gut health and weight management but it also works to balance blood sugars, reduce excess estrogen levels, and enhance immunity. But it's not just about taking a supplement and calling it a day. For optimal benefits you need your Daily 35 grams from diverse sources of fiber! But I've made it so simple. Adopt my Beller Method tips and you'll be sure to reach your goals, which will help fiber work for YOU...to lower risk and support thrivership. And here's the bonus benefit: when you're cleaned up, you feel great.

Fiber Up & Diversify

**FOR HORMONAL BALANCE, IMMUNITY,
GUT HEALTH, AND MORE**

You're probably tired of hearing fiber this, fiber that, and maybe you think you're getting more than enough—you had a couple salads, right?

We all know fiber's good for you, but did you know that adequate fiber is linked to lower breast cancer risk? It's KEY to consistently hit your fiber target—the research is clear that fiber is essential!

Here Are 5 Reasons Why Fiber Is Essential

- Fiber regulates hormones and reduces circulating estrogen

- Fiber supports gut health

- Fiber balances blood sugars

- Fiber supports immunity

- Fiber assists with weight management

All these may reduce your risk of breast cancer.

But I'm not just saying you should take a fiber supplement—getting the right *amount* and *types* of fiber is key for optimal breast cancer risk reduction.

Eat the Right AMOUNT of Fiber

Research has shown again and again that getting at least 30 grams of fiber per day is associated with decreased risk of breast cancer. Here are some of the larger studies that show that the threshold of greater than 30 grams per day is key for a substantial risk reduction:

First I want to discuss one of the most famous, large-scale studies that has been completed in our country: The Nurses' Health Study. Researchers collected nutrition and health information from almost 89,000 women over the span of 18 years. The scientists had women fill out detailed questionnaires about how much and how often they ate different types of foods, five times throughout this timeframe, and from these questionnaires the researchers determined their average fiber intake. In an analysis published in the *American Journal of Epidemiology*, researchers compared fiber intake among women who developed breast cancer to women who did not develop breast cancer. They found that women who ate over 30 grams of fiber per day had a trend toward a 32% decreased risk of breast cancer compared to women who only consumed 10 grams of fiber per day!

A follow-up study called the Nurses' Health Study II looked at a younger population—women completed questionnaires about their typical diet in high school. From this researchers found that fiber intake during adolescence may be especially important for lowering breast cancer risk—a 16% decreased risk was found among women who ate 29 grams of fiber per day in high school compared to 14-15 grams per day.

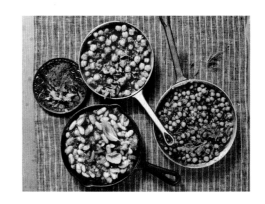

Women who ate over 30 grams of fiber per day had a trend toward a 32% decreased risk of breast cancer compared to women who only consumed 10 grams of fiber per day!

Now let's cross the Atlantic to Sweden. Researchers there followed about 52,000 postmenopausal women for about 8 years. They also measured fiber intake via responses from a food questionnaire and then related fiber intake to breast cancer cases. In their 2007 study published in the *International Journal of Cancer*, they found that women who had about 29 grams of fiber per day tended to have about a 15% lower risk of breast cancer compared to women who only had ~16.6 grams fiber per day (the average American has even less—11 to 15 grams per day).

Those are just a few large-scale studies that demonstrated that high fiber intake may be linked to lower breast cancer risk. In the scientific community we also like to examine overall trends that take into account many different studies—scientists combine data and analyze the outcomes in studies called "meta-analyses." A recent 2020 analysis from the American Cancer Society looked at 20 studies and concluded that high total fiber consumption was significantly associated with an 8% lower breast cancer risk compared to low fiber consumption. And a 2012 meta-analysis published in the *Annals of Oncology* combined data from 16 prospective studies including >500,000 participants and found that every 10 gram increase of fiber eaten in a day was associated with a 5% lower risk of breast cancer. This outcome was also replicated in a 2022 meta-analysis that showed for every 10 gram per day increase in dietary fiber, breast cancer risk decreased by 4.7% (an even greater reduction of 6.3% if you just looked at postmenopausal cases). So this would mean that 30-35 grams of fiber per day would potentially be about 15% lower risk of breast cancer compared to a low fiber diet!

There are so many more studies (this is just the tip of the iceberg).

Bottom line: You need to get at least 30 grams of fiber per day—and I prescribe 35 as insurance.

This seems so effective and so simple—yet unfortunately it's a miracle if the average individual gets even half of my recommended 30-35 grams (again, the average American only gets 11-15 grams of fiber per day). One reason is that many people tend to vastly overestimate how much fiber is in the food they eat. For example, a lot of patients tell me they eat a salad every day during lunch. While this is fantastic on so many fronts, a large leafy salad contains only around 5 grams of fiber. You would need to eat 7 large salads daily to meet your daily 35 grams!

Think of all the breast cancer protection the average American is missing out on! Don't be average—be above average. It's not about getting some fiber—it's about hitting the goal of 30-35 grams of diverse fiber per day.

I'll show you in a bit how to easily get your Daily 35 without worrying about needing to eat multiple huge salads throughout the day. But first, let's learn a little more about the magic of fiber!

Eat the Right TYPES of Fiber— Diversification Is Key!

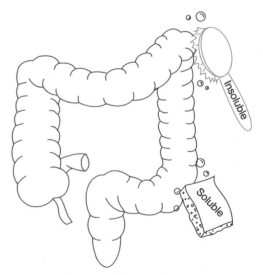

It might be tempting to reach for a fiber supplement to easily meet your Daily 35 grams of fiber. But let me stop you right there—doing so will rob you of the benefits that a diverse range of fiber intake provides.

Similar to how "eating the rainbow" of fruits and vegetables is important to get a wide spectrum of vitamins and antioxidants, diversification of fiber intake ensures you reap the benefits of the many different fibers out there.

Fiber is your gut's cleaning crew

So what is fiber, exactly?

You can think of fiber as the undigested plant parts. It's the parts of vegetables, fruits, whole grains, and legumes that your body doesn't break down for energy. Fiber is shuttled through the stomach, into the small intestine, and then into the large intestine (also called the colon). And that's where fiber's magic happens.

The beauty of fiber isn't just about what fiber gives—it's also about what fiber takes away. No matter how cleanly you think you're eating, your body not only accumulates a lot of junk, but it produces it, too...by-products of metabolism and excess hormones that, if not cleaned up, can lead to inflammation and ultimately may contribute to breast cancer risk. Fiber is the cleaning crew that sweeps your insides clean—talk about a real detox!

There are two main categories of fiber (insoluble and soluble) that work like a tag-team of power cleaners.

Insoluble fiber works like an exfoliating brush, gently scrubbing your intestinal tract and promoting regular bowel movements to speed the elimination of waste and excess hormones from your gut.

Examples: millet, legumes, cabbage, Brussels sprouts, apple skin, cauliflower

Soluble fiber has a soft, gummy texture and dissolves in water. It acts like a sponge that soaks up water and can slow down how fast food leaves your stomach, effectively adding an extra set of brakes on how quickly blood sugar levels rise. Once in your gut, soluble fiber binds to toxins, potential carcinogens, excess bile acids, cholesterol, and excess hormones and shuttles them out of your body.

Examples: oatmeal, beans, peas, citrus fruits, apple pulp

Within the category of soluble fiber are two special types of fibers: prebiotics and beta-glucans. These have unique properties that can support your gut health, immune system, and promote breast health...more on these later!

So while taking a fiber supplement powder may seem like an easy way to get your Daily 35 grams, you'd be missing out on the consumption of a diverse range of fibers in your diet that you'd get if you ate many different types of plant foods. I've described just a few types above, but there are actually many types of fibers in nature from unique plant foods—seaweeds have special fibers that aren't found in kiwis, oatmeal, or kale, for example. By diversifying the types of plants you eat, you'll expand the variety of fibers you get and therefore have a wider range of health benefits that we will explore in a minute. Some research suggests, for example, that eating 30 different types of plant foods and fibers promotes a more diverse (and healthy) gut microbiome.

We've seen that there are different types of fiber and it's essential to hit your Daily 35 grams. Now let's dive into it and explore what fiber can do for you!

How Fiber Can Reduce Your Risk of Breast Cancer

Thousands of studies have explored the relationship between fiber and breast cancer. The relationship is complex but can be broken down into the following concepts.

Remember this list?

Here are 5 reasons why Fiber is Essential

- Fiber regulates and reduces circulating estrogen

- Fiber supports gut health

- Fiber balances blood sugars

- Fiber supports immunity

- Fiber assists with weight management

 FIBER REDUCES ESTROGEN LEVELS

It's well established that high estrogen levels in the blood are one of the strongest risk factors for breast cancer. This is because the hormone estrogen stimulates breast cancer cell growth. While our bodies naturally produce this hormone, excess estrogen over time can build up and increase breast cancer risk. Fiber naturally helps get rid of extra estrogen.

Let me first explain what usually happens with excess estrogen in our body. Excess estrogen is typically released from the bloodstream into the digestive tract and then excreted out of the body through the stool. Ideally the majority of extra estrogen would leave the body, but occasionally too much is reabsorbed back into the body, which raises blood estrogen levels.

Fiber helps make the excretion process efficient and thorough in a few ways:

- Soluble fiber binds to excess estrogen in the intestines and helps shuttle it to excretion.

- Insoluble fiber increases stool bulk and weight. This may shield estrogens from being reabsorbed from the intestines back into your body.

- Fiber nourishes the gut microbiome, which can also lower estrogen levels—more on this in the next section!

All of these activities help remove extra estrogen from the body, effectively lowering blood estrogen concentrations and reducing the risk of breast cancer.

Fiber's role in estrogen removal was illustrated in a simple study published in the *New England Journal of Medicine*. The researchers compared 10 women who ate a low fiber "Western Diet"

(~12 grams per day) with 10 women who followed a higher fiber vegetarian diet (~28 grams per day). They found that the vegetarians had triple (3x!) the amount of estrogens excreted in their stool, as well as 15-20% lower blood estrogen levels. The higher fiber vegetarian diet resulted in way more estrogen excreted. It's not just a theory—it works in a real, measurable way in humans!

 FIBER PROMOTES A HEALTHY GUT MICROBIOME

Trillions of bacteria and microorganisms live inside our digestive tracts—collectively these are called the "gut microbiome." The gut microbiome has a major impact on our health, and scientists have examined how a healthy balance of bacteria in our guts may reduce inflammation and improve conditions such as heart disease and arthritis.

It's not a surprise, then, that the gut microbiome also plays a role in breast cancer risk.

Women with breast cancer have been shown to have dysbiosis, which means their gut microbiome is imbalanced, usually with higher populations of "unhealthy" gut bacteria and overall less diversity. This has the potential to disrupt estrogen metabolism and increase inflammation. Optimizing gut health is essential for those at risk for or impacted by breast cancer.

Foods Rich in Prebiotic Fiber

- Vegetables (e.g., asparagus, mushrooms, jicama, dandelion greens, and artichokes)
- Fruit (pre-ripe bananas, avocados, and apples)
- Soybeans (edamame)
- Garlic, onions, and leeks
- Basil seeds, chia seeds
- Whole grains and oats

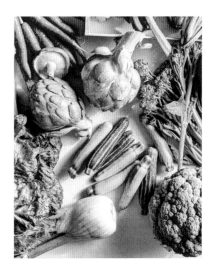

My goal is to improve the health of your gut microbiome—meaning promoting the health of diverse, good-for-you gut bacteria.

Let's briefly think of our gut as a garden. Producing a fruitful harvest of home-grown vegetables doesn't happen automatically—you need to water, fertilize, and nourish a garden so it is robust and productive. Likewise, our gut microbiome needs nourishment. How we feed it determines its health.

How do we nourish our gut microbiome? We feed the microbiome with prebiotic fibers.

The majority of the microbiome lives in the colon, or large intestine. The good-for-you bacteria need food to survive and flourish.

Foods with prebiotic fibers (like vegetables, whole grains, and beans) cannot be fully digested in our small intestine. The prebiotic fiber passes through to the large intestine, where it serves as food for our gut bacteria, which are able to break down the fiber and use it for fuel (yes, even though humans can't fully digest fiber, our gut bacteria can and thrive off of it!). This promotes the growth of a diverse array of beneficial gut bacteria and improves the overall health of the microbiome. Think of a high fiber meal as a feast for your gut bacteria.

Bonus: if you give to your gut microbiome, it gives back! When the gut bacteria break down prebiotic fibers for fuel, they produce metabolic by-products called "short chain fatty acids," or SCFAs for short. SCFAs nurture and repair the inner lining of your digestive tract, improve immunity, and decrease inflammation by down-regulating cellular inflammatory signals throughout the whole body. There's even research that suggests that SCFAs may help with weight loss, lower cholesterol, and improve memory!

On the flip side: when you eat foods without fiber, such as refined white grains or meats, the nutrients (carbs, proteins, and fats) are broken down and absorbed in the small intestine, before they even reach the large intestine. No fiber = no food for the good bacteria = dysbiosis. A diet that is super low in fiber essentially starves the microbiome.

We've seen how fiber promotes a healthy gut microbiome, and that a healthy microbiome is associated with lower breast cancer risk. There are a couple mechanisms that explain *how* this happens.

One way is that a healthy gut microbiome can help balance estrogen levels. As we've learned, usually some estrogen is reabsorbed from the gut back into the bloodstream. This occurs through the activity of an enzyme called *beta-glucuronidase,* which is found in certain types of gut bacteria. If an overabundance of beta-glucuronidase is present, then more estrogen is reabsorbed back into the bloodstream, which can raise blood estrogen levels. We don't want this—we ideally would like to have lower beta-glucuronidase activity. Research has shown that beta-glucuronidase activity can actually be modulated by the gut microbiome.

When there is dysbiosis, there tends to be more beta-glucuronidase activity, which sends more estrogen back into the bloodstream. This raises blood estrogen levels, leading to higher breast cancer risk.

When the gut microbiome is fiber-fed and healthy, there are more good gut bacteria that have less beta-glucuronidase enzyme activity. Thus, less estrogen is reabsorbed, and the excess estrogen is shuttled out of the body via the stool. This removal of excess estrogen contributes to breast cancer risk reduction. So by eating prebiotic fibers we may reduce beta-glucuronidase activity and therefore reduce risk!

Another way that a healthy gut microbiome helps reduce breast cancer risk is by activating beneficial plant compounds called **phytoestrogens**. Phytoestrogens are plant compounds (found in foods like soy, flax, sesame, and also in small amounts in fruits and veggies) that are similar in structure to human estrogen. I know you may be thinking, "Wait, don't I want to decrease the amount of estrogen in my body?" Phytoestrogens actually play a protective role in our body. Because they're similar in structure, phytoestrogens may bind to the body's estrogen receptors and prevent true estrogen from binding. This may block the potential carcinogenic effects of excess estrogens in the body.

The microbiome—through its metabolic and processing actions—works to transform plant phytoestrogens into supercharged, more active phytoestrogens. So a healthier gut microbiome results in more phytoestrogen activation, which makes them more effective at reducing the negative consequences of excess estrogen in the body.

In summary, fiber fuels a healthy gut microbiome, which works to reduce breast cancer risk by lowering estrogen levels.

 ### FIBER HELPS WITH BLOOD SUGAR CONTROL

High blood sugars aren't just associated with diabetes—they may lead to increased risk of breast cancer.

Typically, when we eat carbohydrates and sugars our body absorbs the sugar from our digestive tract into our bloodstream, then releases a hormone called insulin that shuttles the sugar from our blood into cells to be used for energy. However, chronically elevated sugar intake can promote insulin resistance—meaning your body is no longer sensitive to normal levels of insulin to help clear out the sugars in the blood, and instead needs to produce more and more insulin. Studies have shown that high insulin levels may *double* the risk of breast cancer—both in normal weight and overweight women. And preliminary research suggests it may have a negative impact on thrivership. We also know that lots of insulin hanging around

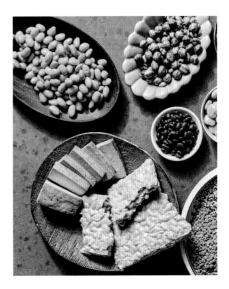

Foods Rich in Phytoestrogens

- Soy foods
- Legumes
- Flax
- Sesame seeds
- Nuts
- Oats, barley
- Yams, carrots, apples, pomegranate, berries

in your body leads to increased levels of a pro-inflammatory hormone called insulin-like growth factor 1 (IGF-1). Studies have shown over and over that elevated amounts of IGF-1 are associated with increased risk of breast cancer.

So—does this mean that women shouldn't eat carbs?

I don't believe so. Carbohydrate-containing foods, specifically complex carbohydrates, are a major source of fiber, which we already know helps balance hormones and maintain the health of our gut microbiome. Many of these foods are also rich in antioxidants and phytochemicals. What you should do is choose the most premium sources of carbohydrates—and focus on getting your daily 35 grams of fiber.

> Fiber effectively adds an extra set of brakes on how quickly your body absorbs sugars, and how fast blood sugar levels rise.

Fiber—specifically soluble fiber—has been shown to improve blood sugar control. This is because the gooey texture slows down how fast food leaves your stomach and moves through the small intestine. Fiber effectively adds an extra set of brakes on how quickly your body absorbs sugars, and how fast blood sugar levels rise. This allows lower levels of insulin to effectively deal with blood sugars, and prevents insulin resistance and elevated IGF-1 levels.

In summary, fiber reduces blood sugars, lowers insulin requirements, prevents insulin resistance, and decreases IGF-1 levels, therefore contributing to reduced risk of breast cancer.

 FIBER MAY STRENGTHEN THE IMMUNE SYSTEM

A healthy immune system is essential to not only fight off disease, but also to identify and destroy cancerous cells. It's important to keep your immune system as strong as you can—and fiber may help you do this.

Beta-glucans (found in foods like mushrooms and oats) are special types of soluble fibers that may enhance the immune system. As beta-glucans move through the digestive tract, they are recognized by receptors located on intestine cells. Once stimulated by beta-glucans, these receptors signal the immune cells to activate. This sets off a chemical cascade that may help protect your body against disease, stress, and cancer cell growth.

Beta-glucans can potentially enhance the immune system and help it better defend the body against fatigue, infection, stress, some radiation treatments, and may also help slow the growth of cancer cells.

BONUS: Beta-glucans also fall within the category of prebiotic fibers that nourish the microbiome.

This effect is so significant that some studies are examining how beta-glucans can be used to modulate the immune system in breast cancer patients to help fight off tumors!

5 FIBER ASSISTS WITH WEIGHT LOSS

As explained in the previous chapter, there's an undeniable connection between higher weight and breast cancer. But the good news is that losing excess body fat and keeping it off can lower your risk of breast cancer. Fiber helps you along this journey.

Studies overwhelmingly show that eating more fiber is associated with healthy body weight. In the Nurses' Health Study, weight gain was associated with high intake of refined grains and low intake of high-fiber and intact whole grain foods. But it's not just an association—research has explored multiple mechanisms for how fiber aids in weight loss:

- **High-fiber foods require your body to work harder** to break them down in your digestive tract, which results in more calories burned during digestion.

- **High-fiber foods tend to have fewer calories**—so you can fill up with larger portions of those foods.

- **The S-word: Satiety.** Satiety is the feeling of fullness. Higher satiety = less hunger = you won't be reaching for snacks so soon after your meals.

How does fiber increase satiety?

- Fiber increases chewing (you especially notice this when you chew on a celery stick!), which on a sensory level makes you feel like you've eaten more, and on a neuronal level gives your brain more time to receive the signal that you've had a satisfactory amount of food.

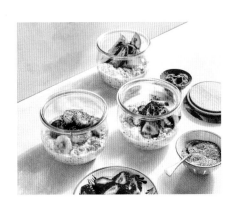

Foods Rich in Beta-Glucans

- Mushrooms, in particular reishi, maitake, shiitake, and oyster mushrooms
- Seaweed and algae
- Barley, oats, and whole grains

- Soluble fiber absorbs water and takes up significant space in your stomach. This contributes to an extended feeling of fullness and more gradual absorption of nutrients.

While there are of course many aspects to losing excess body fat (I will guide you through my tried-and-true tips throughout this method), ensuring you are hitting your fiber goals can help and possibly reduce cancer risk!

Note: Regardless of your receptor status, fiber can help with risk reduction. Fiber intake has been associated with lower risk of *both* ER+/PR+ *and* ER-/PR- breast cancers. Yes, fiber helps reduce the total estrogen load by possibly decreasing circulating estrogen and increasing estrogen excretion—but it may also lower risk via non-estrogenic pathways such as lowering insulin and IGF-1. It also helps keep you full and nourish a healthy microbiome, both of which affect weight management, which in turn is essential even for triple negative breast cancer. High-fiber foods are also rich in phytochemicals such as lignans that may have anti-proliferative, anti-angiogenic, anti-inflammatory, antioxidant, DNA-protecting, and immune-enhancing properties. So Fiber Up, regardless of your age, weight, or receptor status!

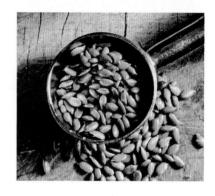

Studies overwhelmingly show that eating more fiber is associated with healthy body weight.

Action Plan: Fiber Up

Now we've seen how fiber works in multiple ways to reduce the risk and fight breast cancer. It really is amazing how something that our bodies don't fully digest is so essential to hormonal balance, our gut microbiome health, immunity, and more. We have our daily goal of 35 grams, and know the importance of diversifying the types of fiber to reap the most benefits. Now—let's put this knowledge to action and Fiber Up!

Remember, we have 2 main goals with fiber:

- Hit your Daily 30-35 grams

- Diversify your fiber intake

Through years of experience educating patients, I've found a few tips that help ensure you achieve your fiber goals.

TIP 1: FRONTLOAD YOUR DAY WITH 10 GRAMS

Breakfast is an excellent opportunity to get your day started out on the right fiber-foot! My easiest tip for getting your fiber fix is to frontload every day with at least 10 grams, which will put you well on your way toward your Daily 35. Whole oatmeal (not instant sugar junk), sorghum, and quinoa are my faves, but even they contain only about 4 grams of fiber, so...

You should include Fiber Boosters.

Think of fiber boosters as the supercharged spoonfuls that will elevate your breakfast! My Starter Kit Fiber Boosters, or "Basic 4," are: chia seeds, basil seeds, whole hemp seeds, and flaxseeds. Adding a spoon or two of any of these will bring up the total fiber content of your breakfast by 4-7 grams—making it easy to hit your AM 10 grams and transform the nutritional power of your meal. It can look like stirring in a tablespoon of chia seeds into your oats, adding some basil seeds to your morning tea, or topping your smoothie with a couple tablespoons of whole hemp seeds or ground flax. And feel free to add other fiber rich ingredients if you feel daring...

- **Basil seeds:** 7 grams of fiber per tablespoon

- **Chia seeds:** 5 grams of fiber per tablespoon, has more omega-3's than basil seeds

- **Whole hemp seeds:** 4 ½ grams of fiber in 2 tablespoons, as a bonus has high protein content

- **Flaxseeds:** 4 grams of fiber in 2 tablespoons, the #1 dietary source of protective lignans

After you've gotten used to a regular rotation of some basic Fiber Boosters, it's time to Level Up and diversify your fiber options, which will add to the health of your microbiome, stooling regularity, and potential cancer risk reduction.

- **Oat Fiber:** 3 grams of fiber per teaspoon, zero calories, a natural gut detox to keep you regular

- **Acacia Fiber:** 5 grams of fiber per tablespoon, is a prebiotic fiber meaning it feeds your gut bacteria

- **Psyllium Husk:** 4-7 grams of fiber per tablespoon, is a prebiotic fiber and can also balance blood sugar levels and decrease cholesterol

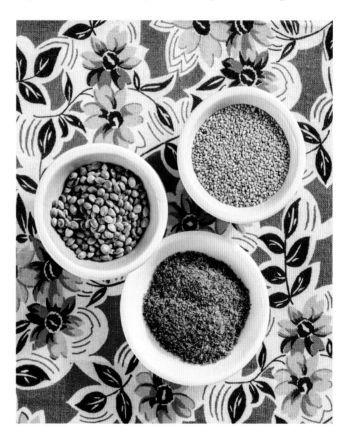

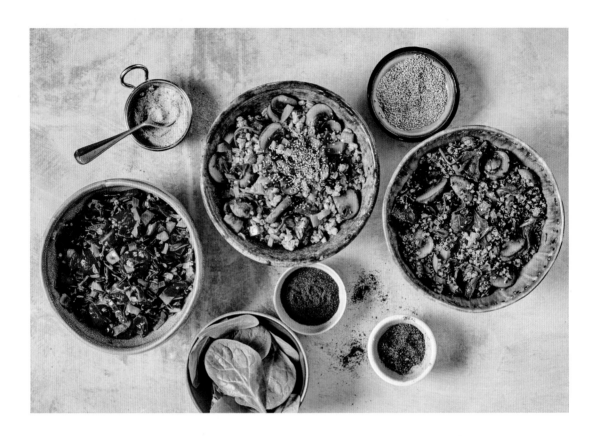

TIP 2: **INCLUDE PREMIUM PLANT-BASED PROTEINS DURING LUNCH AND DINNER**

We'll discuss the most premium proteins for cancer risk reduction in the next section, but including plant-based proteins is going to dramatically boost your fiber intake. A cup of beans or legumes contains anywhere from 15-18 grams of fiber. Compare this to a piece of chicken or fish which, like all animal proteins, has *zero* grams of fiber. A plant-based meal doesn't have to be tedious or fancy—throw some cooked sprouted lentils, edamame or chickpeas atop a salad, in a soup, or with some roasted vegetables. I have tons of easy and delicious plant-based protein recipes for you in the Let's Eat! recipe section.

TIP 3: **APPRECIATE THE POWER OF PRODUCE**

Seize every opportunity to include produce at nearly every meal and snack. It's super simple yet so powerful—eating your fruits and veggies throughout the day helps you pack in diverse types of fibers, in addition to cancer protective vitamins, minerals, and antioxidants. Toss some greens into your breakfast smoothie, top your oats with fresh or frozen fruit, or add leftover vegetables to an AM tofu scramble. Keep pre-cut veggies and fruit in your kitchen for easy grab and go snacks. And include a robust base of low starch veg at lunch and dinner.

TIP 4: WHEN INCLUDING GRAINS, GO THE WHOLE, INTACT WAY

While whole wheat bread has more fiber than white bread, it isn't the top tier when it comes to complex carbohydrates. Limit products made from flours (even whole wheat flour) because flours tend to spike blood sugars. Instead reach for intact whole grains, which are unrefined and have a gentler impact on blood sugars. These are as close to how they're found in nature as possible... examples include barley, millet, buckwheat, farro, wheat berries, spelt, popcorn, and brown, black, and wild rice. Certain products also are made of intact whole grains—check out the nutrition label, the whole grains should be listed as ingredients (i.e., sprouted wheat, barley, millet, etc.) and if possible try to limit products made with "whole wheat flours."

Power Tip: Take it slow! If your baseline fiber intake is low, I recommend gradually increasing the amount of fiber you consume over time. This allows your body to adjust to a higher fiber load and may minimize any GI side effects like gas (normal and harmless, but can be bothersome!). Integrate one tip at a time and be sure to drink enough water along the way to help regulate your stooling habits. Soon enough you'll hit your Daily 35 and you'll feel the difference.

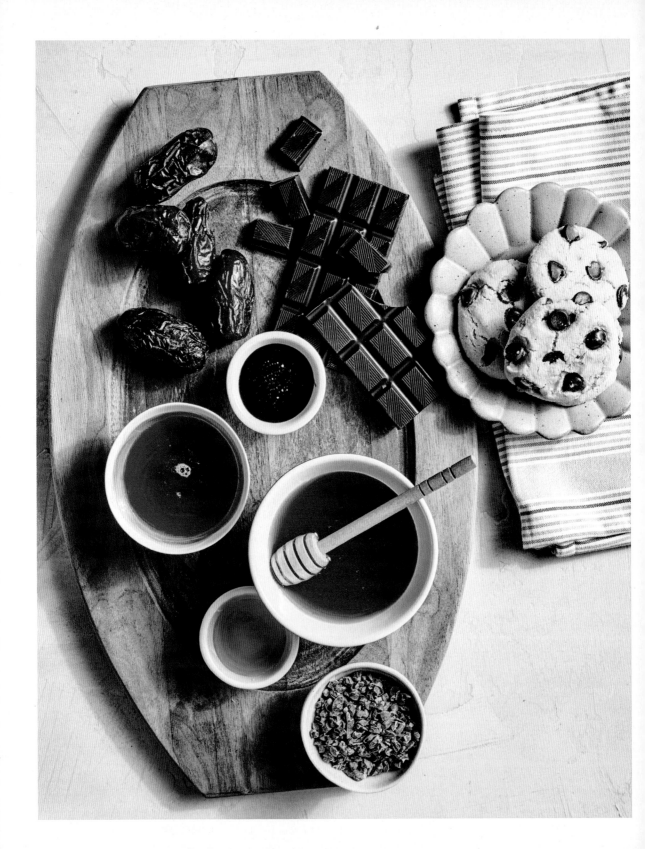

Strike a
Sugar Balance

KEEP YOUR BLOOD SUGAR IN CHECK

Sugars—aka carbohydrates—are necessary fuel for your body's cells. But high amounts of simple sugars can spike your blood glucose levels leading to elevated IGF-1 and increased cancer risk. So be selective and choose complex carbohydrates in appropriate portions and in strategic combinations with other foods. This will help manage blood sugars, balance insulin response, lower IGF-1 levels, and support weight management. Fueling with moderate amounts of wholesome carbohydrates and reducing cravings for ultra-refined foods will help you start thriving on the real deal.

Strike a Sugar Balance

KEEP YOUR BLOOD SUGAR IN CHECK

Oh how sweet it *isn't*! Everyone's finally waking up to all the threats that sugar poses to our bodies, from diabetes to tooth decay to weight gain. And excessive sugar is addictive, too, which is why it can be hard to stop with just one cookie. There's the common claim that sugar "feeds" cancer cells and therefore you need to cut all sugars out of your diet—but simply put, it isn't that simple.

I want to let you in on a little secret: every cell in your body needs sugar to survive.

No, that's not an excuse to go to town on the jelly beans! It just means that you can't cut out ALL forms of sugar, as many of my patients tell me they're doing. While you should absolutely reduce foods with added sugars, you can't afford to eliminate fruits, intact grains, and other phytochemical-rich foods that contain natural sugars. Avoiding them won't stop cancer growth—in fact, doing so will eliminate many nutrients your body needs to fight cancer. And that could ultimately damage your healthy cells.

Here's the sugar scoop. When most people think of "sugar," they are visualizing those sweet white crystals, but "sugar" is actually a general term for the simplest form of a carbohydrate (carb). Through the natural process of digestion, our bodies break down carbs to basic sugars, the most common one being glucose. Glucose fuels the cells of our body, providing energy for essential functions like powering your brain, transporting nutrients, building new cells, and moving muscles. If you don't get enough carbs and glucose in your diet, then your body may start breaking down the all-important proteins (including muscle, hair, and nails) as well as critical fat stores that make up cellular membranes and cushion your organs.

So what's the bottom line? Your body needs a modest amount of carbs—which are broken down to sugar—for optimal function.

However, you can totally overdo the sugar intake, which may lead to increased breast cancer risk! Let me explain.

The Sugar and Breast Cancer Connection

The body has a fine-tuned, delicate system for absorbing and utilizing carbohydrates. After you eat a meal and there's a lot of glucose in your bloodstream, a hormone called insulin is secreted. Insulin acts as a signaling molecule that stimulates your cells to take in glucose, thus lowering your blood sugar levels. Then the glucose is either used immediately for energy or stored away for future use.

If you chronically overconsume sugar, it may result in persistently high blood sugar levels, and you can develop something called insulin resistance. With insulin resistance, your body becomes dulled to the presence of regular amounts of insulin, and requires more and more insulin to be released in order to absorb glucose. Excess glucose and insulin sitting around in the bloodstream can cause the liver to release increased levels of a hormone called insulin-like growth factor 1 (IGF-1).

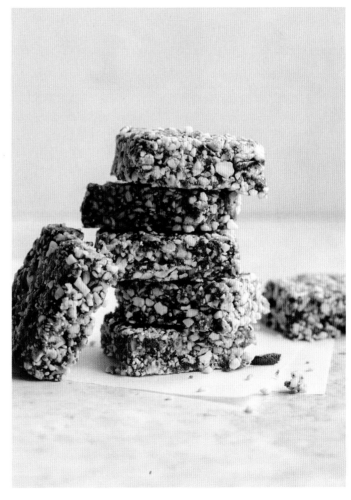

IGF-1 is important in breast tissue growth and development—levels are typically high from birth to puberty, and then decrease with age. High levels of IGF-1 during adulthood are not necessary, and research has shown that elevated levels may trigger a chemical cascade that leads to increased inflammation and breast cancer tumor development, progression, and metastasis. Plus, elevated IGF-1 levels may inhibit cellular pathways that usually protect against tumor development.

So now we know...sugar (or carbohydrate) seems necessary for your body's natural function and health, but high amounts of sugar can eventually lead to elevated IGF-1 and increased breast cancer risk. So how do you strike a balance?

That's where I come in. There are two key concepts when thinking about carbohydrates:

- **Carbohydrate Type:** Not all carbs are created equal—so pick the ones that will help with blood sugar control.

- **Food Balance:** Combine carbohydrates with other essential foods in a way that helps balance blood sugars.

As often as you can, keep these two concepts in mind as you stock your pantry and build your meals.

Carbohydrate Type: Not All Carbs Are Created Equal

Most of us think of rice or pasta when we hear the word "carbohydrate." But in fact sugars—or carbohydrates—come in many foods: added sugars, fruits, grains, starchy vegetables, beans, and legumes for example. Aim to limit added sugars as much as possible as these are highly processed and cause rapid spikes in blood glucose levels. But what about naturally occurring sugars present in foods?

We've heard again and again that you should be choosing whole grains over refined grains, and apples over apple juice. And that's true! That's because the "healthier" options come packaged with fiber, which works to actually improve blood sugar control. Fiber—especially soluble fiber—creates a gooey texture that slows down how fast food leaves your stomach and moves through the small intestine, effectively adding a set of brakes on how quickly sugar is absorbed into the bloodstream. This slower rise of blood sugars allows your body to respond with appropriate levels of insulin and prevents the development of insulin resistance. This halts the cascade of elevated glucose, high insulin, and IGF-1 levels.

WHAT ABOUT GRAINS?

Now I want to take things a step further when it comes to grains—don't just look for "whole grains," opt for intact grains whenever possible. This means that you should be able to see the individual grains intact or cracked into large pieces, rather than ground into a flour. Some examples of intact grains include wheat berries (instead of whole wheat flour); steel cut oats (instead of instant oats); flourless breads (instead of soft whole wheat breads). We don't often see "whole grain" distinguished from "intact grain" in the media, but research has demonstrated again and again that it makes a difference—a 2021 meta-analysis of 16 studies found that intact steel cut oats resulted in lower post-meal blood sugar and insulin levels compared to instant oats. And another study demonstrated that coarse bread made with intact grain kernels resulted in significantly lower insulin release compared to bread made from flour.

Why is this the case? Intact grains retain the tough outer layers of the bran and germ surrounding the starch within. The body needs to work harder to break down and digest these layers, resulting in a slower release of sugar into the bloodstream. This blunts the high blood sugar, insulin, and IGF-1 pathway that has been linked to increased breast cancer risk. On the other hand, when a grain (whether whole or not) is ground into a flour, there is increased surface area for the body's digestive enzymes to work on, which results in a rapid spike in blood sugars.

So rather than avoiding all sugar sources, just choose them wisely. Fiber-rich carbohydrates, including intact whole grains, can improve blood sugar control and work to effectively fuel and strengthen your body while reducing cancer risk. We know that fiber is KEY to optimal breast health (see the Fiber chapter for more information), and these complex carbs not only serve as sources of unique fibers, but they're also rich in phytochemicals and antioxidants that may also have protective properties. And an added bonus is that many complex carbohydrates—such as intact grains, beans, and legumes—include protein, which is another nutrient your body needs.

> Opt for intact grains whenever possible. This means that you should be able to see the individual grains intact or cracked into large pieces, rather than ground into a flour.

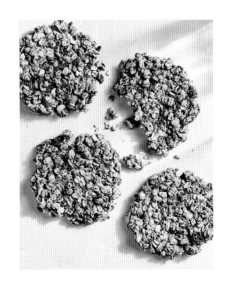

FIBER-RICH CARBOHYDRATES TO INCLUDE WITHIN THE BELLER METHOD:

- **Whole intact grains,** such as amaranth, barley, buckwheat, bulgur, farro, millet, oats (preferably steel cut or rolled), rice (black, brown, wild), sorghum, spelt

- **Flourless and intact grain breads**

- **Fiber-rich starchy vegetables** in moderation: sweet potatoes, yams, corn, potatoes, parsnips, taro, pumpkin, and winter squashes such as butternut, delicata, acorn, etc.

- **Fiber-rich fruits,** such as apple, berries, kiwi, pear, citrus fruits, pomegranate, etc.

- **Low starch vegetables** (quite low in carbohydrate amount)

CARBOHYDRATES TO LIMIT:

- Flours and breads made out of flour (whether all purpose, multi-grain, whole wheat, or rice flour—grains that have been pulverized and finely ground into flour cause rapid blood sugar spikes)

- Refined grains such as white rice, corn grits, cream of wheat, instant oats, pasta

- Crackers, chips, most snacks unless they do not contain much flour or added sugar

- Sweetened beverages including fruit juice, sweet coffee/tea, sodas

- Sweet treats and baked goods

- Milk, ice cream

- Excess added sugars (see page 60 for their undercover names!)

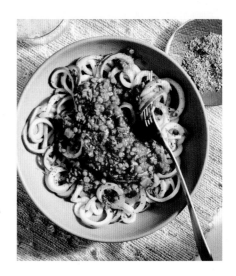

My approach to meal building not only optimizes intake of cancer protective nutrients, but also helps blunt blood sugar spikes.

Food Balance:

INTEGRATE CARBOHYDRATES IN A WAY THAT HELPS MODERATE BLOOD SUGARS

Now we know that certain carbohydrates (such as intact whole grains or fiber-rich starchy vegetables) are okay and even GOOD to include in a breast cancer protective diet. The next step is making sure that you're choosing appropriate portions and combining them with other types of foods. You need glucose, ideally in the form of complex carbs—but too much of a good thing isn't always beneficial.

An entire meal of complex carbs may taste good—but it's essential to keep portions in check and even more importantly, to prioritize the concept of combining different food groups to create a balanced meal. A carb-heavy meal (think a bowl with a base of brown rice) will not keep your blood sugars as stable as a meal that has a base of low starch vegetables with a smaller portion of carbohydrate, along with proteins and fats.

My approach to meal-building not only optimizes intake of cancer protective nutrients, but also helps blunt blood sugar spikes. How? Protein, fat, and fiber take longer to digest, which slows down the rate at which your stomach empties the meal into your intestines.

This means that the rate of sugar digestion and absorption of sugar into your bloodstream is also slower—allowing your body to have an appropriate insulin response. Let's go back to the analogy from before: if choosing a whole intact carbohydrate is similar to adding a set of brakes on how quickly blood sugar spikes, you can think of constructing a meal with my method below as upgrading to a stronger set of brakes!

Protein and fat also activate a variety of hormonal cascades that work to prepare your body to most optimally digest the food, shuttle food through the intestines, and regulate satiety (fullness) signals. So for ideal digestion, weight management, and blood sugar control it is vital to create a meal with the appropriate proportions of low starch vegetables, premium proteins, healthy fats, and complex carbohydrates.

THE POWER OF 3:

Here's my basic method for a meal building strategy for lunches and dinners that will support both long-term weight and blood sugar management: **The Power of 3.** These three components below are essential, non-negotiables for each meal. First prioritize building your meal with these three power players.

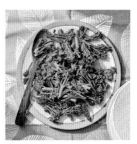

- **Low Starch Vegetables:** This is your base of the meal. Low starch veg are rich in fiber, antioxidants, and cancer protective phytochemicals, are gentler on your blood sugars, and are lower in calories compared to high starch vegetables.

  Aim for at least 2 cups of low starch vegetables as your base—but have more if you wish (see page 66 for a list of low starch veg).

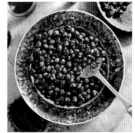

- **Premium Protein:** 1 serving (see Go Pro Protein chapter)

  1 serving = typically ¾ cup—1 cup of a plant-based protein

- **Beneficial Fat:** 1 serving, often added or used in cooking the vegetable and protein (see the Oil Change chapter)

  1 serving = about 1 tablespoon oil, 2 tablespoons of dressing/nuts/avocado

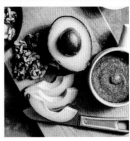

The Power of 3 ensures that you have a solid foundation to your meal. If you have The Power of 3, your meal is balanced, supportive of weight loss goals, and appropriate for breast cancer risk reduction. Nailing this concept has been very successful for my patients—it's a simple way to structure your meal whether at home or at restaurants with minimal measurements or counting.

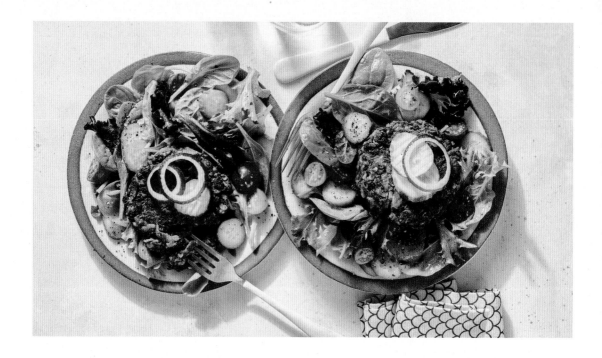

You can build upon the foundation of The Power of 3: If you are not actively on a weight loss journey, you have the option of adding a high starch fiber-rich carbohydrate to your meal. These can be part of a healthy cancer-protective eating pattern, but keep the portion to 1 serving per meal (about the size of your fist). Examples include:

- 1 slice of flourless intact grain bread

- ½ cup cooked wild, black, or brown rice, farro, millet

- ½ cup cooked soba noodles

- 1 sweet potato or yam

- 1 cup cooked butternut, acorn, or delicata squash

- ½ cup corn

BALANCED MEAL IDEAS:

- A warm bowl of low starch vegetable soup with ¾ cup white beans and topped with a drizzle of pesto

- 2 cups of low starch vegetables roasted in olive oil (red bell peppers, mushrooms, and broccoli) with 1 cup of chickpea pasta and marinara sauce

- Mexican fajita bowl: 2 cups of lettuce with fajita vegetables (multi-color bell peppers and onions) with 1 cup black beans and 2 tablespoons of guacamole

- 2 cups of vegetables (onion, garlic, snow peas, spinach) sautéed in avocado oil and 1 cup marinated tofu

- 2 cups chopped cucumber and tomato salad with spiced olive oil dressing and parsley, topped with 1 cup of mixed quinoa and garbanzo beans

- See the Complete Meals (pp. 188–229) and Mix & Match Meals (pp. 230–263) for many more!

What's key here: the base and highest volume component of the meal is the low starch vegetables, and including a premium protein and power pantry fat are non-negotiables. High starch vegetables and carbohydrates occupy a smaller volume than what we've come to expect at least in American restaurants, and can even be optional for some meals if you have a goal of losing excess weight. But meals don't often end up being zero-carb. If you are following the Beller Method then most likely the Premium Protein you are including will be a plant-based option, which contains protein, fiber, and some wholesome carbohydrates (beans, lentils, and edamame, for example).

It's important to not just balance meals, but to also balance your snacks! Let's consider an apple. Yes—it's rich in nutrients and fiber, but you can take it to the next level and upgrade your snack by sprinkling it with ground hemp seeds. The hemp seeds contain fiber, protein, and fat, which further modulate blood sugars. Another example

Power Spicing

Some spices may have blood sugar balancing properties. It's still important to keep in mind the type and amount of carb—but sprinkle on these spices to give your body a little "boost" in managing blood sugar spikes.

- Allspice
- Basil
- Cacao
- Cayenne
- Ceylon Cinnamon
- Cilantro
- Cloves
- Coriander Seed
- Fenugreek
- Garlic
- Ginger
- Nutmeg
- Orange Peel
- Oregano
- Parsley
- Rosemary
- Saffron
- Sumac
- Turmeric

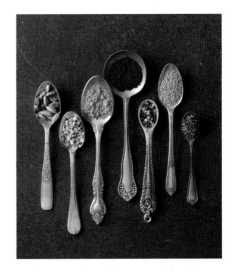

is a banana—it contains natural sugars and fibers, but by adding some nut butter (as in my Frozen 'Nana "Sandwich" on page 273) you further blunt the rise in blood sugars and provide your body with the protein and fat it needs to stay full for longer. And if you want an extra upgrade: consider adding a power spice blend that has potential blood sugar regulating effects.

Managing Sugar Cravings

How do you manage your sweet cravings? Moderation, moderation, and more moderation. The more you indulge in sugar, the more your body wants. It's been shown that sugar is addictive—when you eat it, it activates similar areas in your brain that an addictive drug would! And given the amount of hidden sugar in our diet, it's no surprise that we've been wired to crave sugar.

Beware of Hidden Sugars

While complex carbs can be included in a balanced meal, we want to of course limit refined carbs that don't offer nutrition and spike our blood sugars.

Look out for hidden sugars—added sugars are hiding in 74% of packaged foods! They're not just in cookies and candies—they're slipped into salad dressings, crackers, hummus, yogurts, and more.

For items that you're consuming on a regular basis, try to choose options that don't contain added sugars. Of course you can't avoid all added sugars, especially when dining out, on vacation, or for special treats! But it's what you do most of the time that matters for your long-term health. So when you're doing your routine grocery shopping, look out for some sneaky added sugar names:

- Agave nectar
- Barley malt
- Beet sugar
- Brown sugar
- Cane juice
- Cane sugar
- Caramel
- Carob syrup
- Coconut palm sugar
- Corn sweetener
- Corn syrup
- Date sugar/syrup
- Dehydrated cane juice
- Dextrin
- Dextrose
- Evaporated cane juice
- Fructose
- Fruit juice/ concentrate
- Glucose, glucose solids
- High fructose corn syrup (HFCS)
- Honey
- Malt syrup
- Maltodextrin
- Maltose
- Mannose
- Molasses
- Rice syrup
- Sucrose

But slowly you can break that addiction to sweet flavor.

I'm not a fan of simply replacing sugars with sugar alternatives (sugar alcohols like erythritol, sorbitol, and mannitol, or even large amounts of stevia and monk fruit). Even though you're not getting the calories from sugar, you're still feeding your brain's addiction to the sweet flavor! Plus, some individuals may experience gastrointestinal discomfort from sugar alternatives.

Of course, there are times when some sweetness is okay, but overall it is important to break the sweetness addiction. If you train your taste buds that "a little is enough," they eventually learn to adapt. It may be hard at first but your tastebuds literally regenerate every couple weeks so you will adjust—I promise—and when it happens you will feel empowered! So start to cut down on sweetness and your cravings will slowly fade.

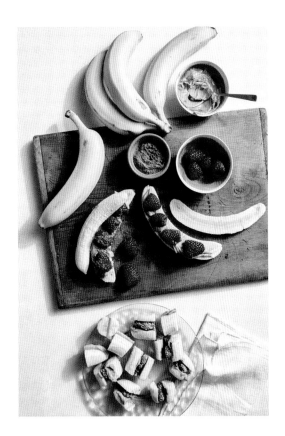

Here are a few tips:

- Dilute your sweet drinks slowly over time by adding more ice, or cutting with plain sparkling water.

- Reduce the sugar in your coffee or tea by ¾ the amount for one week, then to ½ for one week, then to ¼ for one week...then to none as your taste buds adjust.

- Instead of automatically reaching for a sweet treat, opt for a piece of whole fruit with a bit of protein such as a few nuts—this will provide an energy boost and may halt your sweet cravings.

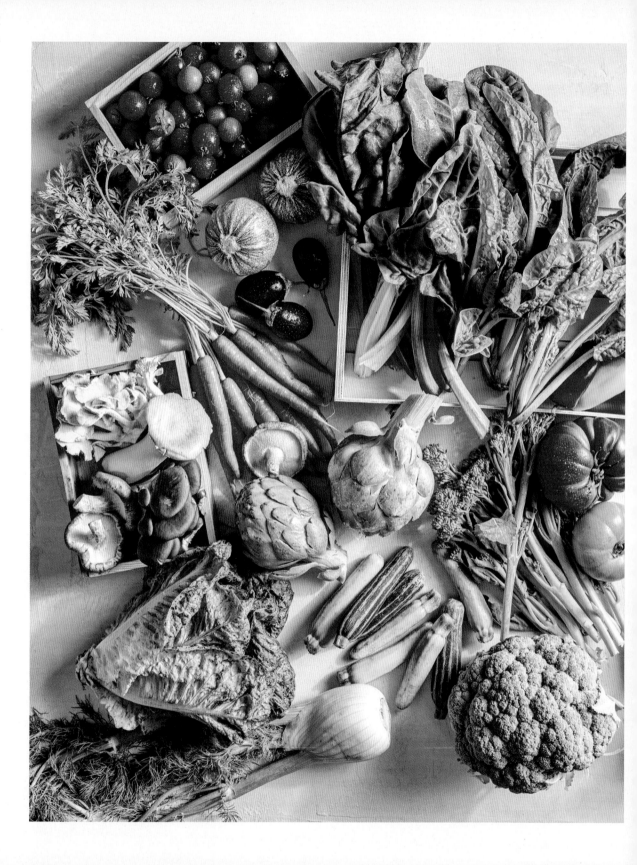

Veg Out

WITH ANTI-CANCER FOODS

Diversity of vegetables is key! Flood your insides with protective phytochemicals and load up on my top-of-the-line cancer-fighting choices: cruciferous, alliums, carotenoid-containing, and prebiotic-rich veg. Veg are deserving of the spotlight—so elevate them and make them the base of your meals. Get at least 2 cups (minimum!) of low starch veg per meal as part of the Beller Method to optimize antioxidant intake, fuel your microbiome, and moderate blood sugars.

Veg Out

WITH ANTI-CANCER FOODS

Maybe you're already eating cleaner and greener for cancer protection and weight management—let's say fruit for breakfast, a salad for lunch, and some roasted veg for dinner. That's a great start, but the Beller Method isn't just about including some vegetables in your diet...veg should be the BASE of your lunch and dinner. It seems so obvious, but years of experience show me that people often fall short of their daily veg requirements. Let's transform how we think about vegetables and not underestimate their importance. And it's not just about getting any veg. I'll share my top-of-the-line cancer-fighting favorites that you should be incorporating on a daily basis.

Research actually links high vegetable intake to decreased breast cancer risk. A 2018 study published in the *International Journal of Cancer* analyzed data from 182,000 women from the Nurses' Health Study. Researchers found that after 24 years of follow-up, women who ate more than 5 ½ servings of fruits and vegetables every day had an 11% lower risk of breast cancer compared to those who ate 2 ½ servings or less. One serving is a cup of leafy greens or about ½ cup of other raw or cooked veg. Now, the effects were especially marked among those who regularly incorporated cruciferous and yellow and orange vegetables. More on those in a bit.

So how do we ensure we're getting enough? For years, I've taught my patients to build their meals with a base of vegetables—that is, their first priority is to load up their plate (or bowl) with at least 2 cups of low starch veggies. Why is this essential? Vegetables...

- **Deliver phytonutrients:** It's not just about vitamins and minerals. Vegetables are absolutely packed with plant-based chemicals (phytonutrients) that have antioxidant and anti-inflammatory properties. Research has also shown that some phytonutrients may halt the formation of carcinogens in the body, prevent carcinogens from attacking healthy cells, and boost our body's ability to fend off any cancer-like changes. Getting a diverse range of veg is simply the best way to ensure you're getting a broad spectrum of phytonutrients. A simple carrot has more than 100 phytonutrients...talk about a power food! Scientists estimate that there are more than 10,000 phytochemicals that we've already identified (likely many remain unknown), but we've only studied about 150 in-depth. Consider all the potential cancer-fighting properties you're getting when you Veg Out. You can't replace this nutritional diversity with a supplement!

- **Help detox your system:** Vegetables are packed with fibers of all types—soluble fibers, insoluble fibers, prebiotic fibers, beta-glucans...the list goes on. As we learned in the fiber chapter, fiber helps scrub your insides to stimulate elimination, and sucks up carcinogens, toxins, and excess hormones to then shuttle them out of your body. A natural detox!

- **Power your gut health:** Your gut is home to billions of bacteria collectively called the gut microbiome. These bacteria are fed and nourished by prebiotic fibers, which are abundant in so many vegetables. The microbiome, in turn, helps balance estrogen levels which may lower risk for breast cancer. A healthy microbiome also may enhance immunity—70% of your immune system is based in your gut (it's called gut-associated lymphoid tissue)! Bonus: when your gut is well-fed with a veg-rich diet, it produces metabolic by-products called short chain fatty acids (SCFAs for short). SCFAs have whole body-wide effects and may help with weight loss, reduce inflammation, and lower breast cancer risk.

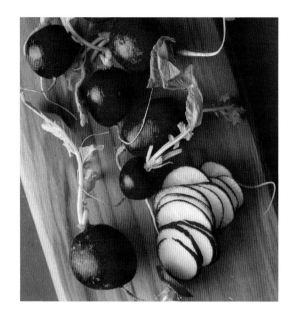

Women who ate more than 5 ½ servings of fruits and vegetables every day had an 11% lower risk of breast cancer compared to those who ate 2 ½ servings or less.

- **Fill you up—for very few calories:** Low starch vegetables are dense in nutrients, but low in calories. That means you'll max out your nutrients and can eat a substantial volume— all while staying on track with your weight loss goals. A review of 13 research studies with over 3,600 people found that eating foods with lower calorie density was linked to increased weight loss.

- **Balance your blood sugars:** High blood sugars are linked to diabetes, inflammation, and breast cancer risk (see the previous chapter for more details). Vegetables not only contain fiber, which works to blunt blood sugar spikes, but they also contain many phytochemicals that have potential blood sugar-lowering properties.

Now, like fiber, diversity is key. It's not enough to just eat 5 cups of romaine lettuce every day, or subsist off of an all-broccoli diet. Different veg contain various types of phytonutrients, fibers, and vitamins that can work to fight cancer from multiple fronts...and switching things up keeps things interesting! Aim to have a variety of veg flavors and colors at your meals, not just to make them more enjoyable, but to diversify your cancer-fighting nutrients.

Beller Action Plan for Veggies

Enjoy your veg any way you like them: raw, in a soup or salad, lightly roasted, blanched, or sautéed. In fact, I encourage you to eat both raw and cooked veg on a regular basis, as certain phytonutrients like lycopene in tomatoes are more biochemically active when cooked, but other nutrients like vitamin C are deactivated in cooking and are best eaten when raw.

Low Starch Vegetables

Low Starch Veg—2 cups minimum as the base of your meal (but eat all you want!)

Load up on any of the low starch veg from below—they're going to be the "main event" of your meal for all of their amazing benefits.

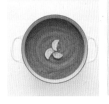

- Artichoke
- Arugula
- Asparagus
- Bamboo shoots
- Bell peppers
- Bok choy
- Broccoli
- Brussels sprouts
- Cabbage
- Carrots

- Cauliflower
- Celery
- Chard
- Collard greens
- Cucumber
- Eggplant
- Fennel
- Green beans
- Horseradish
- Jicama

- Kabocha squash
- Kale
- Kohlrabi
- Lettuce (all types)
- Mushrooms
- Okra
- Onions
- Radish
- Rhubarb

- Rutabaga
- Spinach
- Sprouts
- Summer squash
- Swiss chard
- Tomato
- Turnips
- Watercress
- Zucchini

Top-of-the-line Cancer Fighting Veg

I know I just told you that variety is key and to choose from any of the low starch veg. That's true...but I want you to really hone in and make sure to include one or more of these TOP cancer-fighting categories with most of your meals. And have diversity within each category—while broccoli every day is good for you, I'd argue that rotating through the different cruciferous veg and incorporating several types is even better as you'll get a range of nutrients, fibers, and flavors.

CRUCIAL CRUCIFEROUS:

Arugula, bok choy, broccoli, broccoli sprouts, Brussels sprouts, cabbage, cauliflower, collard greens, horseradish, kale, mustard greens, radishes, rutabaga, turnips, watercress

Cruciferous veg are especially amazing at fighting breast cancer because they're a rich source of sulfur-containing phytochemicals called glucosinolates. Once in the body, glucosinolates are broken down into metabolites including the super-potent isothiocyanates, indole-3-carbinol, and sulforaphane...these compounds have been shown to fight cancer by enhancing our body's natural detoxifying and antioxidant enzymes, which then work to neutralize and remove carcinogens. Research indicates that they may induce cancer cell death, prevent growth of tumors, and have major antioxidant and anti-inflammatory properties. A meta-analysis compiled data from 11 epidemiological studies and found that high intake of cruciferous vegetables is associated with 15% lower risk of breast cancer!

Tip: While cruciferous veg are good to eat no matter how you cook or eat them, I'll let you in on a trick of the trade that will maximize the bioavailability and efficacy of their cancer-fighting compounds! Let me explain: the glucosinolates in cruciferous vegetables need to be broken down by an enzyme called myrosinase in order to be transformed into the active metabolites. When cruciferous vegetables are intact, prior to being chopped, glucosinolates are actually separated from myrosinase. But when the vegetables are chopped or chewed, the myrosinase is released, comes into contact with the glucosinolates, and catalyzes a transformation into their active, powerful metabolites. But cooking deactivates the

High Starch Vegetables

We're letting the low starch veg be the main event, and the high starch veg will be a secondary player. These veg can still be rich in antioxidants, vitamins, and phytonutrients, but they contain more carbohydrates and are more calorie-dense. So if you opt to include them, keep them to more moderate portions on your plate (about the size of your fist), especially if weight management is your goal.

- Corn
- Parsnips
- Potatoes (any kind)
- Sweet potatoes and yams
- Pumpkins
- Taro
- Winter squash (acorn, butternut, delicata, hubbard)

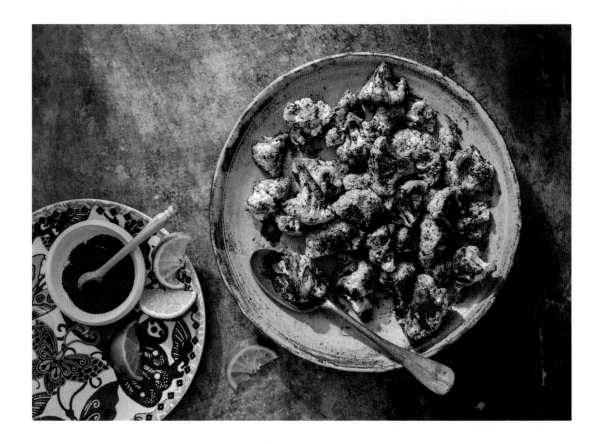

myrosinase so the glucosinolates aren't transformed into those active compounds. So...what do we do? Three options:

- **Eat them raw,** as chewing well will release the myrosinase and allow it to react with the glucosinolates.

- **If cooking: use this technique:** Chop, then Pause. Cut up your veg and let them sit for about 10 minutes to let the myrosinase transform the glucosinolates prior to cooking.

- **If eating pre-cooked cruciferous**—sprinkle on and mix in some mustard seed powder after cooking! Mustard seed contains myrosinase, which can help break down glucosinolates.

GO ALL IN FOR ALLIUM:

Onions (yellow, white, sweet, red), garlic, leeks, scallions, chives, shallots

Alliums are particularly rich in organosulfides (alliin and gamma-glutamyl cysteine peptides), which have been shown to potentially fight breast cancer by protecting from DNA damage, inhibiting tumor growth, and preventing cancer cells from spreading. Plus, alliums contain at least 50 different types of flavonoids including quercetin, zeaxanthin, and anthocyanins. These compounds are powerful anti-inflammatory and antioxidant agents in the body.

Similar to cruciferous, you should Chop, then Pause in order to activate alliin into its active form. When you crush, chop, or chew garlic, for example, you release an enzyme called alliinase which then reacts to form the more biochemically active allicin. Not only will this release a more delicious flavor, but it'll result in even more powerful health benefits. So again, chop, then wait 10 minutes (prep other components of your meal or do a quick chore around the house) before cooking to fully activate the alliin.

MAKE ROOM FOR SHROOMS:

Beech, button, chanterelle, crimini, enoki, lion's mane, maitake, morel, oyster, porcini, portobello, reishi, shiitake, trumpet, turkey tail (fresh, dried, or powder form)

Mushrooms are one of my key veg in reducing breast cancer risk! A recent study published in the *International Journal of Cancer* followed over 2,000 women and found that those who ate the most mushrooms were 64% less likely to be diagnosed with breast cancer compared to those who didn't eat mushrooms. Similar results have been seen in other studies—mushroom intake was consistently related to lower breast cancer risk and cancer risk in general (a 17-study meta-analysis published in the journal *Nutrition* by researchers at Penn State found a 34% decrease in cancer risk among several cancer types).

Why are mushrooms so mighty? First of all, mushrooms contain beta-glucans, which are special types of fibers that may enhance immunity, nourish your gut microbiome, and help level out blood sugars—all of which may contribute to lower breast cancer risk. Mushrooms also

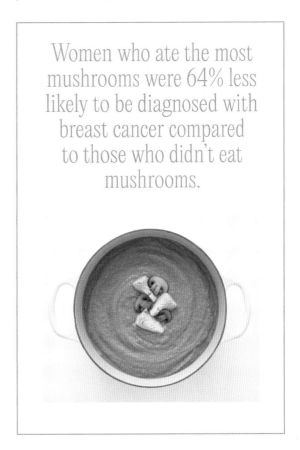

Women who ate the most mushrooms were 64% less likely to be diagnosed with breast cancer compared to those who didn't eat mushrooms.

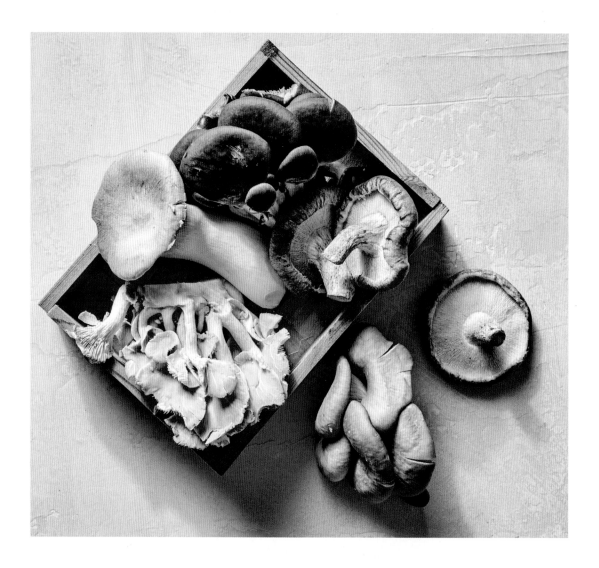

have been shown to decrease the activity of an enzyme called aromatase, which tumors use to produce estrogen. So eating mushrooms can potentially help lower estrogen levels in the body—which may help reduce the risk of breast cancer. Some anti-cancer drugs also target aromatase, and very few foods are natural aromatase-inhibitors—so mushrooms are a unique anti-breast cancer power food!

- The common white button mushroom has measurable aromatase-inhibiting activity that may suppress breast tumor proliferation—they're a staple in my kitchen. But I always encourage my patients to diversify when they can, as different mushrooms contain various types of prebiotic fibers and may have other health benefits! Less common types including reishi, maitake, turkey tail, and shiitake mushrooms are excellent to include to ensure you get a wide range of anti-cancer compounds. This is where dried mushrooms come into play—you don't always have to get the fancy fresh varieties to reap the benefits. The dried organic varieties are super versatile and amazing to keep in your pantry (see Power Up chapter).

24-CAROTENOID GOLD:

Bell peppers (red, orange, and yellow), carrots, dandelion greens, kale, mustard greens, pumpkin, spinach, sweet potato, tomatoes (especially dried tomatoes), winter squash varieties (delicata, acorn, butternut, hubbard, kabocha). Yes, green vegetables can also be rich sources of carotenoids although the green pigment chlorophyll hides the yellow-orange color.

Carotenoids are yellow, orange, and red pigments naturally present in plants. The most common carotenoids include beta-carotene, beta-cryptoxanthin, lutein, lycopene, and zeaxanthin. These carotenoids are major antioxidants, and may be associated with lower breast cancer risk due to their antioxidant activity and inhibition of breast tumor cell growth. The Women's Health Initiative found that among over 5,400 women, those with higher levels of blood beta-carotene had up to a 22% lower risk of breast cancer. The Nurses Health study found a 28% lower risk, the EPIC study found a 60% lower risk (for ER- breast cancers), and pooled analyses have found about a 20% decreased risk.

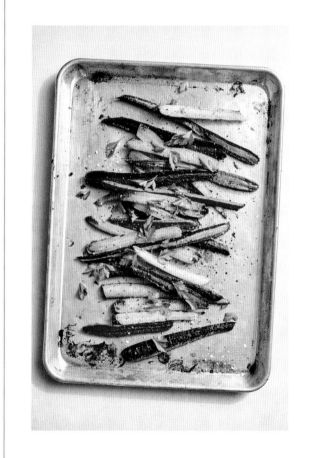

The Women's Health Initiative found that among over 5,400 women, those with higher levels of blood beta-carotene had up to a 22% lower risk of breast cancer.

Now, I don't want everyone to go out there and start taking supplements—there's evidence that supplementation with isolated beta-carotene, for example, may have some health risks! Red-orange vegetables are the best natural sources of carotenoids and are what I want you to be incorporating into your diet on a regular basis.

The body doesn't always absorb carotenoids easily, as they're typically trapped between cell walls and are released when chopped and cooked. What can help: enjoy your carotenoid-rich veg with a dose of healthy fat in the same meal. This may boost their absorption because carotenoids are largely fat-soluble. So drizzle some olive or avocado oil over that roasted tomato or carrot salad to optimize carotenoid absorption!

POWER YOUR GUT WITH PREBIOTICS:

Certain veggies are rich in prebiotic fibers, which are fuel for the beneficial bacteria in our gut—and a healthy gut microbiome may help reduce the risk of breast cancer. Prebiotic fibers are fermented by the microbiota and produce short chain fatty acids, which in turn may improve gut function, enhance immunity, and have anti-inflammatory benefits throughout the body.

Some of the top prebiotic vegetables include but are not limited to:

Asparagus, artichoke hearts, burdock root, chicory root, dandelion greens, garlic, Jerusalem artichoke (sunchoke), jicama, leeks, mushrooms, onions, seaweed and algae, shallots

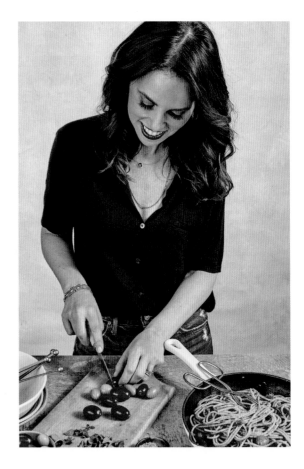

Rachel's Veg Tricks of the Trade

How to Veg Out with style and flavor— no boring steamed spinach in sight!

- **Shop in-season** for best prices, flavors, and peak nutritional value. Peruse the stalls at your farmers market to see what's fresh.

- **Make it easy:** it's okay to take shortcuts. Pre-chopped veg and frozen veg are good options if you're short on time—

just get the veg in as your base! Bonus: frozen veg are picked at their peak nutritional value so they may have high antioxidant and vitamin levels.

- **Prep ahead of time:** to save time on weeknights, wash and chop veg in the beginning of the week so you can quickly cook up or add to your meal base when needed.

- **Variety in preparation can help keep things interesting and fresh.** Vegetables in all types of dishes count toward your 2 cups: crudités, salads, lightly steamed, sautéed or grilled, chopped into a bean salad, blended in a smoothie, or in a soup.

- **Don't forget about breakfast:** add veg whenever you can—sautéed in a tofu scramble, atop an intact grain avocado toast, shredded in a wholesome muffin recipe, or blended in a smoothie.

- **Spice them up!** Rotate between spice blends to change up the nutrient and flavor profile—while of course dramatically elevating the nutritional value of the dish.

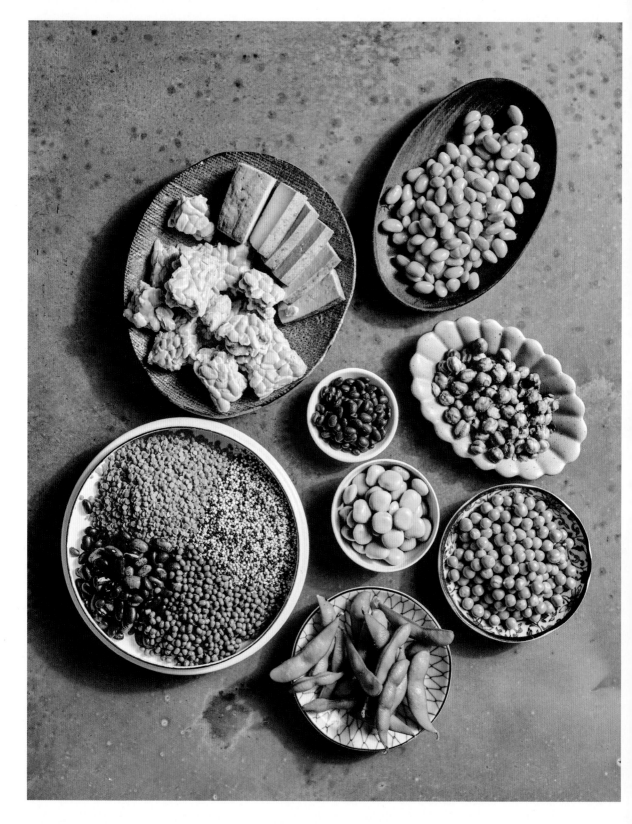

Go Pro with Premium Proteins

WITH BENEFITS FOR CANCER RISK REDUCTION AND BEYOND

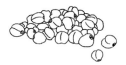

Protein is a key component of your diet—but one of the most common questions I get is "which proteins should I include for optimal cancer risk reduction?" Plant-based proteins are the preferred choice when it comes to reducing cancer risk due to their phytochemical and fiber content, benefits for gut health, and anti-inflammatory properties—plus they don't contain hormones that may potentially increase risk. That's why the Beller Method is built around these premium options. While I know that transitioning to a more plant-based diet can sometimes be overwhelming, it can absolutely transform the way that you feel.

Go Pro with Premium Proteins

WITH BENEFITS FOR CANCER RISK
REDUCTION AND BEYOND

If you think you can live on salad alone, think again. You NEED protein, which helps your body recover, repair tissue, and maintain a healthy immune system. Protein also keeps you satisfied and energized for hours, which means less snacking and optimal weight management.

The challenge for most women: knowing which proteins support cancer risk reduction, particularly in a world of conflicting information. It's not easy to navigate these choices. I'll show you the way, first by explaining the science and then by giving you a step-by-step guide to choosing the best protein options within the Beller Method.

Plant-based is my recommended protein route—years of research confirm that a primarily plant-based diet is most beneficial for cancer risk reduction, cardiac health and more.

What is protein, anyways? Protein is one of the three major macronutrients that are essential for our body to survive (the other two are carbohydrates and fat). Amino acids are molecules that are combined to form proteins, and are the "building blocks" for every cell in our body. Our hair, bones, muscle, skin, and organs are built with protein, and proteins make up the enzymes that carry out the hundreds of chemical reactions in our bodies. Now, protein is present in many types of foods and most of us here in America can easily get adequate amounts of protein with every meal.

But the type of protein that you fuel your body with is essential. Some high protein foods are packaged up with anti-inflammatory and antioxidant compounds. Other protein-rich foods can potentially lead to increased inflammation, higher IGF-1 levels, and elevated cancer risk. So the source matters! I recommend building your protein foundation on the premium options that provide the most protection.

I'm always asked: How much protein do I need? While I'd love to give you a simple number, the answer is...it depends on so many factors. Most women need a minimum of 0.8 grams per kilogram body weight; for a 140-pound (63.6 kg) woman this would be about 50 grams per day. Women who are pregnant or breastfeeding, or elderly need more than this minimum (closer to 1-1.3 gm/kg so for our example that would be around 70 grams), and women who are undergoing active cancer treatment may need more!

Here Are the Different Protein Options

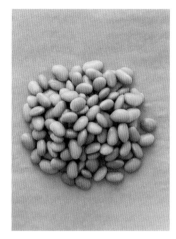
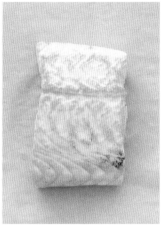
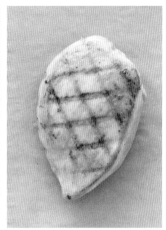

Preferred choice: Plant-based proteins, including beans and legumes, peas, quinoa, edamame, tofu, and tempeh, have amazing cancer protective perks!

Second choice: Omega-3 rich fish confer some anti-cancer benefits but not to the same extent as plant proteins.

Least preferred: Organic poultry, grass-fed meat, and organic eggs are low return proteins.

What I can tell you is this: the majority of Americans are getting plenty of protein in their diets—we're far from protein-deficient! Most people don't need to shovel down chicken breasts or scoops of protein powders to hit their goals—many foods have protein even if we don't typically consider them to be "protein rich" (did you know a cup of oatmeal has 6 grams?). If you're aiming to get one serving of protein-rich food with each meal and snack, you're likely to hit your protein goals, no problem.

I want to reiterate here that a nutrition plan that emphasizes breast cancer risk reduction will be based upon premium, plant-based protein choices. These should be your foundational, "workhorse" choices that are present on a daily basis. While I believe that the most benefits do come from a plant-based diet, if you do opt to include meat, poultry, fish, eggs, or dairy, I'll give some tips for the best options that you can modestly sprinkle into your nutrition plan.

Premium Proteins: Plant-Based

Years of research has shown that by choosing plant proteins, you may lower your risk of developing breast cancer, reduce your risk of recurrence, support weight management, and optimize your gut health.

Let's look at the science—don't just take my word for it!

There are dozens of studies that link plant-based proteins with lower cancer risk. One study followed 91,000 women and found that a plant-based diet was associated with a 15% reduction in breast cancer risk. That's right—a 15% lower risk due to choosing plant-based proteins! The researchers noticed that this effect was even stronger for those with estrogen-receptor negative and progesterone-receptor negative (ER-/PR-) tumors, indicating it's not *just* due to the anti-estrogenic effects of plant proteins that I'll discuss in a few pages.

Another study from Loma Linda found that among 69,000 individuals, those following a vegan diet had about a 33% lower rate of breast, cervical, and ovarian cancers. And a recent 2022 study coming from Oxford included 470,000 participants and found that being a low-meat eater, a fish-eater, or vegetarian was associated with a lower risk of all cancers compared to people who regularly ate meat! Vegetarian women in particular were observed to have a 12% lower risk of breast cancer compared to those who ate animal proteins (though the vegetarians in this study did have lower weight, which also contributes to reduced cancer risk). Impressive numbers all around.

But it's not just about limiting meat, it's about choosing nutritious, minimally processed

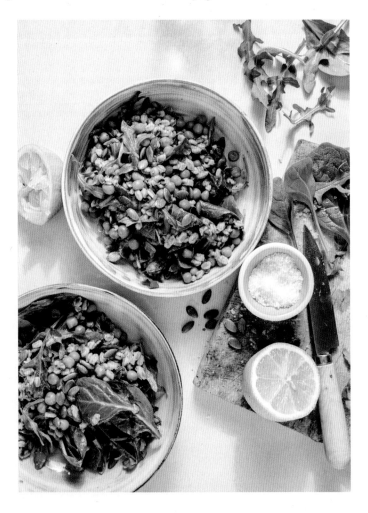

plant foods. 2022 research based in France tracked over 65,000 women for two decades and found that a healthy plant-based diet reduced breast cancer risk by 14% (healthy meant their intake was primarily fruits and vegetables, whole grains, nuts, legumes, tea, and coffee, with occasional meat sprinkled into the equation). But they found a 20% increased risk of breast cancer among the women whose diet was full of unhealthy plant-based foods (refined grains, juice, and desserts). And a 2021 study published in the journal *Nature* found that women who followed the most healthy plant-based diets ("healthy" defined similarly to the previous study) were 36-67% less likely to have breast cancer compared to women following unhealthy diets.

> It's not just cancer risk—research also supports a plant-based diet for prevention of heart disease, diabetes, inflammatory disease, and more!

All this evidence has resulted in leading cancer organizations providing recommendations for a primarily plant-based diet for optimal cancer risk reduction. The Beller Method's preference for plant-based protein falls in line with the American Institute for Cancer Research's primarily plant-based diet recommendations, and the American Cancer Society's statement that a diet rich in plant-based foods may reduce the risk of cancer. And it's not just cancer we're concerned about—research also supports a plant-based diet for prevention and treatment of heart disease, diabetes, inflammatory disease, and more!

SO HOW DO PLANT PROTEINS REDUCE BREAST CANCER RISK?

Here are a few of the perks that plant proteins offer:

- **Plant proteins are fiber-rich.** Just 1 serving (¾ cup) of legumes contains about 10 grams of fiber—this meets nearly 30% of your daily fiber goal! Research has suggested that for every 10 grams of fiber—or 1 serving of legumes—you may lower your risk of breast cancer by about 5%. So pile on those plant protein servings! Fiber also works to help balance estrogen levels, lower blood sugars, and help with weight loss. How much fiber do animal-based proteins have? None at all.

- **Plant proteins boost gut health:** Your gut microbiome primarily is fed with prebiotic fibers that are only found in plants—it's not fed with animal-based proteins. If you don't eat prebiotics, you're starving your gut microbiome. Some key prebiotics are uniquely found in plant-based protein sources such as legumes or quinoa—you simply can't obtain them by just eating vegetables and fruits. By primarily choosing plant proteins, you are optimizing your gut microbiome health; if you primarily choose animal-based proteins, you're missing out on gut health benefits. And as we've learned in the fiber chapter, a healthy gut microbiome assists with reducing estrogen levels, strengthening immunity, decreasing inflammation, and even enhancing weight loss.

- **Plant proteins may assist with weight loss:** For many people, plant proteins keep you full and more satisfied than meat, meaning you may eat less at the next meal! A study published in *Food and Nutrition Research* had participants eat a meal high in animal protein and another high in plant-based protein. The researchers found that the participants felt the *most* satisfied and full after eating the plant-based meals compared to the animal protein meals—regardless of whether the plant-based meals were high or low in protein content. This may be due to the fact that plant-based proteins contain fiber, which helps activate satiety signals. Fiber also requires the body to "work" a little harder to break down the food, therefore increasing the calories that the body burns in the process of digestion.

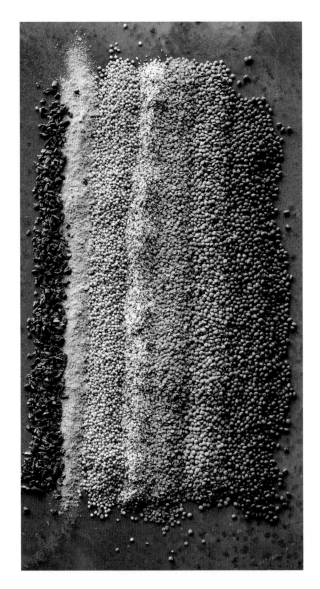

- **Plant proteins may help reduce inflammation:** Plant-based proteins contain many anti-inflammatory compounds that are not present in animal protein sources. Numerous studies support this—one analysis of 2,000 people in the Framingham Heart Study found that replacing animal protein with 10 grams of plant protein per day was associated with a beneficial decrease in inflammation. Plus, plant-based proteins are rich in phytochemicals, which have been shown to have anti-inflammatory benefits.

- **Plant proteins appear to lower IGF-1 activity:** IGF-1 (insulin-like growth factor-1) is a hormone that has been linked to breast cancer development (see the Strike the Sugar Balance chapter and also pages 89-90 for more). Studies have found that plant protein sources such as beans and soy appear to lower IGF-1 activity, thus reducing cancer risk. Another reason to power up with plant-based proteins.

- **Plant proteins contain cancer-fighting phytochemicals** such as saponins, protease inhibitors, and phytic acid. Research shows that these compounds may inhibit cancer cell growth and reproduction, and may even contribute to tumor cell death. They have been shown to have antioxidant properties as well, which may help reduce cellular and DNA damage that may lead to cancer development. These phytochemicals are *only* found in plant proteins—they're not present in animal-based proteins.

Note: What about anti-nutrients? Saponins, protease inhibitors, and phytic acid are known as "anti-nutrients," and some people claim that you shouldn't eat them because they can block the absorption of minerals like calcium, zinc, and iron. I say—still include these foods because of their potential anti-cancer properties! If you include a wide variety of plant foods in your diet, you should be getting enough nutrients to not have to worry about the small effect of "anti-nutrients."

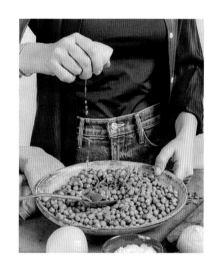

Just 1 serving of legumes contains about 10 grams of fiber—this meets nearly 30% of your daily fiber goal!

And what about lectins? Lectins are a family of protein compounds that bind carbohydrates and are found naturally in humans, animals, plants, and fungi. Some foods have higher amounts of lectins including beans and legumes as well as eggs, tomatoes, cow's milk, eggplant, fruit, and grains. Recent diet trends promote eliminating all high-lectin foods, claiming they are inflammatory, damage the gut, and overstimulate the immune system. While there are a handful of test tube studies from the 1970s–80s that associate lectins with disease development, there aren't good human studies that would convince the world's top scientists, doctors, and dietitians to encourage removing lectins from our diets. On the flip side, lectins and high-lectin foods such as legumes and whole grains have actually been suggested to have cancer-protective properties similar to other "anti-nutrients." And hundreds of studies show us that legumes and their fibers are beneficial for your gut microbiome and have been associated with positive health outcomes and long life.

So long story short: plant foods rich in saponins, protease inhibitors, phytic acid, and lectins should not be avoided! They're an essential part of a cancer protective eating plan!

- **Plant proteins contain phytoestrogens**: Some plant proteins (lentils, soy, and nuts for example) contain phytoestrogens, which are plant compounds that protect breast tissue from the potentially carcinogenic effects of excessive estrogen in the body (they're anti-estrogenic). These phytoestrogens are only present in plant foods!

TO SOY OR NOT TO SOY?

Whether or not to include soy foods is one of the top questions I get as a dietitian specializing in breast cancer risk reduction. Although soy can be a hot topic, the great news is that soy actually may *help* women survive breast cancer and avoid its recurrence!

I believe that women should consume soy, especially to replace meat dishes! But choose the best soy foods: I recommend wholesome soy like sprouted organic tofu, edamame, tempeh, and miso. Go for organic whenever possible since conventional soy tends to be highly sprayed with pesticides. I do not recommend highly processed soy products, such as soy protein powders and soy snacks.

Soy Science: Research indicates that women who regularly consumed soy foods when they were younger (especially during puberty) had less than half the risk of breast cancer of women who didn't. Studies also show that even in women with BRCA gene mutations who are genetically inclined to get breast cancer, eating 4-5 servings of soy foods per week may reduce breast cancer risk by up to 73%! Important note: the same study on BRCA and soy found that eating 3-10 servings of meat per week nearly *doubled* the risk of cancer for women with BRCA mutations, while increasing the risk by 41% for those with normal BRCA genes. Another analysis found that women who ate more than

> Scientists from the American Institute for Cancer Research state that soy may reduce recurrence and increase breast cancer thrivership.

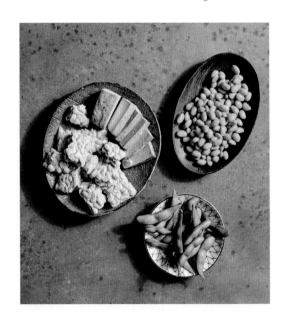

10 milligrams soy isoflavones per day (about ⅓ cup edamame or ½ serving of tofu) had a 25% lower risk of breast cancer recurrence than those who averaged less than 4 milligrams per day.

The evidence stacks up. Experts from the American Cancer Society have concluded that soy is not harmful for breast cancer thrivers. And scientists from the American Institute for Cancer Research state that soy may reduce recurrence and increase breast cancer thrivership.

So why do people fear soy? It has to do with estrogen. Normal breast cells as well as breast cancer cells have estrogen receptors. When estrogen in our blood attaches to these receptors, it triggers these cells to undergo a variety of responses, including cell growth. It's been shown that excessively high estrogen levels can increase the risk of breast cancer.

Now soy contains phytoestrogens, which are plant compounds that are structurally similar to but different from human and animal estrogens. On a cellular level, soy phytoestrogens interact with our body in an opposite manner than human estrogens do.

- There are two different kinds of estrogen receptors in our bodies: Alpha receptors (ER-α) and Beta receptors (ER-β). These receptors have opposite cellular effects in breast tissue... when ER-α is activated, it signals cancer cells to multiply and divide. However, ER-β activation results in anti-growth properties...it opposes cancer cell growth and therefore has an "anti-estrogenic" effect.

- Human estrogen binds with ER-α and stimulates a growth response. This is why excess estrogen has been linked to higher breast cancer risk.

- Soy phytoestrogen primarily binds with ER-β rather than ER-α. When soy binds to ER-β, it tells the breast cell not to multiply. Thus, soy phytoestrogens have an anti-proliferative, anti-growth effect against tumor growth.

In summary, soy phytoestrogens are NOT the same as human estrogens, nor do they act like human estrogens. They actually have an anti-estrogenic effect and may be protective against breast cancer! Plus, soy has antioxidant properties, essential minerals like magnesium, iron, copper, and potassium, and fiber.

PREMIUM PLANT PROTEIN SOURCES: THE BELLER METHOD

Let's put this into action! Here are my quick and easy pantry plant protein suggestions:

A typical serving is ¾ cup—1 cup cooked, except for hemp hearts and seeds, which have a smaller portion size.

- **Legumes:** Legumes are an excellent source of plant-based protein, and research shows they provide just as much (if not more!) post-meal satisfaction as beef. Plus, a ¾ cup serving gets you to about one-third of the way to your daily 30-35 grams of fiber.

Legumes have specifically been linked with a reduction in breast cancer risk: A Harvard study including over 88,000 women found that those who substituted just one serving of legumes for one serving of meat per day had a 15% lower risk of breast cancer. Women had a 24% lower risk of developing breast cancer if they ate beans at least twice a week compared to those who ate them less than once a month.

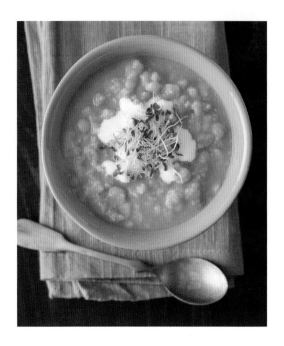

Common legumes: black beans, lupini beans, black eyed peas, cannellini beans, chickpeas, Great Northern beans, kidney beans, lima beans, pinto beans, fava beans, navy beans, adzuki beans, mung beans, lentils (any type)...the list goes on!

Shopping tips:

Dried legumes: If you have the option, purchase sprouted varieties of lentils, mung beans, and other legumes, as these have increased bioavailability of nutrients and phytochemicals.

Pre-cooked legumes: If possible purchase in BPA- and BPS-free containers including tetra packs, glass jars, and pouches.

- **Whole organic soy:** Opt for sprouted organic tofu, edamame, and tempeh.

- **Quinoa:** This gluten-free ancient seed is a complete vegan protein—meaning it contains all the essential amino acids (building blocks) that your body needs. It has an impressive 8 grams of protein and 5 grams of fiber per cup, which will limit spikes in blood sugars—in addition to the crucial minerals magnesium, manganese, phosphorus, copper, iron, folate, B vitamins, and zinc. Quinoa also contains the flavonoids quercetin and kaempferol, which have potential antioxidant, anti-inflammatory, and cancer-fighting properties.

- **Protein pasta:** When it comes to cooking for the whole family, boiling a pot of water is about as easy as it gets! Chickpea, black bean, edamame, or lentil protein pastas are readily available at health food stores and contain about 13 grams of protein in a 1 cup serving.

- **Hemp hearts:** These light, nutty inner parts of hemp seeds are a good plant source of anti-inflammatory omega-3 acids and are rich in protein—10 grams per 3 tablespoons. I sprinkle them atop smoothies, salads, and plant-based yogurts.

- **Watermelon seeds:** Just ⅓ of a cup has 13.5 grams of protein. That's almost twice the protein found in almonds! The kind I recommend is shelled so that they are easy to digest, deliciously crunchy, and ready to add to just about any meal or snack.

- **Pumpkin seeds (aka Pepitas):** With about 7 grams of protein per ¼ cup, they're a nutrient-dense addition to your pantry. Bonus: Sprouted pepitas may have more bioavailable nutrients such as iron and zinc!

- **Nuts and nut/seed butters:** They are all packed with anti-inflammatory fats and phytonutrients. Keep portions in check as they are calorically dense—I think of them as delicious toppers or stirred into oatmeal, salads, or a crunchy addition to a snack.

Power Tips to Alleviate the Typical Side Effects When Eating Beans

Let's be real, eating beans and legumes may definitely cause you to pass some extra wind, so here are some tricks to help alleviate this:

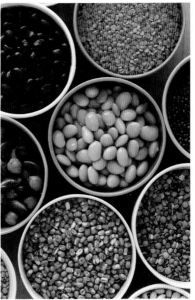

- Choose sprouted options for improved digestibility and enhanced bioavailability of nutrients.

- Soak beans overnight, rinsing them thoroughly before cooking.

- Add anise, fennel seeds, coriander seeds, cumin, caraway, or ginger while cooking.

- Add kombu (a type of dried seaweed) while cooking.

- For packaged cooked beans: drain the liquid and rinse thoroughly before consuming.

- Gradually add beans to your diet, starting with smaller serving sizes and working your way up so your body can get used to digesting them.

- Sip on hot water that's infused with fennel, peppermint, or chamomile during or after meals.

- You can take a supplement called alpha-galactosidase with the first bite of your bean-containing meal. It's the enzyme that helps break down the gassy parts! I don't recommend taking just any digestive enzyme—specifically look for alpha-galactosidase at a dose of about 300 units.

I like to mix up the types of nuts or seeds I choose to get a wide range of benefits...some of my favorites include walnuts, pistachios, almonds, cashews, Brazil nuts, pecans, and baru nuts!

Second Choice: Moderate Return Proteins

OMEGA-3 RICH FISH HAVE ANTI-INFLAMMATORY DHA AND EPA

Fish is an animal protein and does not contain the key fiber or protective plant phytochemicals like our premium plant-based protein options. Fish also has the potential for environmental contaminants and antibiotics, depending on how it's raised or where it's caught.

However, fish can provide a healthy dose of omega-3s, a type of fat that provides a whole-body anti-inflammatory effect. My goal for you is to increase your omega-3 intake to reduce the inflammatory load of your diet. While plant-based sources of omega-3s are healthy and great for you (such as the alpha linolenic acid aka ALA found in flaxseeds, walnuts, and chia seeds), they don't have the same extent of anti-inflammatory activity as the marine-based omega-3s called DHA and EPA. Our bodies can convert some ALA to DHA and EPA, but the rates are relatively low—only 0.1-21% of ALA is converted to DHA and EPA.

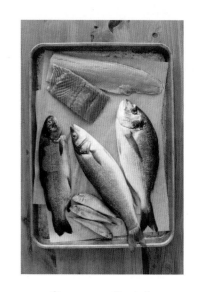

Omega-3 rich foods have an anti-inflammatory effect in the body.

Studies show DHA and EPA may also do the following:

- Reduce the risk of breast cancer: research indicates women with high omega-3 intake tend to lower rates of breast cancer. A meta-analysis that combined the results of 21 prospective cohort studies (overall including 20,900 cases of breast cancer) indicated that the risk of breast cancer was reduced by 5% per 0.1 gram per day of omega-3s—equivalent to about 1 serving of wild salmon per week, for example. Omega-3s have been shown to lower inflammation, prevent tumor cells from proliferating, and cause cancer cells to self-destruct.

- Improve heart health, lowering blood pressure and triglycerides while raising "good" cholesterol.

Where do you get the all-important DHA and EPA other than eating omega-3 rich fish? If you are fully plant-based then I recommend taking an algae-derived omega-3 supplement (of course, check with your healthcare team for any supplement use). Researchers have shown that the DHA in the supplements made from microalgae are biologically equivalent to those from fish oil.

In summary, omega-3 rich foods have an anti-inflammatory effect in the body and are important in breast cancer risk reduction. You can opt to take a microalgae supplement, or if you are not ready to dive 100% into a solely plant protein lifestyle, sprinkle in some low mercury, omega-3 rich fish such as wild salmon, herring, black cod, branzino, mackerel, low mercury tuna, or sardines to supplement your plant-based protein foundation.

Least Preferred: Low Return Proteins

GRASS-FED MEAT, ORGANIC POULTRY, AND EGGS

I can't tout anti-cancer benefits for poultry, meat, and eggs. These proteins don't offer the protective benefits of fiber or phytochemicals like plant-based proteins, and don't have high levels of omega-3 fats such as the moderate return proteins.

Scientific literature as a whole supports reducing meat consumption for optimal cancer risk reduction. A large study published in the *British Journal of Cancer* with over 35,000 women found that meat and processed meat intake increased the risk of breast cancer by 20-40%—the exact numbers vary on the type of meat: high total meat intake increased risk by 34%; red meat by 41%; processed meat by 39%. And we saw earlier that subbing out meat for a plant-based protein source can reduce risk—just subbing 1 serving of legumes for 1 serving of red meat per day resulted in 15% lower breast cancer risk!

> I can't tout anti-cancer benefits for poultry, meat, and eggs. These proteins don't offer the protective benefits of fiber or phytochemicals like plant-based proteins.

Of course, we're always awaiting more research on this topic. But based on the strong suggestive literature that already exists as well as some basic science and logic, I recommend gradually reducing and phasing out these animal-based proteins as part of the Beller Method for optimal breast cancer risk reduction.

WHY ARE ANIMAL PROTEINS THE LEAST PREFERRED OPTIONS FOR BREAST CANCER RISK REDUCTION?

All animal proteins have naturally occurring hormones: Estrogen is naturally produced in the animal body, regardless of whether the animal is treated with hormones or not. Of course, hormone-treated animals are even less ideal (cattle and sheep treated with estrogen naturally have been shown to have higher levels of estrogen compared to non-treated animals). No studies have specifically looked at the risk of breast cancer between women who eat meat from hormone-treated animals compared to those who eat meat from untreated animals. But logically hormone-treated animals would have more estrogenic effects.

Now, the big question is—does the estrogen in meat, poultry, eggs, and dairy actually increase your body's estrogen levels and raise risk of breast cancer? This is hard to study—especially if the potential effects are subtle and cumulatively add up over years. There are no scientific studies on the effects of long-term consumption of excess hormones from animal protein consumption...but there is research that suggests that even low levels of hormones can have effects on the body.

There is evidence in men and children that drinking cow's milk causes blood levels of estrogen to spike. Women are harder to study because the body produces higher and fluctuating levels of natural estrogen than men and children, but we do have some research with women. It has been shown that women who eat plant-based proteins with minimal meat intake have lower estrogen levels than those who ate a diet higher in animal proteins.

One thing we do know—conventionally raised cattle in the US are administered a synthetic estrogen chemical called zeranol as a growth promoter (it accelerates the growth of a calf to a full-grown cow ready for slaughter). Zeranol is a potent growth hormone that's found in human food and in lab studies may have up to 100,000 times the estrogenic effects of the plastic bisphenol A (BPA), though specific effects in humans remain to be studied.

Our goal is to minimize estrogen exposure, as lifetime exposure to estrogen has been linked to higher breast cancer risk. If you are being careful with estrogenic effects of plastics and medications, it makes sense to be mindful with estrogen-containing proteins.

Meat, poultry, and eggs have a poor fatty acid profile:

Meat, poultry, and eggs contain saturated fats and cholesterol, which may be linked to higher rates of breast cancer and heart disease. There is suggestive evidence that cholesterol may stimulate growth of human breast cancer cells. Additionally, a metabolite of cholesterol called 27-hydroxycholesterol may have estrogenic properties and may cause breast cancer cells to multiply and migrate. Saturated fat contributes to increased blood cholesterol (particularly LDL cholesterol, or "bad cholesterol") and also induces chronic inflammation, which may lead to the progression of tumor development.

We know that high total fat intake is linked with increased breast cancer risk, so the limited fat you do eat should be good-for-you fats rather than potentially harmful sources. There seems to be ongoing associations between saturated fat, cholesterol, and increased breast cancer risk, so it is best to minimize intake for optimal risk reduction.

> If you are being careful with estrogenic effects of plastics and medications, it makes sense to be mindful with estrogen-containing proteins.

Meat and poultry also have low levels of anti-inflammatory omega-3 fatty acids and higher levels of pro-inflammatory omega-6 fatty acids. If our goal is to lower the total amount of inflammation in the body, it makes sense to reduce the amount of meat we're consuming. Now, does grass-fed make a difference? Not too much. Yes, there are slightly more omega-3s in grass-fed meat; however the amount is still minimal when compared to the levels in fish and algae. According to the USDA, grass-fed beef top sirloin contains about 65 milligrams of omega-3 fatty acids per 100-gram serving. This amount seems meek compared to wild salmon, which clocks in at around 1,200-3,600 milligrams per 100-gram serving.

Animal proteins negatively affect the gut microbiome:

A healthy gut microbiome can help balance estrogen levels and therefore contribute to breast cancer risk reduction. It's important to nurture an environment that encourages the growth of healthy gut microbes...and research shows that meat can quickly and significantly affect the gut microbiome (in a bad way) in as little as one day! A diet rich in meat has more saturated fat than a plant-based diet. The saturated fat in meat requires increased levels of bile acids for digestion...and an environment rich in fat and bile acids encourages the growth of unhealthy bacteria in your gut. This state is called "dysbiosis" and dysbiosis has been linked to increased risk of breast cancer.

Why? Unhealthy gut bacteria, which may be sustained by a meat-rich diet high in saturated fat, may contain high levels of an enzyme called beta-glucuronidase, which actually causes the body to retain and recirculate excess estrogen instead of getting rid of it. We don't want excess estrogen, as this has been linked to breast cancer risk. Contrast this to plant-based proteins which, due to their fiber content, promote a healthy gut microbiome and reduce the excess estrogen in the body! It's pretty clear which is more advantageous for health.

Animal proteins may increase IGF-1 levels:

Insulin-like growth factor 1 (IGF-1) is a hormone that signals our cells to grow and multiply. While IGF-1 is needed for normal growth and development in children, it's typically not needed in large amounts as we age—our adult bodies don't need the signal to grow, grow, and grow! So levels of IGF-1 naturally decrease in adulthood. It's been observed that excessive IGF-1 in adults can actually have negative effects—in fact, high levels of IGF-1 have been linked to increased breast cancer risk.

In a recent 2020 study published in the *Annals of Oncology*, researchers looked at the blood levels of IGF-1 among over 206,000 women. The researchers found that women with the highest levels of IGF-1 were 25% more likely to develop breast cancer than those with the least amount of IGF-1. Why would this be? It's thought that excess IGF-1 ends up telling tumor cells to grow, potentially stimulating tumor cell proliferation, that, in turn, may lead to more estrogen activity.

A study from Oxford with 292 women found that IGF-1 was 13% lower in vegans compared to meat-eaters. They did not see any difference in IGF-1 levels based on the *amount* of protein consumed—but they did see a difference in IGF-1 based on the *source* of protein. Animal protein seemed to increase IGF-1 levels, and plant protein seemed to decrease IGF-1 levels.

Why is this? Not all protein is created equal! Yes, the protein from animals and the protein from plants both include all nine essential amino acids, which are necessary for carrying out important functions in the body, such as building muscles and transporting nutrients. However, the difference between the two is that the proportions of amino acids in animal proteins more closely resemble the proportions in our body's human proteins, compared to those from plants. When the liver responds to ingestion of animal protein, it quickly releases a flood of IGF-1 because the proteins are easily recognizable and broken down for use. On the other hand, plant sources of protein have more dissimilar ratios of amino acids, so they don't result in such a quick flood of IGF-1. Eating meat seems to signal our body to produce and release more IGF-1, and eating plant proteins instead may decrease IGF-1 levels.

> It's been observed that excessive IGF-1 in adults can actually have negative effects—in fact, high levels of IGF-1 have been linked to increased breast cancer risk.

In summary, even if you eat the same amount of protein (20 grams of meat versus 20 grams of a plant-based protein) your body is going to react to and process it differently—so when it comes to cancer risk reduction, plant-based is the way to go.

Animal proteins can produce carcinogenic compounds: Heterocyclic amines (HCAs) and polycyclic aromatic hydrocarbons (PAHs) are chemicals that are formed when animal meat is cooked over high temperatures—like pan frying, grilling, and smoking. A particular HCA called PhIP has been shown to fuel the initiation and growth of breast cancer in a similar way to estrogen. The National Cancer Institute has recognized that these chemicals can cause DNA mutations that may increase cancer risk.

A NOTE ON EGGS

It seems like the "expert recommendations" on eggs are changing every five years—it's confusing for sure! Let me shine some light on how eggs are potentially connected to breast cancer.

The body of literature is limited, but growing, in regard to eggs and breast cancer. There were two meta-analyses published in 2014 and 2015, along with a pooled cohort study that showed moderate trends toward increased breast cancer risk with egg consumption.

The 2015 study concluded that eating greater than 5 eggs per week was associated with moderately increased risk of breast cancer compared to women who didn't eat eggs. The researchers primarily attributed this elevated

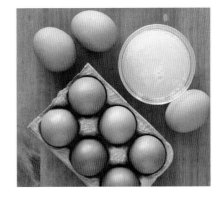

Researchers attributed this elevated risk in breast cancer to two nutrients found in eggs: cholesterol and choline. There is clinical data suggesting that cholesterol may contribute to breast cancer growth.

risk to two nutrients found in eggs: cholesterol and choline. There is clinical data suggesting that cholesterol may contribute to breast cancer growth, possibly due to the estrogenic effects of 27-hydroxycholesterol. As for choline, new research suggests that the nutrient in excess may possibly increase proliferation of cancer cells and increase inflammation. The gut bacteria break down the choline producing an inflammatory by-product called TMAO. Harvard researchers have linked the TMAO production from just 2.5 eggs per week to an increased rate in prostate cancer—it's possible the same inflammation could also contribute to breast cancer risk. Therefore, some experts suggest individuals with hormonally responsive cancers (such as breast, ovarian, and prostate cancer) exercise caution in regards to their egg intake.

While more research is still needed, I believe it's prudent to minimize egg consumption—logically there may be some potential risks that come along with eggs linked to hormonal and inflammatory effects.

WHAT ABOUT DAIRY?

In addition to soy, dairy is one of the foods my patients ask me about the most...for good reasons!

Studies that have examined the relationship between dairy and breast cancer are convoluted. There are many different dairy types—fermented, high-fat, low-fat, etc., and the findings of each and the impact on breast cancer risk rates of various breast cancer subtypes is difficult to research. Traditionally, large studies have not found a link between dairy products and breast cancer—though a well-known cohort from the Nurses' Health Study II found that higher fat dairy products (such as full fat milk and butter) were linked to breast cancer risk. But a 2020 study published in the *International Journal of Epidemiology* found that among a group of Seventh Day Adventists, all types of milk intake were significantly associated with an increased risk of breast cancer—even just ⅓ cup per day may increase risk!

The big question is: can the hormone level in a cup or two of milk actually hurt you? Nobody really knows—population-level studies are unclear and nutrition studies are hard to conduct, especially if the effects are subtle and cumulatively add up over the years. According to a 2021 meta-analysis that evaluated 36 articles with 1,019,232 participants, there is a trend toward

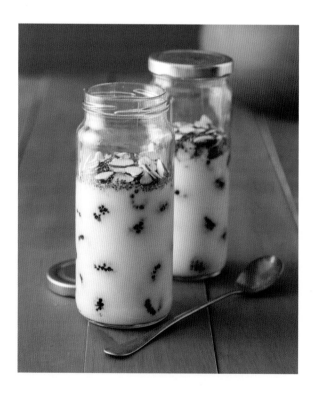

Getting Enough Calcium

Calcium intake is important to help maintain strong bones. Of course, dairy is the first thought when it comes to a calcium source, but there is also calcium in some plant-based foods such as whole soy foods, dark green leafy vegetables, cruciferous vegetables, kelp noodles, beans and legumes, and calcium-fortified plant-based milks to name a few. Some individuals may find it helpful to augment their calcium intake with supplements to help meet the Recommended Dietary Allowance (RDA) of calcium—consult with your doctor to see if this would be appropriate for you.

high-fat dairy possibly elevating breast cancer incidence, however more research is needed.

But let's think about the science and approach this from a logical perspective.

Dairy—like all animal products—contains naturally occurring hormones. Dairy cows persistently have high levels of hormones in their bodies as they are constantly producing milk—up to 20 times the normal amount, even without added hormones. One study has shown that estrogen levels in men and children spike just hours after drinking milk. Research has also shown that vegetarian women have lower hormone (specifically estrogen) levels than women who include meat and dairy in their diets. Additionally, milk naturally contains the growth hormone IGF-1, saturated fats, and cholesterol.

> The best tip I give my patients is to not focus on what you are trying to remove from your diet (animal proteins), but instead start being more inclusive of plant-based proteins.

With all of this information, my advice (knowing that the research is still not 100% conclusive) is to play it safe and err on the side of caution, and phase out dairy or keep to an occasional treat *especially* if you are at higher risk for breast cancer. Even the researchers conducting some of the above studies recommend caution with dairy milk. There are other ways to get your calcium and vitamin D, with less potential risk.

Let's Recap:

Meat, poultry, and eggs don't have nutrients that offer cancer protective benefits, and in fact may increase breast cancer risk in all the ways listed above. For optimal breast cancer risk reduction and as part of the Beller Method, I recommend greatly reducing or eliminating this category of protein. However, I understand that it can be a big transition to reduce intake—so if you are still including them, here are some tips to help work your way toward phasing them out:

- **If opting to eat red meat:** go with organic and grass fed—these varieties don't include "extra" hormones (though they still contain naturally occurring hormones) and tend to be leaner. They have slightly more omega-3 content but nothing to write home about. Also, avoid using high temperature cooking methods (>300 degrees) and if possible marinate with rosemary, garlic, and onion to help reduce some of the HCA formation.

- **Avoid all processed meats**: The World Health Organization classifies them as a carcinogenic food. Processed meats are those that have been preserved or changed by smoking, curing, salting, canning, or adding preservatives. This includes ham, bacon, sausage, pepperoni/salami, luncheon meats, prosciutto, smoked meats/salmon, hot dogs, and bratwurst.

- **If opting for poultry:** choose organic to avoid antibiotics. Choose leaner cuts and remove the skin to reduce saturated fat intake.

- **If opting for eggs:** choose, organic, omega-3 rich eggs. They come from hens fed a diet containing flaxseed or fish oil, resulting in higher omega-3 content. However, I wouldn't rely on eggs for omega-3s. A 4-ounce piece of salmon will give you 6-7x more omega-3s than two omega-3 eggs. I recommend boiling, poaching, or scrambling eggs instead of frying to avoid HCAs and PAHs. You can also consider opting for egg whites more often than the yolks to reduce cholesterol and choline intake.

- **If opting for dairy:** choose unsweetened varieties that also contain probiotics that may benefit gut health, such as kefir and yogurt. There are many dairy alternatives on the market today, including plant-based products made from nuts and seeds without highly processed additives (see page 109 for plant-based milk alternatives).

Select Premium Proteins

	PREFERRED CHOICE: Plant Protein	SECOND CHOICE: Fish/Seafood Microalgae Supplement	LEAST PREFERRED: Meat, Poultry, Eggs, Dairy
Contains cancer fighting phytochemicals	✓		
Rich in fiber	✓		
Boosts gut health	✓		
Is anti-inflammatory	✓		
Good source of DHA and EPA omega-3 fatty acids		✓	
Harmful carcinogenic HCAS are produced during cooking			✓
Contains naturally occurring hormones		✓	✓

Here's the Takeaway:

I've summarized the pros and cons of each protein category in the chart on the left. It's pretty clear—plant-based proteins are the clear winners and take the hat when it comes to breast cancer protective benefits. That's why the Beller Method is built around these premium protein options. And I've made it so simple with recipes that are easy to integrate seamlessly into your routine.

I recognize that the transition to a more plant-based diet can be a daunting one—but it's so beneficial for risk reduction and can really transform the way that you feel. The best tip I give my patients is to not focus on what you are trying to remove from your diet (animal proteins), but instead start being more inclusive of plant-based proteins. By doing so, you naturally start to phase out and reduce intake of animal proteins in a way that feels very comfortable and natural. Focus on adding more good!

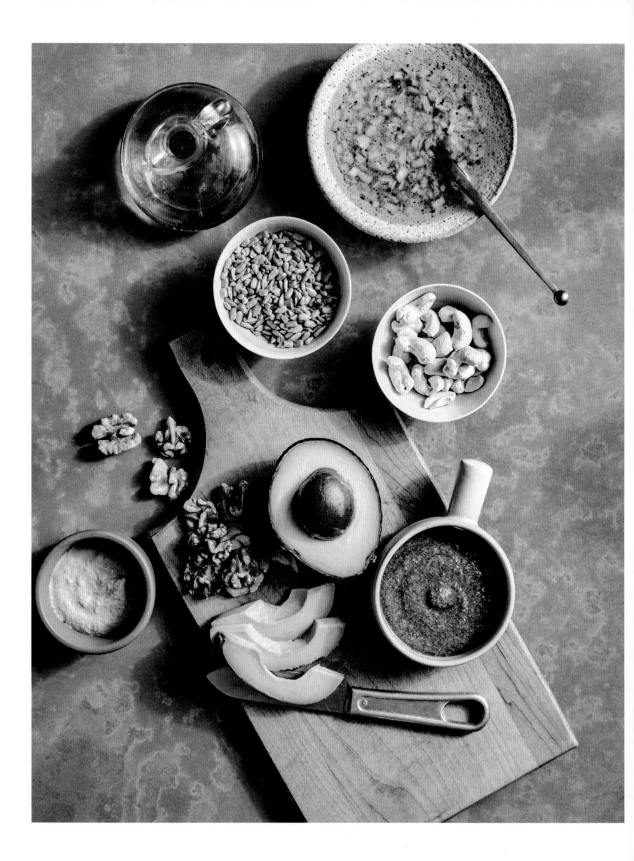

Get an Oil Change

HEALTHFUL FATS ARE A MUST!

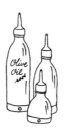

A lower-fat diet has been associated with reduced risk of breast cancer. We all need some fat in our diet, so stock your pantry with the best types of fats (Premium Power Pantry oils, nuts, seeds, and avocados) for optimal benefits including anti-inflammatory and antioxidant properties, while limiting ultra-processed options that have been linked to poor outcomes. It's okay to be picky with your fats!

Get an Oil Change

We now know the truth: fat in our food isn't the villain it was framed to be for decades. As it turns out, some kinds of fat are actually good for us—and some are even *essential*. Fat improves skin and hair, helps us absorb nutrients, and keeps our immune systems strong. For optimal breast cancer risk reduction, a moderate amount of the RIGHT kinds of fat is necessary. But before we get into the specifics, let's take a look at the research about fat and breast cancer.

What the Research Says About Fat and Breast Cancer

Since the 1970s, scientists have hypothesized that high fat intake increases breast cancer risk, but recent studies have shed more light on this issue.

One of these was the EPIC study, which followed more than 300,000 women across Europe. Researchers concluded that women who ate the most fat (equivalent of 4 tablespoons of oil per day) had a higher risk of breast cancer compared to those who ate a third of that amount. Women who ate the most saturated fat in particular had about a 30% higher risk of ER+/PR+ and HER2-negative breast cancer. This was similar to findings in a few other major research projects: Women's Health Initiative and Nurses' Health Study.

The above studies suggested a link between high fat intake and increased breast cancer risk, but they were observational studies—meaning that they're looking at associations, not cause and effect. To learn about cause and effect you need to conduct the gold standard of scientific research: a randomized control trial. That's what I worked on for 10 years as the Site Coordinator at Cedars Sinai Medical Center and Providence Saint John's Health Center for the Women's Intervention Nutrition Study (WINS). In this study, we assigned 2,400 women with early-stage breast cancer to either a control group or a dietary intervention group. The women in the intervention group were given 8 counseling sessions with a dietitian to help them reduce their fat intake. Not only did these women lose about 6 pounds, but they lowered their fat intake by about 10 grams per day. After 5 years of follow-up, there were 24% lower breast cancer relapses in the intervention group compared to in the controls. After 10 years, there were 59% fewer deaths in the ER-/PR- patients in particular. Wow!

There haven't been other large scale randomized control trials examining the role of fat intake on breast cancer risk and thrivership—we're still waiting on more research. But collectively research seems to suggest a correlation between a higher fat diet and increased risk—and it does make sense on a cellular level.

WHY: Fat and Breast Cancer, Explained

Eating high amounts of fat increases the size of fat cells in the body. After menopause, these fat cells become estrogen factories, churning out additional hormones daily. And we know that higher estrogen levels increase breast cancer risk (ER+/PR+).

But it's not just about the estrogen! A low-fat diet also seems to work in an estrogen-independent way, as the WINS study found significant benefit of a lower fat diet among ER-negative patients. How? It's thought that excess fat tissue accumulation can lead to insulin resistance—the state where the body is less sensitive to the effects of the hormone insulin. And chronic insulin resistance activates a chemical cascade in the body that leads to an increase in insulin-like growth factor 1 (IGF-1), which in turn may promote tumor growth. Therefore, a lower-fat diet could potentially help restore the body's insulin sensitivity and reverse insulin's tumor-promoting effects. Additionally, extra fat cells can trigger chronic low-grade inflammation in the body, which can set off a cascade of chemical reactions that cause the immune system to stimulate breast cancer cell growth.

> After menopause, fat cells become estrogen factories, churning out additional hormones daily.

So in summary—large scale studies on fat intake and breast cancer are mixed, but experimental research suggests that a lower-fat diet may reduce risk. In general, experts tend to recommend a lower-fat diet for optimal protection, ideally in a range of just 20% of calories from fat. What's essential is the TYPE of fat you're choosing.

Be Picky with Your Fat

Not all fats are considered equal. Not by a long shot! If we're going to be limiting our fat intake to a moderate amount, then it's essential to stock our pantries with the best of the best—the right types of fats that have so many benefits, from optimizing nutrient absorption to reducing inflammation, modulating immunity, keeping your skin healthy, and potentially decreasing cancer risk. Shop for and cook with my Power Pantry fats on a daily basis so that your overall diet consists primarily of anti-inflammatory and antioxidant-rich options for optimal breast cancer risk reduction.

FATS TO EMBRACE:

- **Omega-3 fatty acids** have been shown to have a protective effect on breast cancer, largely due to their anti-inflammatory effects. Eating omega-3s inhibits inflammatory chemicals and decreases signaling of growth receptors in the body—they act in opposition to omega-6s (which you'll read about in a minute). The omega-3s found in fish and microalgae in particular may cause cancer cells to self-destruct. Plus, they can help with insulin sensitivity, which we know is tied to lower risk. There are two main types of omega-3 fatty acids:

  – **Eicosapentaenoic acid (EPA) and docosahexaenoic acid (DHA)** come mainly from fish and algae. These are the most potent anti-inflammatory and anti-cancer fats—a meta-analysis of studies found that higher consumption of these fats was found to decrease the risk of breast cancer, with a 50% decreased risk observed for every 1 gram per day intake of marine omega-3s! This is why I recommend an algae-based omega-3 supplement. Or, if you do choose to include fish I consider omega-3 rich fish to be a moderate return protein.

  – **Alpha linolenic acid (ALA)** is found in nuts, flaxseeds, flaxseed oil, chia seeds, and leafy vegetables. ALA is great and the foods that contain them are healthy—but they aren't the best type of omega-3s. As we've discussed in the protein chapter, the body can only convert 0.1-21% of these fats to the more potent omega-3s: EPA and DHA. So eat up—but don't rely on them alone for optimal benefits.

- **Monounsaturated fats** found in certain plant foods (olive oil, avocados, nuts, and seeds) have been linked to significantly decreased breast cancer risk. How? Potentially due to lowering inflammation and improving insulin sensitivity.

  Olive oil in particular is rich in oleic acid, a monounsaturated fat that has been linked to lower breast cancer risk. Its benefit may possibly be related to improving insulin resistance, or potentially due to olive oil's rich polyphenol content.

PREMIUM POWER PANTRY OILS

These are rich in anti-inflammatory monounsaturated fats and omega-3 fatty acids and should be your basic go-to's to use for cooking.

- **Cold-pressed (unrefined) extra-virgin olive oil:** My go-to oil. It has at least 30 plant-based phytochemicals, which account for its antioxidant, anti-inflammatory, and potential anti-cancer effects. It has a low smoke point, so it's best for salads, dressings, and cold dishes.

- **Extra-virgin (refined) olive oil:** It's a little less flavorful than unrefined extra-virgin olive oil, but it has a bit higher of a smoke point, making this oil is best for medium-heat cooking such as baking, braising, or a gentle sauté.

- **Avocado oil:** It adds a slight buttery flavor to foods and has a high smoke point for high-heat cooking and searing. Purchase unrefined and cold pressed for the highest levels of antioxidants and phytochemicals. Bonus: It's also rich in heart-healthy monounsaturated fats!

- **Walnut oil:** It has a rich, nutty taste, and is high in beneficial omega-3 fatty acids. Walnut extract has also been shown to possibly decrease breast cancer cell proliferation. While you can use it for medium-heat cooking, walnut oil's flavor is best showcased in cold dishes and salads.

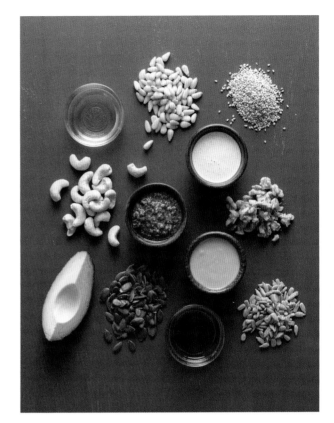

- **Almond oil:** It's rich in monounsaturated fat and the antioxidant vitamin E, and adds a slight sweet nuttiness but isn't as earthy as walnut oil. Purchase a cold-pressed variety and use over salads, cold dishes, and baking.

- **Flaxseed oil:** It's rich in plant-based omega-3s and lignans, which have potential anti-cancer benefits. Make sure to purchase cold-pressed oil in a dark bottle and use relatively quickly, as it may develop a bitter taste. Use on cold dishes and for salad dressings.

OTHER POWER KITCHEN FATS

- Avocados

- Nuts: such as almonds, hazelnuts, pecans, and walnuts

- Seeds: pumpkin seeds and pepitas, chia seeds, sesame seeds

- DHA/EPA rich foods have particularly potent anti-inflammatory omega-3s (see protein chapter for more information): Algae oil or omega-3 rich fish

FATS TO LIMIT:

Omega-6 fatty acids: High intake of omega-6 fatty acids have been linked to higher breast cancer risk. Now, omega-6 fats are essential in small to moderate amounts. But in our Western diets there tends to be an *over-balance* of omega-6s in our diet (compared to omega-3s), possibly leading to increased cellular damage and inflammation. Elevated amounts of omega-6s have been shown to potentially cause an up-regulation of pro-inflammatory chemicals like COX, LOX, prostaglandins, and leukotrienes. Again, most people eat too many of these fats!

The following oils tend to be highly processed, lower in nutrients, and higher in omega-6 fats compared to my Power Pantry fats. I recommend limiting these when it comes to purchasing products and cooking.

- Vegetable oils:
  - Soybean
  - Canola/rapeseed
  - Grapeseed
  - Corn
  - Safflower
  - Sunflower
  - Partially hydrogenated oil (of any kind)
  - Any butters/margarines/spreads with the above

Oils in packaged and restaurant foods

Whenever possible, look for pre-made snacks made with olive or avocado oil. And even better yet, I'd rather you have a whole-food snack that includes healthy fat options like avocado or nuts, or opt for one of the Power Snack recipes later in this book.

Many restaurants tend to use these highly processed oils—you can't always know or control the fat sources when you're out! That's why it's essential to opt for Power Pantry fats in your home kitchen and with products you're purchasing—you leave room for the unknown when you are enjoying meals away from home.

Saturated fats: Due to scientific findings, I recommend limiting saturated fats, found in animal foods like dairy and meat. Harvard scientists found that high intake of animal fat—which contains saturated fat—was associated with increased risk of breast cancer. And a meta-analysis of 15 studies found that high saturated fat intake was associated with an increase in breast cancer mortality rate. Why? This may be due to saturated fat contributing to elevated serum cholesterol, and one of the metabolites of cholesterol may contribute to the proliferation of breast cancer cells. There's also evidence that saturated fat may increase insulin resistance, thus possibly contributing to breast cancer risk (as mentioned in the protein chapter).

Examples of foods high in saturated fat include:

- Meat: beef, lamb, pork, poultry—especially with the skin

- Butter

- Cream

- Baked goods made with a lot of butter

- Cheese

- Coconut and palm oils

A note about coconut:

Coconut and palm oils are also high in saturated fats. I know there's been a big push on coconut oil recently—but we don't yet have the research to say that it's beneficial or harmful in regards to breast cancer risk. Yes, it may not have the same health implications as animal fats due to it being a plant source, and there's preliminary data about lauric acid in coconut oil improving quality of life during chemotherapy, but until more research comes out it's not something I routinely recommend as a daily fat source in your Power Pantry. Some people tout the benefits of medium-chain triglycerides (MCTs) present in coconut oil—but MCTs only make up about 15% of coconut oil as a whole. Coconut oil is 80-90% saturated fat, which has been shown to potentially increase cholesterol levels, both the good and bad cholesterol. I advise my patients to err on the safe side and use coconut oil sparingly and occasionally in recipes that call specifically for that coconut oil flavor—otherwise, stick to my recommended Power Pantry oils.

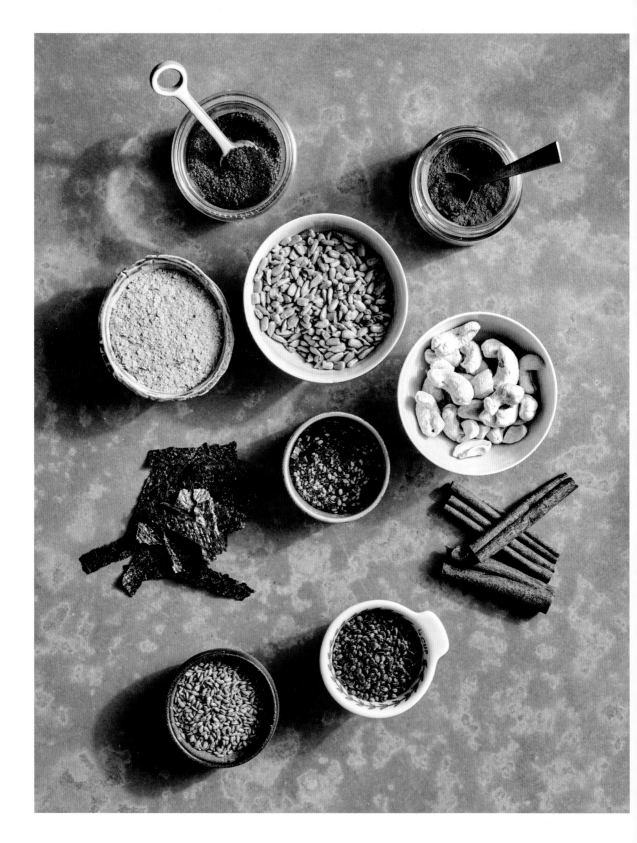

Power Up
Your Pantry!

LEVEL UP YOUR NUTRITION

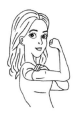

Once you have built a solid foundation and have gotten the hang
of the nutritional principles of the Beller Method, I encourage
you to accessorize and add some outstanding Power Up
ingredients. Of course, these ingredients alone do not make up
an optimal cancer fighting strategy—the other pillars of the Beller
Method do that for you. But Power Ups can truly elevate your
meals and make a difference in the overall nutritional profile of
your diet. Stock your pantry with a few to start—
there's something for everyone's budget and flavor palate.

Power Up Your Pantry!

LEVEL UP YOUR NUTRITION

Now that you've got some core Beller Method strategies under your belt, it's time to learn about my favorite nutrition heavyweights I call "Power Ups" that take your meals from good to great. They come swinging when it comes to antioxidant, anti-inflammatory, or potential breast cancer fighting properties. And the best thing about them: they're not supplements. Yep, they're real wholesome foods—many of which you can find at your local supermarket or online. Just small additions of these foods can make a BIG impact and dramatically elevate the nutritional value of what you eat and drink.

The following are some of my favorite starter items to add to your *SpiceRack* kitchen. You don't have to get them all at once—even a few can make a difference.

Power Pantry Difference Makers

Your pantry isn't just for flour and sugar. Include these incredibly nutritious ingredients so they're readily available for you to incorporate on a regular basis.

Amla powder: Otherwise known as Indian gooseberry, amla has been shown to have potential anticancer properties. Amla is rich in phytochemicals including ellagic acid, gallic acid, quercetin, pyrogallol, and corilagin—and using the powder as opposed to eating the berry gives you a concentrated form of these phytochemicals. Studies suggest that not only does amla have antioxidant and anti-inflammatory effects, which may be protective, but that it also may augment the action of some liver enzymes that assist with carcinogen detoxification. Amla has been shown to also have anti-tumor activity—it may inhibit growth of breast cancer cells while leaving regular cells alone.

Uses: The flavor is slightly bitter and sour, which can sometimes make it a challenge for my patients to integrate with consistency. I've found it's most easily integrated into smoothies.

Black cumin: Also known as nigella seeds, black cumin seeds are rich in a compound called thymoquinone, which has potent anti-inflammatory, antioxidant, and digestion-stimulating properties. It's been shown to potentially halt breast cancer tumor cell growth and spread. Plus, it has liver-protective effects and may help boost some of the liver's natural detoxifying enzymes.

Uses: They have a flavor that slightly resembles cumin or oregano, or that of toasted seeds atop an Everything bagel. Sprinkle these little black seeds on any savory dish, mix into quinoa, or add to dressings. My favorite way to use them is in a soothing tea (see page 147) that supports digestion.

Cacao powder: Cacao powder is a minimally processed form of chocolate and is the closest you can get to the raw cocoa bean in powder form. Because cacao is made at very low temperatures, the final product retains a high concentration of enzymes, vitamins, and nutrients. Cacao powder is packed with polyphenols (primarily epicatechin and catechin)—twice as many polyphenols as red wine and three times as many polyphenols as green tea! Lab studies show that these polyphenols might inhibit cancer cell growth and proliferation and may encourage cancer cell death. They may also boost your body's natural antioxidant enzymes, which help protect your cells against damage.

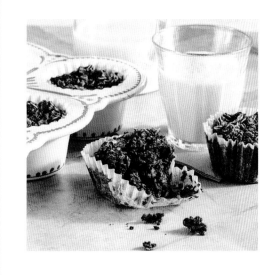

Cacao powder is packed with polyphenols (primarily epicatechin and catechin)—twice as many polyphenols as red wine and three times as many polyphenols as green tea!

Uses: Feel free to use cacao whenever you're craving a chocolatey flavor—I routinely add it to smoothies, tea, oatmeal, nut butters, lattes, and baked goods.

Hemp hearts: Shelling the hemp seed isolates the tender hemp heart. Think of these as protein powerhouses rather than fiber boosters—one 3-tablespoon serving has a whopping 10 grams of protein.

Uses: The hearts have a subtle nutty flavor and can either be eaten raw or cooked. Top a salad, add to yogurt or oats, blend into a smoothie, or stir into your quinoa or other plant-based protein.

Hibiscus flower powder: The hibiscus flower is rich in antioxidants including beta-carotene, vitamin C, and anthocyanins. Anthocyanins in particular may have cancer-protective benefits—they have been shown to have potential anti-mutagenic, anti-proliferative, and anti-metastasis effects. Hibiscus may also help with fat loss and weight management. The powder is a concentrated source of hibiscus flower that is typically used in tea, so you are likely getting even more potency!

Uses: It has a tart flavor, similar to cranberry. You can use the powder to make a hot or cold tea (see Black Cumin Ruby Tonic on page 147), or blend into a smoothie.

Matcha: Green tea contains the potent antioxidant epigallocatechin gallate (EGCG for short), which has been shown to possibly inhibit breast cancer by restricting cancer cell growth and encouraging tumor cell apoptosis. But studies have shown that the best effects may be seen with up to 5-10 cups of green tea per day—who has time for that? Matcha solves the problem! You actually drink the high-quality green tea leaves that are dried and ground up, rather than steeping them. Matcha has up to 137 times greater concentration of EGCG compared to regular green tea. Bonus: EGCG has also been shown to aid with weight loss, which of course also supports risk reduction.

Uses: Of course this makes a delicious latte (see Matcha Latte recipe on page 148)—but I also love using matcha for an afternoon tonic, adding to a smoothie, and stirring into oats or yogurt.

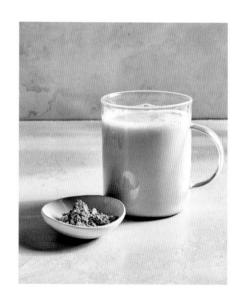

Dried mushrooms and mushroom powder: Mushrooms are rich in aromatase inhibitors, which may reduce the activity of an enzyme that produces estrogen, thus reducing estrogen levels. Mushrooms also contain beta-glucans, which are a special type of prebiotic fiber that may support the immune system. There are so many types of mushrooms out there and they ALL have benefits! Yes, there are exotic varieties such as maitake, shiitake, reishi, and turkey tail. But don't forget about crimini, porcini, shiitake and portobellos—even the humble white button mushroom has been shown to inhibit breast cancer proliferation.

Dried mushrooms: Use my spaghetti prep method to prepare: boil in water for 30 minutes to re-hydrate, then cook as you would any fresh mushroom.

Mushrooms are rich in aromatase inhibitors, which may reduce the activity of an enzyme that produces estrogen, thus reducing estrogen levels.

Mushroom powder: Using powders is a great way to get more exotic mushrooms that may not be readily available in fresh form. Mushroom powders are easy to add into coffee, tea (see Golden Mushroom Latte recipe on page 143), smoothies, marinara sauce, salad dressings, and soups for an extra nutritional boost.

Nori: Nori is a dried seaweed (think: the outside of a sushi roll) that is one of my secret ways to diversify your fiber intake! Not only is it packed with vitamins and minerals (I call it one of nature's multivitamins), but it also contains unique marine prebiotic fibers which may help reduce estrogen levels. A study published in the *British Journal of Nutrition* found that a single sheet of nori per day was linked to a lower risk of breast cancer, possibly due to its fibers, antioxidants, and polyphenols. Bonus: Nori is budget friendly—on average, just $3 per pack of organic nori, which averages out to about 25 cents per sheet!

Uses: Try making quinoa sushi—or roll nori and vegetables into a nori burrito! You can also tear some up and use on top of soups and salads.

Nutritional yeast: Nutritional yeast is an inactive yeast called *Saccharomyces cerevisiae*. Though it may sound odd, it's quite delicious! Nutritional yeast (as well as other yeasts and fungi) contains beta-glucans, which are specific types of fibers that may enhance your natural immune system. In addition, it's a complete protein meaning it contains all nine amino acids that are necessary for life—and a couple of spoonfuls may add 8-10 grams of protein.

Shopping Tips: Nutritional yeast is available in flakes or powder form—either is fine as they taste the same, they just have slightly different textures.

Uses: With its nutty, cheesy flavor, it's often used as a cheese substitute in vegan dishes. Mix into a creamy dressing (like tahini and cashew cream), add into marinara sauce, or season roasted veg, tofu scrambles, soups, pasta—anytime that you'd use a bit of Parmesan. Or, sprinkle onto fresh popcorn with a spritz of olive oil and a dash of garlic.

Plant-based milks: Many recipes utilize plant-based milk—there are a variety of types with different flavors and benefits. My suggestion is to ideally look for options that have a short ingredient list (e.g., just water, the nut, seed, or soybean, and a touch of salt). Many alternative milks contain gums, oils, and other fillers—if possible go for choices that are simple and wholesome. I generally reach for organic soy, cashew, and pistachio milks due to their higher protein content compared to other plant-based milks.

Plant-based protein powders: While they're not a necessity, a protein powder can level up the total protein content of a meal or snack if you need an extra boost. I recommend single-ingredient nut powders, such as almond, pumpkin, watermelon seed or hemp powders. Look for products made without excess fillers, gums, sweeteners, vitamins or flavorings. Almond protein powder in particular tends to mix well into a variety of recipes with a neutral flavor and no chalky texture.

Sesame seeds and tahini: Sesame seeds are the #2 dietary source of lignans (after flaxseeds)—lignans are phytoestrogens that have been shown to have anti-breast cancer, anti-inflammatory, and antioxidant properties. Tahini paste is made out of ground sesame seeds. It's a major ingredient in hummus and is also used to make tahini sauce and dressing.

Uses: Sprinkle sesame seeds as a meal topper (on salads, soups, or quinoa for example). I love using tahini paste to make a simple creamy tahini dressing or sauce (see page 297).

Tart cherry powder: Tart cherries aren't just packed with vitamins A and C—but they are also rich in phytochemicals called anthocyanins. In fact, they may have up to 200% more anthocyanins than their sweet cherry cousins, and 90% more than raspberries! Anthocyanins are powerful antioxidants and have been shown to have anti-inflammatory and potential anti-cancer properties. Tart cherries also contain melatonin, which is a hormone that helps promote better sleep.

Uses: Use in an evening tea (my Bedtime Tonic, page 151), or add to yogurt, oats, or smoothies.

Young barley grass powder: This is made of the ground leaves of young barley grass, about 10 days old, picked at peak nutritional value. Barley grass is rich in flavonoids, antioxidants, and may even have anti-cancer properties—studies have shown it may reduce proliferation of breast cancer cells. It's about 30% fiber (about 3 grams of fiber per tablespoon) and contains some beta-glucans, which have potential prebiotic and immune-enhancing properties. As a bonus: it contains GABA, which is a neurotransmitter that helps relax, alleviate anxiety and pain, and regulate sleep.

Uses: The flavor is mildly sweet and smoother than matcha. Add to water or a plant-based milk for a warm latte (see page 153), or add to a smoothie.

SPICES:

Of course spices are major players in all the recipes—but I want you to always be thinking of how to Power Up and consider using Power Spice Blends liberally throughout your day.

When shopping for spices, I recommend choosing organic, as conventional spices are often sterilized by fumigation or irradiation which may introduce chemicals and also cause loss of nutrients. Organic spices may cost a few dollars more but they are worth the investment, especially since they're a pantry item that you will regularly use over the course of months. Also, read the label and avoid spice blends with a lot of added salt, sugars, or fillers because those dilute the nutritional value—you want the pure spice! Once you open the package, spices tend to last for about 6-12 months. Take a sniff—if there's a potent aroma you're good to go. If the scent is faint, it's time to replace.

Once you've stocked your power pantry with individual spices and synergistic spice blends, you'll be ready to get cooking...and also shake spices on top of your foods and stir into others!

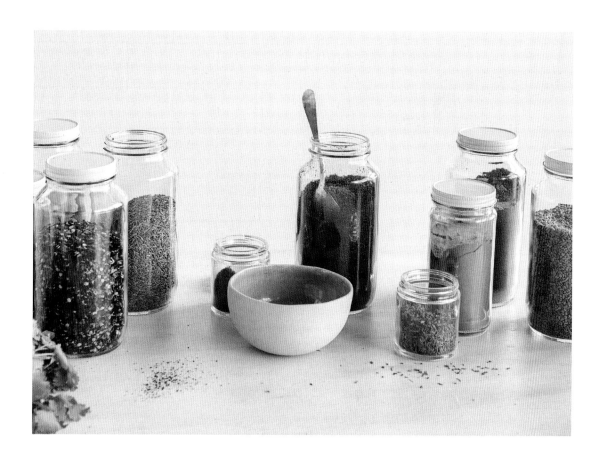

Power Spice Blends: Power Spicing is a pillar to the Beller Method as it dramatically multiplies the antioxidant, anti-inflammatory, and possible anti-cancer benefits of a meal with just a few pinches. While single spices are amazing and I definitely recommend having them on hand, I have found that utilizing balanced, tasty spice blends is an incredibly useful tool to incorporate Power Spicing daily. It simplifies the recipes and streamlines the cooking process (so much quicker to add a teaspoon of a blend instead of pulling out and measuring five separate spices).

So keep your Power Spice Blends handy! I recommend having at least a few blends in your kitchen—some that you can reach for in the morning for breakfast-type or sweet foods, and some savory all-purpose blends that you can rotate between and use for vegetables or protein dishes. I even leave a couple blends on the kitchen table so my family can sprinkle atop any meal. I formulated my Power Spice Blends to optimize their spice synergy and flavor in order to harness some of the most potent spice synergy combos out there (see pages 19–25 in the Spicing chapter for more details and specific ingredients). You can purchase these blends at bellernutrition.com and several other online retailers. Of course you can use alternatives and I've offered some approximations within the recipes.

- **Vegitude Power:** This is my carefully formulated blend for breast cancer risk reduction and can be used in almost any savory dish. It's great with veggies, of course (roasting, sautéing, grilling), but also is great on any proteins, in soups, added to salad dressings and mixed into spreads like hummus and tahini.

- **Everything Savory:** An all-purpose blend with balanced flavors that's easy to incorporate to elevate the nutritional power of dishes, with major flavor notes of paprika, cumin, and turmeric. Add to anything and everything savory—season any protein, mix into a quinoa or bean salad, add to vegetables.

- **Savory Sizzle:** Crank up the heat, flavor, and nutritional power of your dish—this is great on marinades, roasted chickpeas, chili, proteins, and hummus.

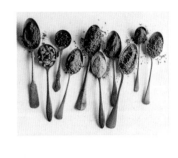

Utilizing balanced, tasty spice blends is an incredibly useful tool to incorporate spicing daily.

- **Tex Mex:** Sprinkle on some south-of-the-border flavor that's more savory than spicy. Use in chili (of course) as well as any protein dish, vegetables, warm bean or grain salad, hummus, or a tofu scramble.

- **Cinnapeel Spicer:** True Ceylon cinnamon is complemented with granulated orange peel and ginger for a bright yet grounded flavor that's great with anything sweet—oatmeal, nut butter, smoothies, yogurts, and baked goods.

- **Golden Breakfast:** This blend takes chocolate to the next level with a few key ingredients that spice up the sweetness and add complexity and depth. I love using it for a golden matcha latte, but it's also great blended into smoothies, mixed into nut butters, stirred into oatmeal, or added to any healthy muffin or baked treat recipe.

- **Morning Boost:** Think apple pie mix...but Power Spicing style. This blend adds a warm, spiced flavor to any sweeter breakfast option—or snack, latte, smoothie, or dessert!

- **Other spice blends you can incorporate** include Italian seasoning blend, curry blend, garam masala blend, and za'atar.

Mustard seeds and mustard seed powder: Mustard seeds come from a cruciferous vegetable and are rich in anti-cancer nutrients called glucosinolates. They also contain an enzyme called myrosinase and this is KEY to harnessing the power of cooked cruciferous vegetables (broccoli, Brussels, cabbage, for example). The glucosinolates in cruciferous veg need to be broken down by myrosinase in order for their cancer-fighting properties to be maximally effective. Unfortunately, cooking the vegetables for a long period of time deactivates the myrosinase—so sprinkle some mustard powder or seeds on top of the cooked veg to re-introduce that enzyme and boost the nutritional power of your cruciferous.

Spice Up Everyday Foods

I get it—we all need a few shortcuts to keep a healthy lifestyle sustainable! But pre-packaged foods don't have to be boring. Level Up! Grab your Power Spice Blends and stir in some spice to these items on your grocery list (and more)...a few pinches of spices will take them from plain to powerful!

- **Marinara sauce:** Add in ½–1 teaspoon per cup of an Italian herb blend or any combination of the following: dried thyme, rosemary, basil, parsley, or oregano.

- **Nut butter:** Stir in 1 teaspoon of one of the sweet Beller Nutrition Power Blends such as Cinnapeel Spicer or Golden Breakfast, or a similar blend of choice. Alternatively, sprinkle some spice on top of nut butter.

- **Hummus:** Stir in any of the following: Vegitude Power blend, Everything Savory blend, Savory Sizzle blend, Tex Mex blend, paprika (sweet or smoked), za'atar, sumac, or turmeric.

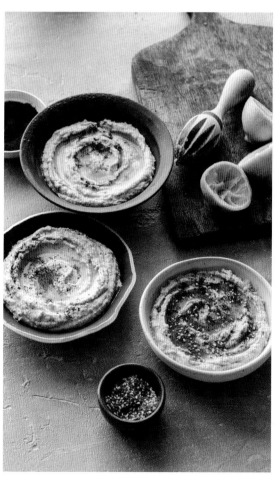

- **Salad dressings and dips:** Don't hesitate to shake in any dried herb or ½-1 teaspoon of a savory spice blend.

- **Coffee:** Add some Cinnapeel Spicer blend, Morning Boost blend, Ceylon cinnamon, or even some ground ginger for a powerful twist.

- **Popcorn or popped sorghum:** You can go savory (nutritional yeast, cayenne, or any savory spice blend) or sweet (Ceylon cinnamon)—just toss the popcorn with a hint of walnut, olive or avocado oil and the spices and enjoy!

- **Whole grains (cooked):** Turn bland into grand by stirring in any savory spice or spice blend with a bit of oil. Bonus points if you add some fresh chopped herbs.

- **Oatmeal or hot cereal:** Don't miss out on this opportunity to majorly boost the antioxidant content of your breakfast—add any sweet spice blend or Ceylon cinnamon, clove, and cardamom to dial up the nutrition.

- **Plant-based yogurt:** Add any of the spices you'd add to your oatmeal here as well!

FIBER BOOSTERS:

Pick from these (or choose a few) to add to your breakfast to get your AM 10 grams of fiber! But don't stop there—add to some of your meals (and beverages) throughout the day and remember to rotate them for enhanced fiber diversification.

Chia seeds: Chia seeds are my classic fiber booster—readily available in most supermarkets now, they're an easy way to upgrade your meal! These little seeds absorb water and form a gel-like consistency, indicating they're rich in soluble fiber (about 5 grams of fiber per tablespoon, which is more than an apple!). This soluble fiber may help soak up and expel excess estrogen and toxins, keeps you regular, and may help with weight management. Bonus: chia seeds are richer in plant-based omega-3s compared to basil seeds.

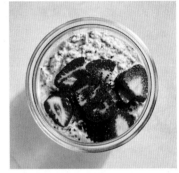

Uses: Blend into smoothies, stir into oatmeal, use to make breakfast cookies, top plant-based yogurt, or make chia seed pudding.

Basil seeds: These are one of my fave fiber boosters—they have a whopping 7 grams of fiber per tablespoon! They may help you excrete excess estrogen, regulate blood sugars, and keep you full for longer. Like chia seeds, basil seeds are neutral in flavor and gel in water, but they only take 1 minute to reach desired consistency.

Uses: Blend into smoothies, top your oatmeal, or stir into a tea or tonic for a major fiber boost.

Flaxseeds: Flaxseeds are a breast cancer power player—they're the #1 dietary source of lignans. Lignans are phytoestrogens that may work to reduce breast cancer tumor growth and spread. A study published in the *Clinical Cancer Research Journal* gave 32 women with breast cancer either a daily ground flaxseed muffin (containing about 2 tablespoons of flaxseed) or a placebo muffin, then took biopsies 1 month later to look at tumor cells. The women who ate the flaxseed muffins had significantly reduced tumor cell growth, indicating that flaxseeds may be protective even in regular, small doses!

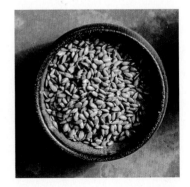

Bonus: Whole flaxseeds have about 3 grams of fiber per tablespoon and they're high in anti-inflammatory omega-3s.

Uses: *Add to oatmeal, baked goods (breakfast cookies, muffins, or pancakes), sprinkle on top of some plant-based yogurt, or add to smoothies.*

Tips: If available, purchase flaxseeds sprouted and ground. Sprouting improves digestibility and enhances nutrient absorption. Grinding the flaxseeds also improves their tolerance and nutrient accessibility—but grinding can cause oxidative damage if it's not packaged correctly. So look for a product that's in an opaque, air-tight package. Store the ground flaxseed in the refrigerator and use it within 4–6 months.

Whole roasted hemp seeds: Hemp seeds come from the hemp plant (but a different variety than cannabis—no psychoactive properties here). The whole seed is rich in fiber and protein—2 tablespoons contain 4½ grams of fiber and 4 grams of protein. It has both soluble and insoluble fiber, making it a well-rounded booster for your gastrointestinal tract. Bonus—hemp seeds also contain omega-3s, have anti-inflammatory properties, and may benefit cardiovascular health.

Uses: *Whole or ground roasted hemp seeds add a nice crunch and slightly nutty, toasted flavor. Add on top of hot cereal or to a homemade granola.*

Psyllium husk: Psyllium is a prebiotic, soluble fiber that's made from the seeds of an Indian shrub. It may help build a healthy gut microbiome (which we know is essential for breast health), and it can balance blood sugar levels as well as decrease cholesterol. There's also substantial research for psyllium husk helping with regularity and digestive symptoms.

Uses: *Mix 1 tablespoon with about 8 fl oz of water, or add to a smoothie.*

Tip: Whole psyllium husk has a more grainy texture and is less dense (3 ½ grams of fiber per tablespoon). The psyllium husk powder has a smoother texture than the whole husk, but is more concentrated (7 grams of fiber per tablespoon). I recommend starting with a small amount and working your way up!

Oat fiber: We all know oats are rich in fiber—but did you know that the oats at the store (yes, even steel cut oats) are actually missing their outermost shell called the hull? They of course have a multitude of benefits, but here's a secret to reap even more from oats: use oat fiber! Oat fiber is made from the ground hull. It is an insoluble fiber that may act as a natural gut detox and help with stool bulking and regularity. It adds 3 grams of fiber (but essentially zero calories) per teaspoon.

Uses: *Mix 1 teaspoon into oatmeal, smoothies, or my Fiberized Breakfast Cookies (see page 167).*

Acacia prebiotic fiber powder: There are tons of fiber powders out there—but many of them (like inulin and wheat dextrin, for example) can cause uncomfortable bloating. I generally recommend acacia fiber—it is a prebiotic, soluble fiber that comes from the sap of an African tree. It can help with regularity and is typically well-tolerated (read: no bloat!). One tablespoon has about 5 grams of fiber. Acacia powder is unflavored and doesn't gel, so it dissolves well without any thickness or grit.

Uses: Stir into smoothies, iced tea, or add to oatmeal.

Fridge Difference Makers

Broccoli sprouts: Broccoli is rich in glucosinolates, a precursor to sulforaphane which is a phytochemical that has been shown to potentially inhibit breast cancer cell growth. But wait till you meet these little guys—broccoli sprouts are 3-5 day old broccoli that contain up to 100 times more sulforaphane than mature broccoli! Just 2 tablespoons of broccoli sprouts has as much sulforaphane as 2 pounds of mature broccoli. You can purchase broccoli sprouts from health food stores or some farmers markets.

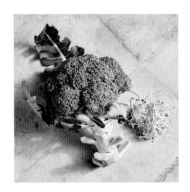

Uses: Add to a salad or sandwich, or blend into a smoothie.

Fresh herbs: Add to salads, soups, and recipes that call for a fresh zing of flavor. While they are all amazing and add nutritional value, one that I'll highlight is parsley—not only does it have benefits for breast cancer risk reduction due to its key phytochemical apigenin, but it's widely available, budget friendly, and has a versatile flavor that is easy to integrate into a diverse range of dishes.

Uses: Add fresh herbs to salads (including quinoa and bean salads), sandwiches, pasta dishes, soups, dressings, and dips.

Ginger root: Researchers have identified over 60 phytonutrients in ginger. Many of these are powerful anti-inflammatory and antioxidant compounds that have been shown to potentially decrease breast cancer cell proliferation and alter gene expression. In addition, ginger may help with weight loss by suppressing fat cell creation, increasing the number of calories your body uses to burn food, and helping you feel full after meals. It can also aid digestion and benefit overall gastrointestinal motility.

Shopping tips: Look for shiny, taut skin that is thin enough to nick with your fingernail, not thick and fibrous. Also avoid ginger with soft spots, as this is an indication that it's been sitting on display way too long.

Uses: Add to smoothies for a spicy kick, add in or grate over a bowl of soup, or brew some fresh ginger root tea, or prepare our Anti-Cancer Debloat Tonic (page 140).

Horseradish: I bet you didn't know this root is part of the cruciferous family. And even more so—did you know that it contains 10 times more glucosinolates than broccoli? Remember, glucosinolates are anti-cancer phytonutrients that get converted to breast cancer-fighting compounds in your body. Specifically, horseradish is rich in a phytonutrient called allyl isothiocyanate, which has been shown to lower the activity of the aromatase enzyme, which in turn may lower estrogen levels.

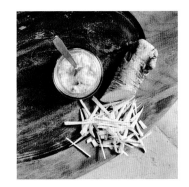

Shopping tips: Check the label on any jarred horseradish and select an option that does not contain added sugars.

Uses: It's not just a condiment for a steak! You can buy the root whole and grate it onto a salad for a spicy kick. Or, use jarred horseradish and stir into hummus, mustard, or salad dressings (my favorite to stir into hummus or tahini sauce). Just remember—a little goes a long way!

Kimchi: Like sauerkraut, kimchi is made of fermented, raw cabbage—but it's got some extra ingredients mixed in, most notably Korean red pepper flakes (antioxidants), ginger (anti-inflammatory), and garlic (anti-viral). Like sauerkraut, kimchi is rich in probiotics and fiber, which nourish your gut microbiome.

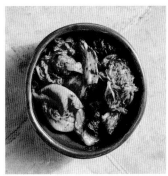

Uses: Add to grain bowls or nori wraps for a probiotic boost.

Lacto-fermented "true" pickles: Most people don't know that true pickles aren't made by adding vinegar to cucumbers! Instead, true pickles are actually made when cucumbers (or another vegetable) are sprinkled with salt and then slowly fermented by lactic acid bacteria. They are rich in probiotics and therefore may be beneficial for gut health. The fermentation process may also improve the nutritional values of the vegetables.

Shopping tips: Most pickles in the grocery store are not true pickles! First, pass up the shelf-stable options and head to the refrigerated section. Then look at the ingredients—true pickles are *not* made with vinegar—the only ingredients should be the vegetable, salt, and perhaps some spices and herbs. Sometimes the label touts they contain "live and active cultures."

Uses: Top a salad, slice on your savory breakfast, or mix into bean or lentil salads.

Microgreens: Meet microgreens—baby greens harvested when they are 7-21 days old, before their mature leaves develop. You'll find them in the refrigerated section of the grocery store (or fresh at the farmers market)—typical varieties include arugula, broccoli, and kale. It's been shown that these young plants may have anywhere from 2-10 times more phytochemicals and antioxidants (such as vitamin C, phenolic acids, flavonols, anthocyanins, and carotenoids) than their mature adult counterparts.

Uses: Add to a salad or sandwich, top a soup, or blend into a smoothie.

Miso: Miso is a Japanese ingredient that is made from fermented soybeans. A Japanese study found that women who drank 3 cups of miso soup per day were 40% less likely to develop breast cancer compared to women

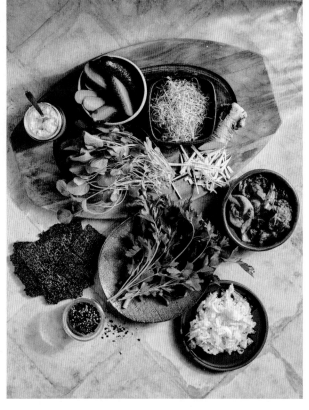

who drank less than a bowl, and there's evidence in laboratory research that miso may suppress breast tumors. Miso has been shown to have antioxidant properties and is also rich in probiotics, which may help maintain a healthy gut microbiome. Bonus: the fermentation process of the soybeans tends to improve their digestibility and slightly increase the protein content.

Shopping tips: Miso has a savory umami and salty flavor. There are three main types: white (mildest with a slightly sweet flavor), red (fermented the longest—from 1-5 years—and has the strongest flavor), and yellow (in the middle!). You can find miso in the refrigerated section.

Uses: Add to marinades, roasted vegetables, salad dressings, stir-fries, and of course—miso soup! When cooking with miso, add it at the end of the cooking process and immediately remove the food from heat as high heat may destroy the probiotics.

Sauerkraut: Sauerkraut is fermented cabbage. It's rich in probiotics and high in fiber, making it excellent for gut health. Probiotics may also help deactivate carcinogens in the gut and improve estrogen metabolism. And eating three servings per week of sauerkraut has been shown to potentially reduce breast cancer risk.

Shopping tips: The good stuff is in the refrigerated section—the probiotics are live and active if kept cold! Avoid the shelf-stable jars as these have been pasteurized and don't contain live probiotics.

Uses: Add a forkful to your salads, or alongside some roasted veg for a bright flavor twist.

Turmeric root: Fresh turmeric contains oils and volatile compounds—notably an aromatic called tumerone, which has been shown to inhibit inflammation as well as migration of human breast cancer cells in the laboratory. And of course, you're still getting the benefits of curcumin, the anti-inflammatory, anti-cancer compound that turmeric is famous for (though the dried spice has higher concentrations of curcumin). Fresh turmeric has an earthy, slightly citrusy, and a slightly bitter taste, but warning—it can stain, so wash up quickly!

Shopping tips: Pick firm roots with taut skin, and avoid shriveled, soft, or dried ones.

Uses: Grate over salads, soups, stir-fries, add to marinades, cook into soups, blend into smoothies, or steep and make a tea.

Watercress: The Centers for Disease Control (CDC) ranked watercress as the #1 most nutrient-dense vegetable. In addition to vitamins and minerals, it's rich in indole-3-carbinol, a phytonutrient that may fight breast cancer by enhancing the body's natural detoxification processes. Bonus: it's a natural diuretic that may help de-bloat and keep you feeling comfortable.

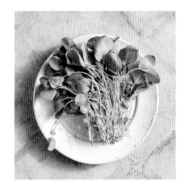

Tip: Don't cook it! Eat watercress raw to maximize its benefits, as cooking may decrease the enzyme that activates the cancer-fighting compounds—possibly reducing its overall nutritional value.

Uses: Add to salads, smoothies, and wraps.

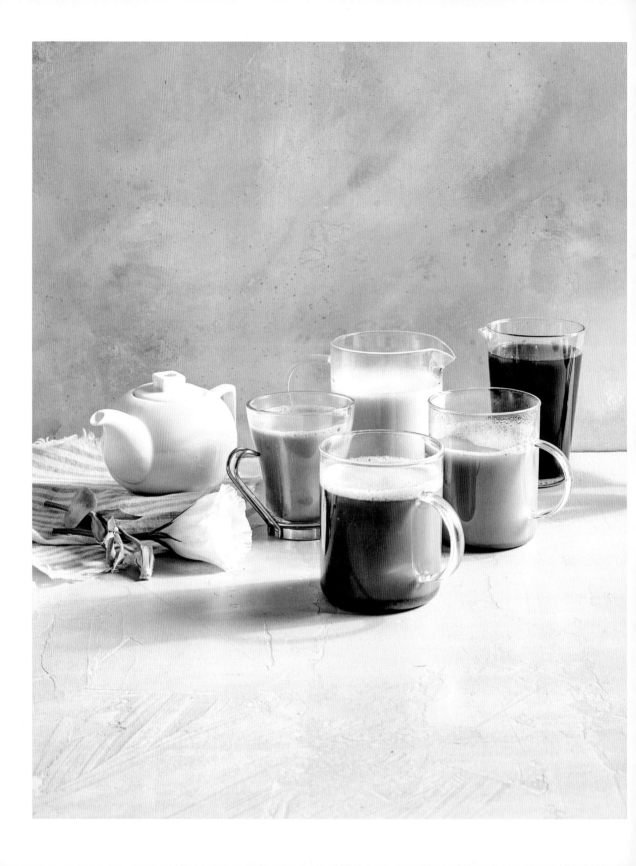

Reconsider that Drink

SIP YOUR WAY TO SUCCESS AND RISK REDUCTION

Research has shown that alcohol intake—even at low levels—
may contribute to increased breast cancer risk due to alcohol's
potential effects on estrogen metabolism and DNA damage.
I suggest limiting alcohol and opting for a dry option whenever
possible. But rather than just avoiding alcohol, I want you
to revamp how you think about beverages. Take every
opportunity to sip on Power Beverages from AM to PM to
contribute to risk reduction. Trust me—you'll experience a
positive shift that you won't think twice about!

Reconsider that Drink

SIP YOUR WAY TO SUCCESS AND RISK REDUCTION

Drinking responsibly isn't just about avoiding DUIs or other misbehavior. There's a connection between alcohol and seven different cancers, including breast cancer risk and development...and I'm here to help you understand what that link is.

Alcohol and Breast Cancer—What's the Connection?

"The more you drink, the higher your risk," says Walter Willett, chair of the Nutrition Department at the Harvard School of Public Health.

That's quite a statement, so I searched the science to uncover the truth.

What did I find? Study after study has linked alcohol to increased breast cancer risk—meta-analyses have pooled data from individual trials and have come to similar conclusions. Here are a few of the big hitters:

The famous Nurse's Health Study found that among 105,986 women, having 3-6 standard alcoholic drinks per week was linked to increased breast cancer risk, and the highest risk was among women who drank regularly from a young age. A similar amount of alcohol intake (about ½ of a standard drink per day) was also linked to increased breast cancer recurrence rates in a 2009 analysis. A summary of 53 studies with over 58,000 women published in the *British Journal of Cancer* showed that just 10 grams of alcohol per day (about ¾ of a standard drink) was associated with a 7% increased risk of breast cancer. And another analysis pooled data from 118 individual studies and found that even light drinkers (one or less standard drink per day) have increased risk of breast cancer compared to non-drinkers—and the risk is greater for moderate and heavy drinkers. Experts estimate that breast cancer risk increases about 10% for each additional drink that women have per day!

So all in all, epidemiologic studies (research of how often diseases occur in different groups of people and why) have consistently found an increased risk of breast cancer with increasing alcohol intake—small amounts of alcohol can potentially affect risk, even if you aren't drinking heavily. These studies were all correlational, meaning that they showed *links* between alcohol and breast cancer but not necessarily proving that alcohol causes breast cancer. It is important to note that the alcohol type does not matter; wine, beer, spirits, hard-cider...if the drink contains alcohol it comes with increased risk.

However, there are logical reasons that explain *why* alcohol could potentially increase breast cancer risk.

First of all, alcohol may change the way a woman's body metabolizes estrogen, which can then raise blood estrogen levels. It's been shown that women who drink alcohol have higher estrogen levels compared to non-drinkers, and we know that higher blood estrogen levels may increase breast cancer risk. Alcohol can also contribute to chronic inflammation, which isn't ideal for risk reduction. It's also the opposite of an antioxidant—alcohol increases the amount of chemically reactive molecules that can potentially damage DNA and other cellular components through a process known as oxidation.

> Alcohol may change the way a woman's body metabolizes estrogen, which can then raise blood estrogen levels.

Alcohol can affect cell signaling, which may make cells more likely to divide, increasing chances of cancer developing. It can also impair the body's ability to break down and absorb nutrients that may have roles in cancer prevention, such as vitamins A, C, E, D, and folate. Additionally, we know that alcohol is broken down to a toxic compound called acetaldehyde. Acetaldehyde can damage DNA and proteins and it may also stop our cells from repairing this damage—and damaged cells may lead to cancer development.

There is emerging research on alcohol and its impact on the health of the microbiome. As I discussed in the Fiber chapter, a healthy microbiome plays an important role in our overall health and possible breast cancer risk reduction. Research is now revealing that chronic alcohol consumption may cause intestinal dysbiosis in both rodent models and humans. Alcohol consumption is also linked to higher levels of stress and anxiety, which can lead to elevated cortisol levels (our stress hormone). Elevated cortisol increases our blood glucose, which as we know over time can lead to insulin resistance, increased IGF-1, and also weight gain...all contributing to the risk of breast cancer.

Also—alcoholic drinks aren't calorie-free! We've already discussed how reducing body fat is a key part of breast cancer risk reduction. Here are the approximate calorie counts of common drinks—the numbers can add up quickly and work against weight management and risk reduction goals.

- an average bottle of beer (12 ounces) = 150 calories

- a typical glass of wine (5 ounces) = 120 calories

- a serving of distilled spirit (1.5 ounces) = 65-100 calories

- and margaritas? 200-300 calories...or more!

These are some reasons why the American Institute of Cancer Research (AICR) and the World Health Organization (WHO) recommend not drinking at all, stating that there isn't a "safe" amount of alcohol that doesn't increase the risk of breast cancer. But for women who do drink, they recommend limiting to one drink per day, max. The Mayo Clinic also recommends limiting to one drink per day. Other organizations like the American Cancer Society state that avoiding or majorly cutting back on alcohol may be an important way that women can lower their risk.

Let me address a major FAQ: *"Rachel, what about red wine? Isn't a glass a day healthy?"*

The relationship between red wine intake and cancer isn't quite as clear as it is with alcohol in general. This is because the grape skins used to make wine contain a polyphenol called resveratrol, and in laboratory studies resveratrol has been shown to have antioxidant activities that may work to fight cancer. Keep in mind that the levels of resveratrol used in lab studies were much, much higher than the amount that you'd be able to consume via red wine—you'd need to drink 100 glasses to have the same concentrations of resveratrol, which isn't considered "healthy" in anyone's book! There was a small 2012 study from Cedars-Sinai that found that women who drank about 8 ounces of red wine nightly for a month had *slightly* lower estrogen levels. But before you all go pour a bottle of merlot, mind that this was a very small study among 36 pre-menopausal women and is far from being conclusive!

It is important to note it is the resveratrol from the grapes themselves, NOT the alcohol in the wine, which contains the powerful antioxidants. Other sources of resveratrol include peanuts, blueberries, cranberries, and cacao. These whole foods also contain other antioxidants, phytonutrients, and fiber so are a better choice by far. Overall, red wine's resveratrol content is not enough to support frequent intake as part of the Beller Method when the greater body of scientific evidence points toward the benefits of alcohol reduction. There are so many other ways to reduce estrogen levels from a nutritional perspective—fiber optimization, protein choices, weight management, and healthy fats to name a few.

HERE'S THE TAKEAWAY:

Population-level research has shown that alcohol intake is linked to increased risk of breast cancer. This might be due to alcohol's effect on estrogen metabolism resulting in higher blood estrogen levels, due to its oxidizing or DNA damaging effects. Major health organizations strongly suggest limiting alcohol intake, and I agree. If you aren't currently drinking—keep it that way! And if you do include alcohol, try reducing the amount and frequency, as less is best.

Now, I'm not here to rain on your parade or spoil the party. Limit your alcohol intake to special occasions, and whenever possible opt for a tasty dry option. I want you to reconsider your drink and opt for tasty beverages that feel special—without the added risk! Rethink your weekend refresher or evening relaxer and instead of something alcoholic, pick a drink with nutritional benefits that can potentially reduce risk rather than add to it—think: sparkling seltzer with orange zest, mint leaves, and frozen blueberries or one of our power beverages like a spicy immunity shot.

Embrace Power Beverages from AM to PM

And while we're at it—let's revolutionize the way we think about drinks. It's not just about avoiding the alcohol and being stuck with plain water 24/7. I want you to embrace the concept of drinking Power Beverages *throughout the day*, from your morning routine and afternoon pick-me-up, to your evening wind-down indulgence (don't worry, I have you covered with tons of options in the Recipes section). Take every nutritional opportunity to add more good, not just with what you're chewing, but with what you're drinking. Choose beverages that are packed with antioxidant, anti-inflammatory and anti-cancer benefits, and make a habit of incorporating Power Beverages from AM to PM to further elevate and Spice Up your daily routine— you will feel the difference!

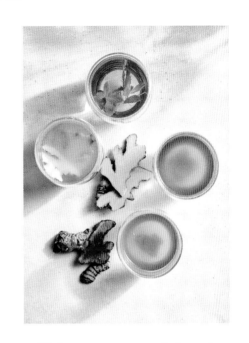

Take every nutritional opportunity to add more good, not just with what you're chewing, but with what you're drinking.

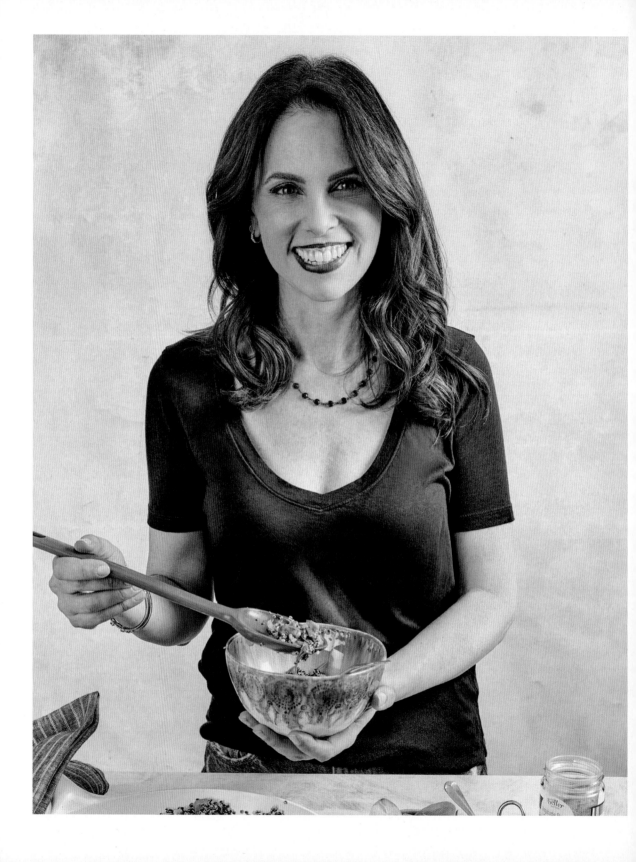

Feel Empowered

USING YOUR BELLER TOOLKIT

Let's take all this knowledge into action. Now, remember that true sustainable change takes time. You may have ups and downs on your weight management and risk reduction journey—and that's totally normal. It's the long-term commitment that matters. From years of experience working alongside patients, I've found micro-SMART goal setting is key for success and accountability. Specific tools, like journaling and a nutrition support system are absolutely essential. These are the difference makers that can really drive you to success. I'm here to guide you through it all—for now and for life.

Feel Empowered

USING YOUR BELLER TOOLKIT

Now that you know what to do, let's talk about how to get started.

The Beller Method gives you evidence-based guidelines and a clear picture of what to eat to provide optimal nutrition, while promoting your long-term wellness and weight management goals. It's a lifestyle, not a fad diet. Let's say that again—this is a lifestyle, NOT a fad diet. This is important to remember because a lifestyle method takes TIME.

This new lifestyle may look different from your current lifestyle—and that's okay! I'm here to tell you that you can make the changes that will help you feel so much better and reduce your cancer risk. It may seem overwhelming at first, but with the right game plan and mindset, you can set yourself up for success. Let's dive in.

Research shows that "motivation" or "willpower" isn't what you need. Trying to incorporate all the recommendations at the same time through brute force and pure will can be stressful—and most importantly becomes unsustainable in the long run. For sustainable change, it's more effective to create actionable goals, have ongoing support and accountability, and remain flexible. That's what this chapter is for: to empower you to implement change and give you tools on how to maintain the change—for now and for life.

It's a Journey—Recognize Where You Are On It!

Nutrition for weight management, breast cancer risk reduction, and long term thrivership are a journey. Each person may embark on it at their own pace—and there is nothing wrong with taking your time! It's totally fine if you're new to these topics and need to pause and process everything before jumping right in. It's also great if you've already made a few nutrition changes, but are looking for a structured and realistic action plan to comprehensively modify your eating habits that is consistent for the long run. The key is to have clarity and confidence with a method that you can trust—of course there will be curves and bumps along the road, and you might regress, but it is crucial to have a system you can jump back on with ease.

Here's an industry secret: dietitians like myself and many other healthcare professionals will often refer to the Transtheoretical Model of behavior change. It's this fancy term for a process that demonstrates how you can move from a state of inaction to action mode.

- **Stage 1:** "Precontemplation." This is when you are not really thinking about making any type of change at all.

- **Stage 2:** "Contemplation." Here is when you start to realize you may want to make a change and are open to learning more, but aren't quite ready to take action.

- **Stage 3:** "Preparation." You're ready to commit to making a change. You've weighed the pros and cons, and are gathering the information and resources you need to succeed.

- **Stage 4:** "Action." This is when you implement the change. It's time to get cooking!

- **Stage 5:** "Maintenance." Once you feel confident about this new change you transition into a "keep going" phase. You feel comfortable with the behavior shift and can keep it up while even focusing on a new goal. Remember that it's normal to slip up and fall back into old patterns at times—but the key is to review what worked and what didn't and keep moving forward.

Remember, this is YOUR journey, and it is as unique as you are; there is no "right" or "wrong" here. If you find yourself in the contemplation stage, then take some time to consider what your long-term goals are and identify barriers that may be standing in your way to getting started. Even reading this book is a step in the right direction—you've acknowledged there is a link between nutrition, weight management, and breast cancer risk reduction. If you're in the preparation stage, perhaps you are gearing up for action—you're bookmarking recipes to try and adding premium proteins, top-tier vegetables, spices, and Power Up ingredients to your grocery list. Or maybe you're in the maintenance phase—you've been following the principles of the Method but need some new products and fresh ideas or motivation to stay inspired.

> The key is to have clarity and confidence with a method that you can trust.

Wherever you are, I applaud you for being present on your journey to better health.

Adopt a Phased Approach with Micro-SMART Goals

At first, it is normal to feel overwhelmed when integrating new lifestyle changes. When faced with change, we tend to look at it as one big hurdle, but in reality it's rarely ever like that. In fact, setting out to implement all of the nutrition changes all at once usually leads to a rollercoaster of "good" and "bad" days. Avoiding this rollercoaster is crucial to long-term success, and leads to more overall satisfaction with the process. People only have so much bandwidth in a day—when work and family become stressful (which they inevitably do), goals that are too lofty will get edged out by more important things.

While there are a few individuals that can completely overhaul their diet in one go, I've found that the majority of people (at least 9 out of 10 of my patients) find this overwhelming and instead, they do better with a phased approach. My patients find more success when they bite off a manageable, achievable section rather than trying to gulp down the whole Method at once. Rather than changing 100% of their nutrition habits immediately, we focus on *one principle at a time*, get used to and comfortable with the principle, and then move on to the next.

Micro goals empower you to make incremental, sustainable changes that add up to macro-level benefits. Micro goal setting is an evidence-based way to achieve sustainable results.

For example, let's start with fiber. The overarching goal is to get your Daily 35 via a diverse range of fibers. That's a great goal, but it's not clear how to get there...I've had many people come to me saying they've tried to up their fiber intake in the past by simply "choosing higher fiber foods," but almost all of them don't consistently get their Daily 35 and they eventually fall off the wagon.

Instead, I may have a patient start with a smaller, more bite-sized "micro goal": just focus on getting 10 grams in before noon on weekdays by incorporating my fiber-filled breakfast recipes. After they have incorporated those breakfast options into their weekday routine, we move on to focus on choosing high fiber protein options for lunches. Then we move on to ensuring dinner time is fiber-rich by incorporating at least 2 cups of non-starchy vegetables. Before long, the diverse Daily 35 is achieved!

So let's work together to break apart the method into manageable pieces. Here are some characteristics of good micro-SMART goals:

- **Micro goals are *Specific*.** Describe exactly what the new habit will be. What will be accomplished? What actions will you take? What foods will you incorporate? Make a list!

- **Micro goals are *Measurable*.** How much will you include with your meal? How many days per week will you do this? Is there a way to keep tabs on this goal?

- **Micro goals are *Achievable and Realistic*.** Make sure you have the tools, information, and ingredients to meet your goal. Is the goal too easy? Too challenging? Ideally a goal should feel like a slight stretch but not incredibly uncomfortable. You should feel confident you can achieve it without feeling stressed—stress around goals is counter-productive.

- **Micro goals have a *Timeframe*:** Goals without a start point are easy to put off! Spell out when you will start and how often you will do it.

EXAMPLE: LET'S LOOK AT REBECCA'S SITUATION:

Rebecca found it challenging to consistently include plant-based protein into her meals. She decided to set a goal: eat 1 cup of plant-based protein, 5 times per week.

- Week 1—she achieved the goal but it was stressful—before setting the goal she was only eating plant-based protein 0-3 times per week.

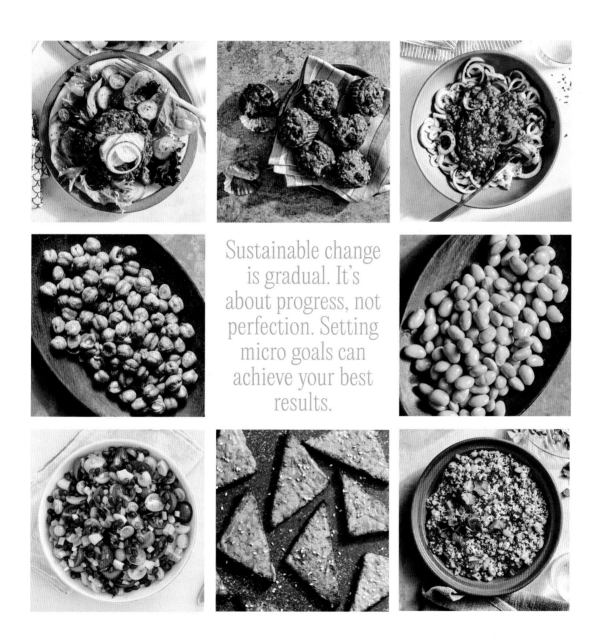

Sustainable change is gradual. It's about progress, not perfection. Setting micro goals can achieve your best results.

- Week 2—she did 4 out of 5 and felt bad about missing the mark. She promised herself that she'd do better next week.

- Week 3—things were really hectic at work and she was only able to do 2 out of 5. She was really feeling guilty about missing her goal once again.

- By Week 4—she felt defeated and didn't even bother to try to meet her goal.

Eating plant-based protein now carried a negative energy for her.

Let's try this again:

Knowing that Rebecca currently only eats 0-3 cups of plant-based protein a week, she and her dietitian decided to set a micro goal: to eat 1 cup of plant-based protein, 2 times per week.

- Week 1—she surpassed her goal! She ate 4 cups and felt successful and confident.

- Week 2—her positive energy carried forward and she ate 5 cups!

- Week 3—things got hectic at work and she was able to eat 2 cups—which was her goal—so she still felt successful.

- Week 4—now she had reached her goal 3 weeks in a row and she was feeling very motivated. Things were still hectic with work but she was able to eat 3 cups of plant-based protein. Yay!

Success breeds more success. Setting goals that are small and realistic helps to build confidence week to week.

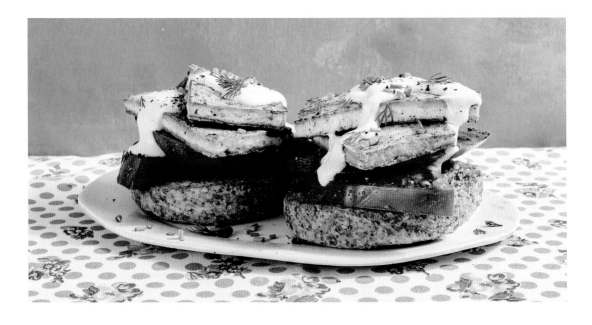

Here are some example micro-SMART goals to get you energized and your mind going on where you wish to start...

- Eat a fiber-boosted breakfast at least 4 times per week

- Switch up your fiber boosters 2 times this week

- Add a Power Up ingredient to dinner 3 times per week

- Eat ¾ cup of beans (legumes) at least 4 times per week

- Follow the Power of 3 meal building strategy when eating out 2 times per week

- Journal your meals 3 times per week, including a weekend day

Remember: sustainable change is gradual and slow. It's about progress, not perfection. Set realistic goals, but if you don't meet that goal one week, it's okay. In fact, it's fairly normal as life can become busy. It doesn't mean you've failed—give yourself grace and understanding as you would give a friend!

Accountability Is Essential

It's one thing to have knowledge. That's what you've gotten from reading the preceding chapters in this book! It's another thing to implement that knowledge and make change—that's where the hard work is.

Research has shown again and again that *the key to successful weight loss (or any nutrition goal, for that matter) is* **accountability**. Accountability is knowing that you are responsible for your choices and staying committed to your goals. Maintaining motivation to continue with change can be challenging in the long run, but having effective accountability can help you achieve your goals.

KEEP YOURSELF ACCOUNTABLE

It's one thing to come up with a list of micro goals in your head. But it's another to see them written down in front of you! That's why I encourage you to actually write those micro goals down—and don't leave them tucked away in a journal. To keep yourself focused, you can even write your micro goal on a Post-it and keep it by your desk or refrigerator.

I also recommend starting a food journal. This means writing down what you eat throughout the day (meals, snacks, and beverages) in order to track the foods and ingredients you're putting into your body. You can do this in a notebook on your kitchen table, logging on your phone, or even using one of the many food diary phone applications available. Journaling increases mindfulness and helps you stay aware of what you're eating. It contributes to you having clarity and confidence. It also helps you keep track of your micro goals—it's not always easy to remember what you ate yesterday, much less remember how many times you may have included a particular Power Food in your diet over the past week! What gets measured gets improved.

Another tip: write down and highlight (or circle in a brightly colored pen) when you've completed a goal. This helps you keep track of what goals you've already accomplished— and can motivate you to keep it up!

Now, you don't need to religiously journal every day, every single week (though if you find it helps you, feel free to). Sometimes it helps to journal for the first couple weeks of a change when you're trying to get used to it, or perhaps if you find yourself deviating from your micro goal.

FIND YOUR TRIBE

Having a support system is a huge difference maker between having knowledge and launching into action mode. Having someone come alongside you who knows what your goals are and is supportive of your nutrition changes is not just encouraging— it's empowering. So I encourage you to find at least one person that you can share your overall and micro goals with: a friend, a family member, a coworker, or a neighbor. Give them the liberty to check in with you and ask how you're doing with your changes. Even better: find someone who also wants to adopt healthy lifestyle habits and you can embark on the journey together!

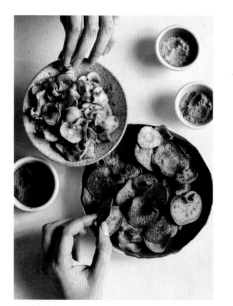

Having a support system is a huge difference maker between having knowledge and launching into action mode.

Alternatively you can find accountability within groups of like-minded individuals: weight management groups, cancer patient networks, or walking groups. Or consider joining the Beller Method Masterclass! Often these groups have online forums where members can post what their goals, progress, or challenges are. It's encouraging to see others make choices that make them feel better about what they put into their bodies—often it sparks inspiration in you, too.

Get Empowered

After years in practice, most of my patients come to me craving a specific, comprehensive, and realistic plan of action to revolutionize their nutrition. I developed the Beller Method to meet this need. I've helped countless women gain clarity and confidence in their food choices, transform the way they think about the power of food, and feel their amazing best. I truly believe that mindfully building habits over time is the key to success—and this leads to true empowerment.

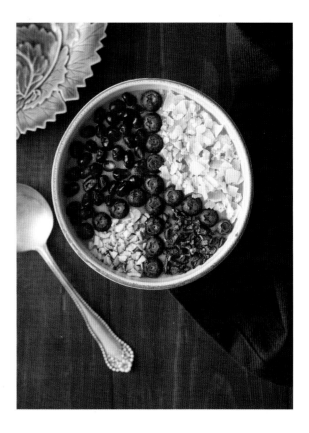

Remember, it's what you do most of the time, not sometimes, that makes a difference when it comes to your long-term health. Regardless of where you are, I'm happy you're here. I am honored to be here to walk with you through the changes and provide the framework and encouragement to help you reach your health goals.

So let's get started!

Let's Eat!

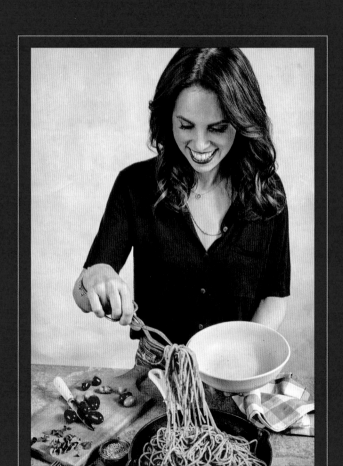

Now that we've gone through the science behind the Beller Method, let's launch into action mode! The recipes on the following pages incorporate all the essential principles of the method: they utilize premium proteins, top-of-the-line cancer-fighting veg, anti-inflammatory fats, Power Up ingredients...and of course are Power Spiced! The flavors are approachable and delicious—making the plant-forward recipes incredibly easy to incorporate into your routine. You and your family will enjoy being inclusive of meals that are centered around premium proteins.

I've included the nutrition facts for each recipe to provide you with knowledge of the details. You will see that I've created the recipes so they are nutritionally balanced with adequate protein, fiber, and fat—so you don't have to keep track. They serve as a solid foundation if you are looking to lose excess body weight and reduce breast cancer risk. And of course, there's flexibility for you to customize the recipes for your individual goals...if you need a bit more protein, for example, feel free to add a protein-rich ingredient like hemp hearts, pepitas, edamame, or a nut or seed protein powder.

I do want to reassure you: fear not the carbohydrates. Fiber is classified as a carbohydrate—so it's included in the total grams of carbohydrate in all the nutrition facts. Naturally a high fiber food will be higher in total carbohydrates—but not all of these carbs are actually going to contribute to calories or spike your blood sugars! This is because fiber passes through your body undigested or partially digested and calories are not released in the same way that they are with sugar or starch.

How do we know that a product or recipe is truly rich in fiber? One way is to use the "5 to 1 Rule." If you divide the grams of total carbohydrates by grams of dietary fiber and the result is less than 5, then the recipe is considered to be rich in fiber. For example: if total carb is 45 grams and fiber content is 10 grams: 45 divided by 10 equals 4.5. This is less than 5, so you're good to go!

Good news: don't sweat when it comes to the recipes in this book—nearly all of them contain at least 10 grams of fiber, and also fit the "5 to 1 Rule."

To get started, pick just a few recipes from each section (beverages, breakfasts, meals, snacks, and desserts) to include on a weekly basis. Be consistent with several recipes—you will taste and feel the difference! Then branch out and cook your way through this book, experiencing the variety of flavors made possible with simple plant-based ingredients, top-of-the-line Power Ups, and of course, Power Spicing. I've kept the ingredient lists simple and the prep times short so that no matter how busy you are, you can feel confident and successful in the kitchen.

I've seen so many of my patients adopt the Beller Method and gain clarity, confidence, and empowerment about the food they choose to eat—for now and for life.

Let's eat!

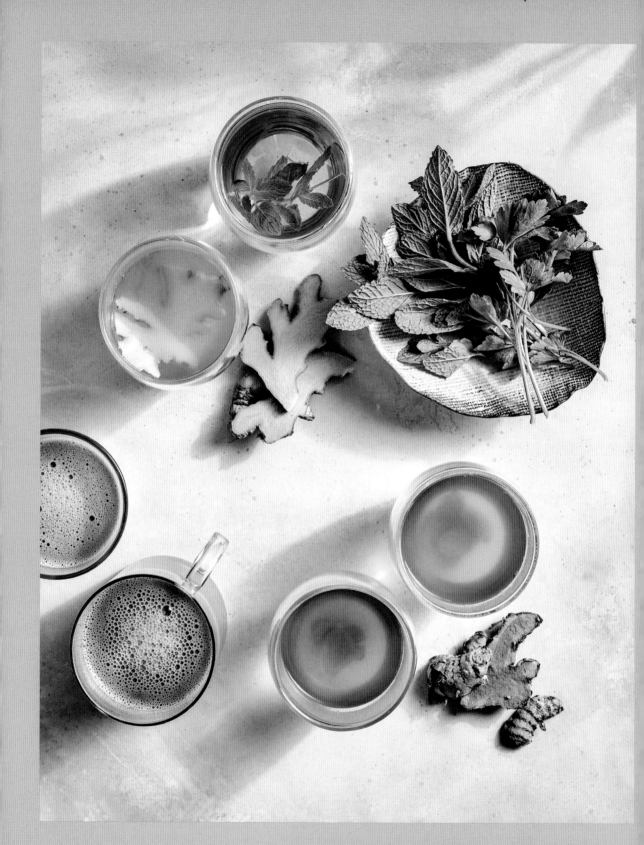

Power Beverages

Raise your glass! My signature power beverages are the perfect mix of fun and function, packing a serious punch of anti-inflammatory and potential cancer-protective properties. They're so easy to make, you'll feel like a mixologist in no time. Whether you need an energizing kick start, a sustaining boost to keep you going, or a calming elixir to help you unwind at bedtime—these drinks have you covered from AM to PM. Cheers—to your health!

Anti-Cancer Debloat Tonic

PREP TIME	**COOK TIME**	**SERVES**
10 MINUTES	10 MINUTES	8

Ingredients

8 cups water

2 fennel tea bags, or
2 teaspoons fennel seeds

2 inches turmeric root,
peeled and sliced into rounds

1 inch ginger root, peeled and
sliced into rounds

1 handful parsley or
dandelion leaves

1 teaspoon Morning Boost
Power Spice Blend*

Sip away the bloat! This morning tonic is the perfect remedy! I use this in my practice for patients who really want support with debloat or discomfort during their day. It features fennel (with its 87 different phytochemicals) and parsley or dandelion leaves, which may help flush excess water from your system for a debloat fix. Plus, the Morning Boost Blend and ginger power up the digestive and anti-inflammatory benefits in this invigorating tonic. Make a big batch and enjoy the flavor and function.

Directions

1. In a medium saucepan over medium heat, stir together all ingredients.

2. Bring up to a simmer, reduce heat to low, and let simmer 8–10 minutes, until the spices are fragrant.

3. Strain, if desired, before serving warm or chilled. Store covered and refrigerated for up to 4 days.

*Substitute spice blend with ¾ teaspoon Ceylon cinnamon, ⅛ teaspoon ground ginger, ⅛ teaspoon nutmeg, pinch of allspice, pinch of ground cloves.

CALORIES: 2 · FAT: 0G · CARBS: 1G · FIBER: 0G · SUGARS: 0G · ADDED SUGARS: 0G · PROTEIN: 0G

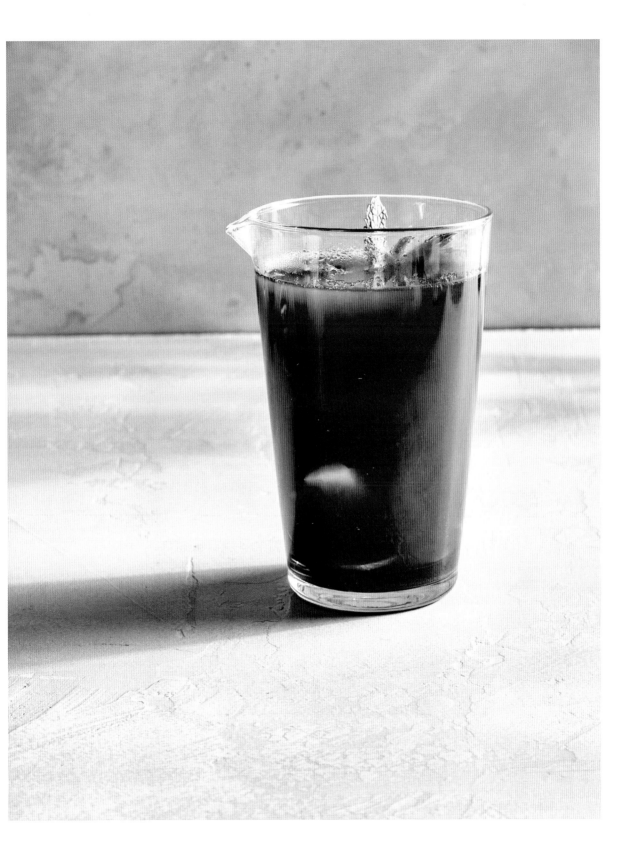

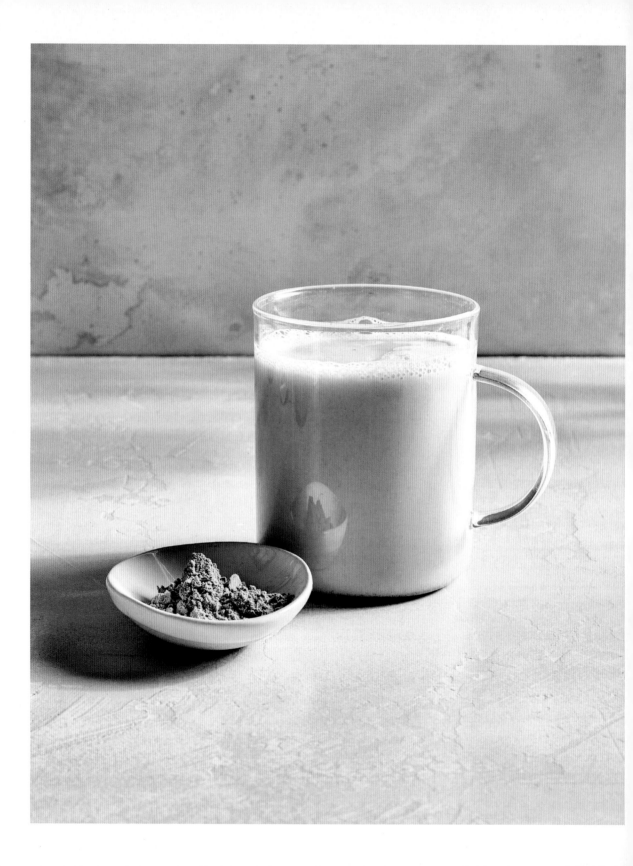

Golden Mushroom Latte

PREP TIME	SERVES
5 MINUTES	1

Ingredients

½ **cup** unsweetened plant milk

½ **cup** water

½ **teaspoon** mushroom powder

½ **teaspoon** Golden Breakfast Power Spice Blend*

1 **teaspoon** date syrup, optional for added sweetness

Feel empowered with this deliciously creamy and powerful anti-cancer beverage. My Golden Breakfast Blend offers a synergistic harmony of cacao and turmeric, which work together to help reduce body inflammation as well as offer cancer protective properties. Loaded with one of my top-tier Power Up foods, mushrooms, this latte offers a concentrated source of aromatase inhibitors that emerging research suggests may reduce the risk of breast cancer. To top it off, mushrooms in powder form are shelf-stable, so you can enjoy the POWER anytime!

Directions

1. Place all the ingredients in a blender. Blend on high 10 seconds (you can also use a handheld frother), until frothy. Heat to desired temperature.

TIP: For a stronger flavor, add black tea or coffee in place of the water.

*Substitute spice blend with ¼ teaspoon Ceylon cinnamon, ¼ teaspoon cacao powder, ⅛ teaspoon ground turmeric, pinch of ground ginger.

CALORIES: 45 · FAT: 2G · CARBS: 3G · FIBER: 2G · SUGARS: 1G · ADDED SUGARS: 0G · PROTEIN: 5G

Morning Boost Latte

PREP TIME	SERVES
5 MINUTES	1

Ingredients

½ cup unsweetened plant milk

½ cup water

1 teaspoon Morning Boost Power Spice Blend*

1 shot espresso, optional

½ teaspoon date syrup, optional

Rise and shine, pumpkin pie lovers! With a blend that includes Ceylon cinnamon, nutmeg, ginger, allspice, and clove, this latte packs a big punch of antioxidant and anti-inflammatory properties that will have you jumping out of bed for that first sip. It's so easy to make—just slip a warm mug of this spicy-sweet drink into your morning routine and enjoy the power within!

Directions

1. Place all ingredients in a blender. Blend on high 10 seconds (you can also use a handheld frother), until frothy. Heat to desired temperature.

2. Optional: For an extra kick, add 1 shot of espresso and ½ teaspoon date syrup to sweeten the espresso.

*Substitute spice blend with ¾ teaspoon Ceylon cinnamon, ⅛ teaspoon ground ginger, ⅛ teaspoon nutmeg, pinch of allspice, pinch of ground cloves.

CALORIES: 45 · FAT: 2G · CARBS: 2G · FIBER: 2G · SUGARS: 1G · ADDED SUGARS: 0G · PROTEIN: 4G

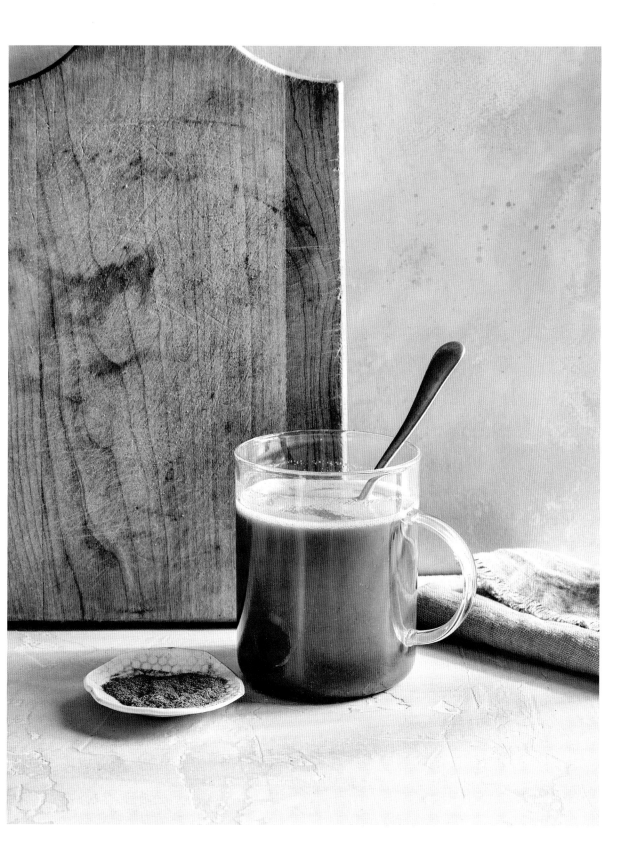

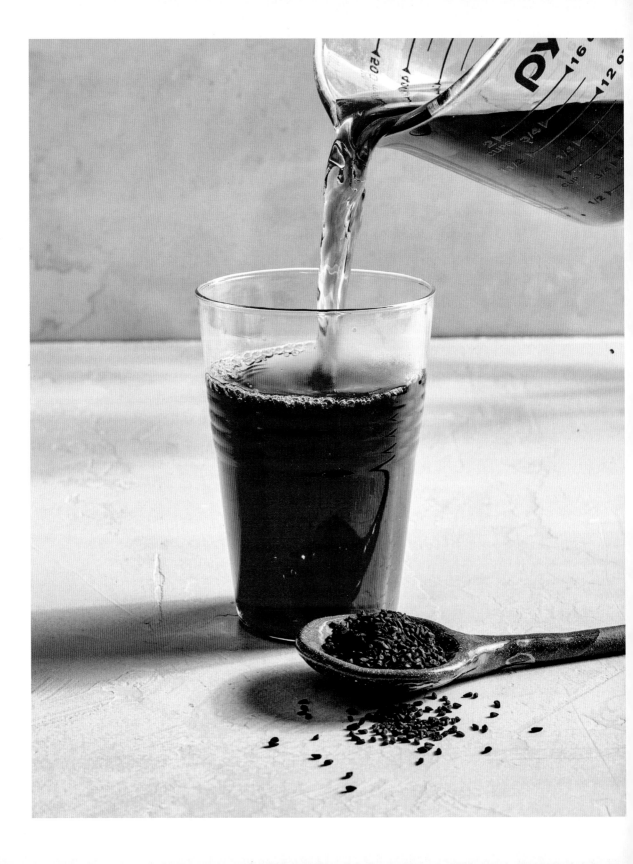

Black Cumin Ruby Tonic

PREP TIME	COOK TIME	SERVES
5 MINUTES	17 MINUTES	2

Ingredients

3 cups water

2 teaspoons black cumin seeds

½ teaspoon hibiscus powder or 2 teaspoons loose-leaf hibiscus tea

½ teaspoon Cinnapeel Spicer Power Spice Blend*

2 teaspoons date syrup, optional for added sweetness

This power-packed drink tastes like a tart Arnold Palmer that's loaded with antioxidants, polyphenols, and potential cancer-fighting properties. Black cumin seeds, also known as the "miracle herb" (unrelated to the cumin in your spice rack), stimulate digestion for GI support. Hibiscus powder is rich in antioxidants and contains anthocyanins, which may have cancer-protective benefits. Sip, savor, and let the health benefits flow!

Directions

1. In a small saucepan over medium heat, stir together all ingredients.

2. Bring up to a boil, reduce heat to low, and let simmer 4–5 minutes. Remove from heat and let steep an additional 3 minutes.

3. Strain and serve warm or chilled.

*Substitute spice blend with ½ teaspoon Ceylon cinnamon, ¼ teaspoon granulated orange peel, pinch of ground ginger.

CALORIES: 5 · FAT: 0G · CARBS: 1G · FIBER: 0G · SUGARS: 0G · ADDED SUGARS: 0G · PROTEIN: 0G

Golden Matcha 2.0

PREP TIME	COOK TIME	SERVES
5 MINUTES	5 MINUTES	1

Ingredients

½ **cup** unsweetened plant milk, heated

½ **cup** water

1 teaspoon Golden Breakfast Power Spice Blend*

½ **teaspoon** matcha powder

1 teaspoon date syrup, optional for added sweetness

A "matcha" made in heaven—this Matcha 2.0 is incredibly powerful and perfect for starting your day off right! It's loaded with anti-cancer properties and brings in some amazing spice synergy. Cacao is rich in quercetin, which may improve the absorption and bioavailability of curcumin, turmeric's powerful anti-inflammatory compound, and EGCG, the major antioxidant found in matcha.

Directions

1. Place all ingredients in a blender. Blend on high 10 seconds (you can also use a handheld frother), until frothy. Heat to desired temperature.

*Substitute spice blend with ½ teaspoon Ceylon cinnamon, ½ teaspoon cacao powder, ¼ teaspoon ground turmeric, pinch of ground ginger.

CALORIES: 40 · FAT: 2G · CARBS: 1G · FIBER: 2G · SUGARS: 1G · ADDED SUGARS: 0G · PROTEIN: 4G

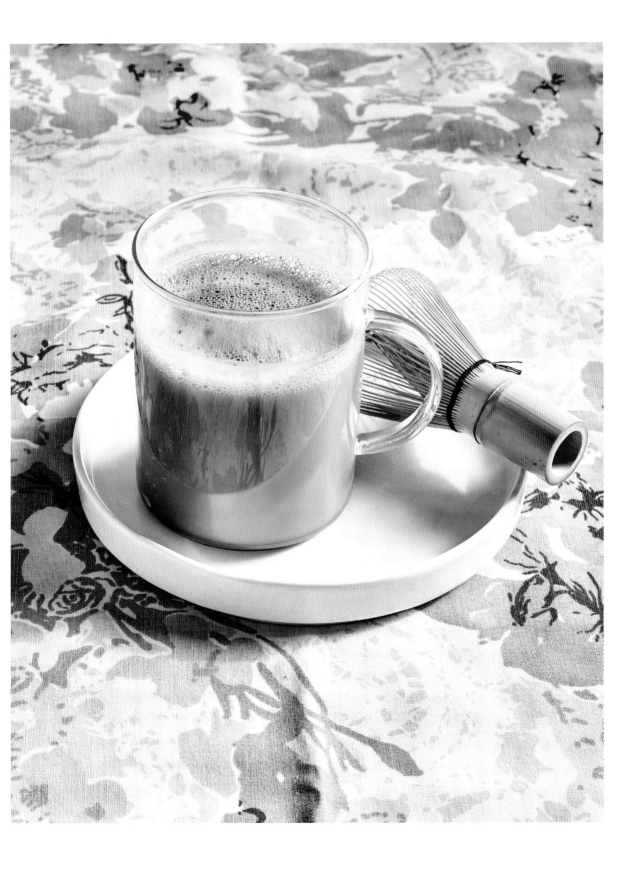

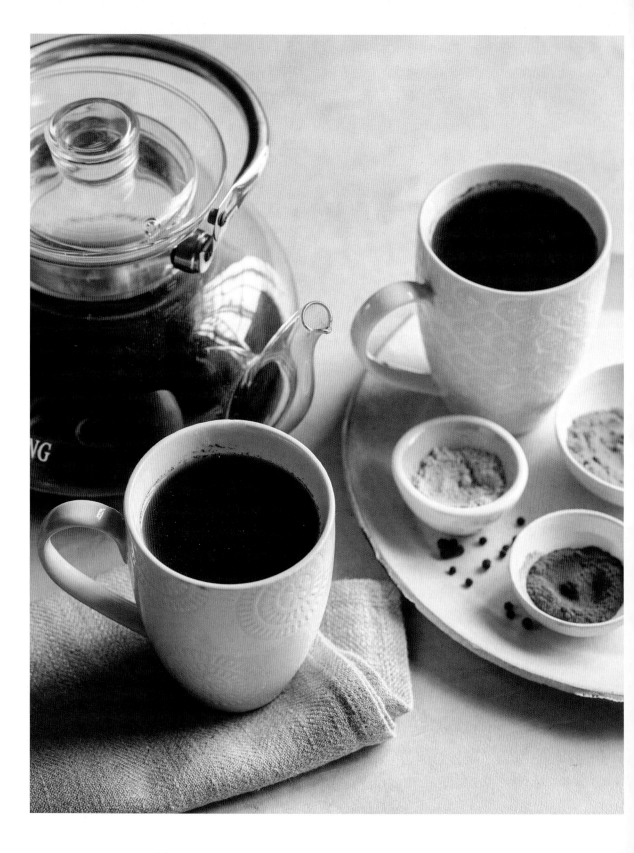

Bedtime Tonic

PREP TIME	COOK TIME	SERVES
5 MINUTES	10 MINUTES	2

Ingredients

2 cups water

2 chamomile tea bags

2 teaspoons tart cherry powder

1 teaspoon Morning Boost Power Spice Blend*

1 teaspoon raw honey, optional for added sweetness

Here's a "cherry" way to drift off to dreamland! This comforting brew features tart cherry powder, which some research suggests may reduce joint/muscle pain and contains compounds like sleep-supportive melatonin and anti-inflammatory anthocyanins. Other anti-cancer and immune-enhancing superstars turmeric, ginger, and Ceylon cinnamon add a soothing fragrance and flavor that will warm up your entire home. Catch some ZZZs with this perfect soothing nightcap!

Directions

1. In a small saucepan over medium heat, stir together all ingredients.

2. Bring up to a boil, reduce heat to low, and let simmer 5 minutes, until the tea and spices are fragrant.

*Substitute spice blend with ¾ teaspoon Ceylon cinnamon, ⅛ teaspoon ground ginger, ⅛ teaspoon nutmeg, pinch of allspice, ground cloves

CALORIES: 5 · FAT: 0G · CARBS: 1G · FIBER: 0G · SUGARS: 1G · ADDED SUGARS: 0G · PROTEIN: 0G

Get Movin' Flax Gel

PREP TIME	COOK TIME	SERVES
1 MINUTE	30 MINUTES	12

Ingredients

3 cups water

¼ cup flaxseeds

1 teaspoon Cinnapeel Spicer Power Spice Blend*

"Re-flax" and smile because this recipe is going to keep you regular. I often recommend this tried-and-true trick of the trade to my patients for optimal digestive health. I've powered it up with my Cinnapeel Spicer Blend for added flavor and potency, and it can be easily added to smoothies, teas, or drunk like a shot. Prepare it in advance and get ready to move!

Directions

1. In a small saucepan over medium heat, stir together all ingredients.

2. Bring up to a boil, reduce heat to low, and let simmer 30 minutes, or until the water begins to thicken.

3. Strain into a glass container or jar (if the gel is too thick, dilute with some hot water). Store covered and refrigerated for up to 5 days.

4. Stir ¼ cup into teas, smoothies, and other foods.

*Substitute spice blend with ¾ teaspoon Ceylon cinnamon, ½ teaspoon granulated orange peel, pinch of ground ginger.

CALORIES: 8 · FAT: 1G · CARBS: 0G · FIBER: 1G · SUGARS: 0G · ADDED SUGARS: 0G · PROTEIN: 1G

Relax-Me Barley Grass Latte

PREP TIME	SERVES
5 MINUTES	1

Ingredients

½ **cup** unsweetened plant milk

½ **cup** water

1 teaspoon barley grass powder

½ **teaspoon** Cinnapeel Spicer Power Spice Blend*

1 teaspoon date syrup, optional for added sweetness

With our busy schedules, it's vital to get a good night's rest; adequate sleep supports weight management, amongst other health benefits. Just a teaspoon of barley grass is packed with phytonutrients and gamma-aminobutyric acid, which may help you to relax and regulate sleep and anxiety. So come and enjoy a cozy latte that may help you relax in no time!

Directions

1. Place all ingredients in a blender. Blend on high 10 seconds (you can also use a handheld frother), until frothy. Heat to desired temperature.

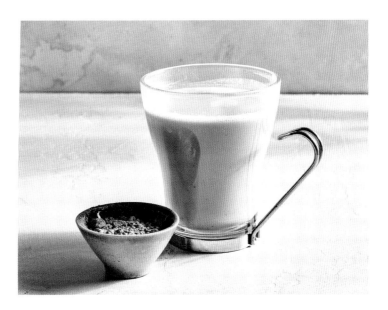

*Substitute spice blend with ½ teaspoon Ceylon cinnamon, ¼ teaspoon granulated orange peel, pinch of ground ginger.

CALORIES: 42 · FAT: 2G · CARBS: 1G · FIBER: 2G · SUGARS: 0G · ADDED SUGARS: 0G · PROTEIN: 4G

Immunity Power Shots

PREP TIME
5 MINUTES

SERVES
2

Ingredients

¼ **cup** coconut water

¼ **cup** water

1 **tablespoon** orange juice

½ **teaspoon** apple cider vinegar

¼ **teaspoon** Ceylon cinnamon

⅛ **teaspoon** ground ginger

½ **teaspoon** raw honey, optional for added sweetness

This zesty concoction of coconut water, orange juice, Ceylon cinnamon, ginger, and apple cider vinegar packs a powerful immune-supporting punch. Sip it straight or spice it up for an extra kick of protection!

Directions

1. Whisk together all ingredients and divide between two shot glasses to serve.

CALORIES: 10 · FAT: 0G · CARBS: 2G · FIBER: 0G · SUGARS: 2G · ADDED SUGARS: 0G · PROTEIN: 0G

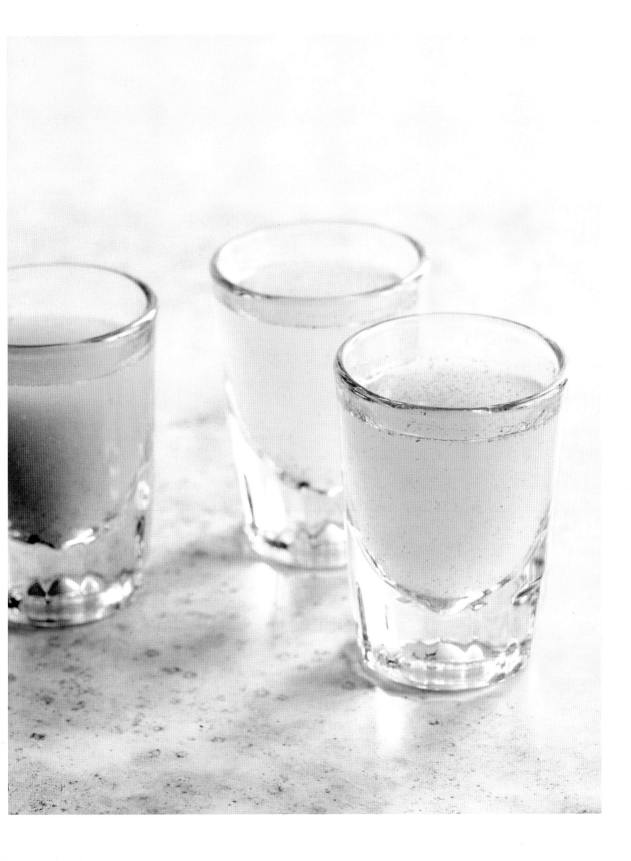

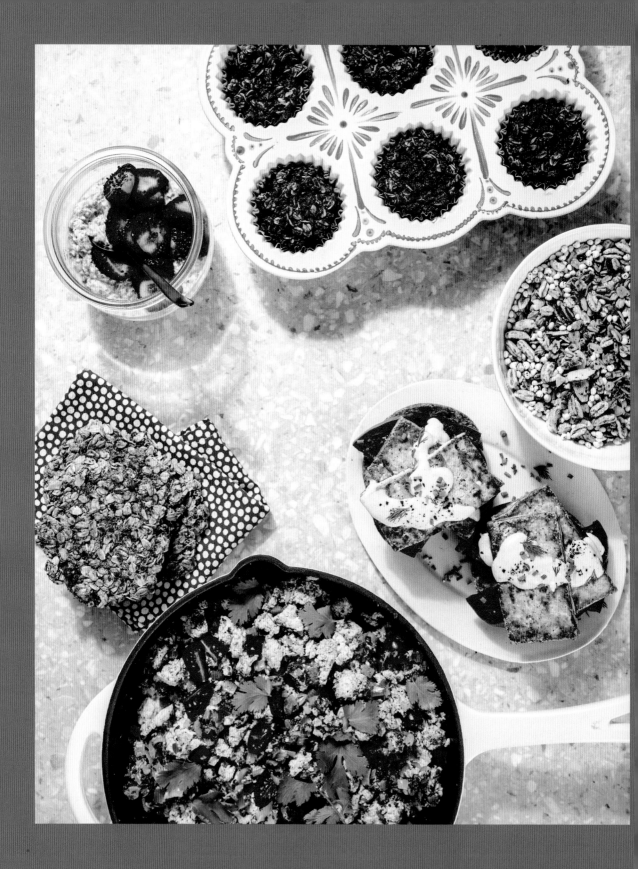

Breakfast

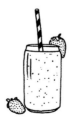

The Beller Method™ AM Blueprint

Breakfast is a golden opportunity to jump-start your day in a way that lowers inflammation, reduces cancer risk, and supports gut health, weight management, and so much more.

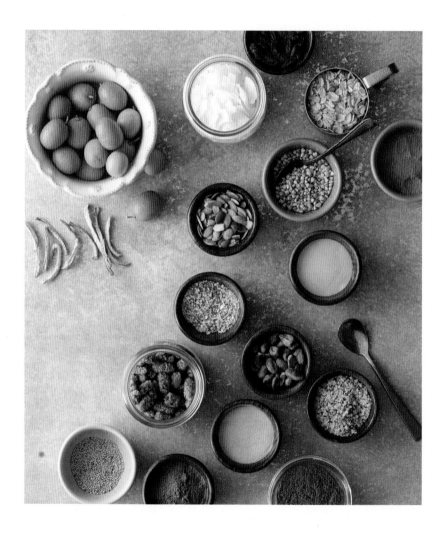

GET YOUR AM FIBER FIX

Your daily fiber goal is **about 35 grams,** which isn't easy unless you have a simple yet super strategic game plan. **The Beller Solution: fuel your body with 10 grams of fiber before noon!**

I've done the behind the scenes work of ensuring your "AM 10"—I've also incorporated Power Spicing, cancer-protective ingredients, and the right combinations of nutrients to keep you full and satisfied.

Start with 2-3 recipes to rotate on a weekly basis (keep it simple!), to get a diverse range of fiber types.

 Step it up! Power it up! Once you feel like you have some of these breakfast options on autopilot...feel free to advance and begin diversifying your fiber and spice intake. Bookmark the Power Up Your Pantry! chapter (page 104) and integrate even more nutrient-dense ingredients to further level up your nutrition—rotate your fiber boosters, add matcha powder to your overnight oats, prebiotic powder to your breakfast cookies, or grated ginger to your smoothies. I've included this symbol for some suggested Power Ups—be creative!

POWER TIP: ROTATE YOUR FIBER BOOSTERS

Explore all of the fiber boosters on pages 114-116.

Think of these as your insurance—with 4-7 grams fiber in just about a spoonful, they supercharge the fiber content of your breakfast so you're guaranteed to meet—or exceed—your 10 gram target. Rotating your fiber boosters supports fiber diversification and the health of your microbiome—and optimal cancer risk reduction.

Vanilla Berry Oatmeal Bake

PREP TIME	COOK TIME	SERVES
10 MINUTES	30 MINUTES	2

Ingredients

Avocado oil spray

1 cup berries, fresh or frozen

⅔ cup rolled oats (sprouted preferred)

⅔ cup unsweetened plant-based milk

2 tablespoons unsweetened applesauce

2 tablespoons chia seeds

1 tablespoon nut or seed protein powder

2 teaspoons pure maple or date syrup, optional

1 teaspoon Cinnapeel Spicer Power Spice Blend*

½ teaspoon vanilla extract

Go "oat" of control with these delightful oatmeal bakes! Bursting with fiber, protein, and a medley of berries—they're a hit with my patients and perfect for changing up your breakfast routine. Bake them in ramekins, leave some in the fridge, and take them on-the-go like a hearty oversized muffin. I'll usually make a few batches for a quick and filling breakfast any day of the week!

Directions

1. Preheat oven to 350°F. Lightly spray 2 large or 4 small ramekins with avocado oil.

2. In a mixing bowl, stir together all ingredients. Divide the mixture evenly between the prepared ramekins.

3. Bake 30 minutes, or until a toothpick inserted into the center comes out mostly clean. Serve warm.

Add before baking: 1 teaspoon prebiotic fiber or mushroom powder.

*Substitute spice blend with ¾ teaspoon Ceylon cinnamon, ½ teaspoon granulated orange peel, pinch of ground ginger.

CALORIES: 266 · FAT: 9G · CARBS: 34G · FIBER: 15G · SUGARS: 5G · ADDED SUGARS: 0G · PROTEIN: 16G

Golden Breakfast Smoothie

PREP TIME	SERVES
5 MINUTES	1

Ingredients

1 sliced and frozen banana

1 cup unsweetened plant milk

1 tablespoon ground flaxseed

1 tablespoon protein powder
(nut or seed)

1 teaspoon Golden Breakfast
Power Spice Blend*

1 tablespoon rolled oats,
optional to top

My go-to breakfast smoothie! It's simple, creamy, and packed with everything I need to start my day off right. And the best part? My signature Golden Breakfast Power Spice Blend simplifies it more by adding cacao, turmeric, and Ceylon cinnamon for nice sweetness with no added sugar. Better yet, studies suggest the quercetin in cacao increases the absorption of curcumin found in turmeric. The rest of the ingredients are all staples of any power pantry and can easily be kept on hand.

Directions

1. Place frozen banana, plant milk, flaxseed, protein powder, and spice blend in a high-powered blender.

2. Blend 2 minutes, just until entirely smooth.

3. Pour into a glass and top with rolled oats, if desired. For more flavor, toast the oats in a dry skillet over medium heat, just until lightly browned and fragrant.

Add to your smoothie:
1 teaspoon prebiotic or oat fiber powder.

*Substitute spice blend with ½ teaspoon Ceylon cinnamon, ½ teaspoon cacao powder, ¼ teaspoon ground turmeric, pinch of ground ginger.

CALORIES: 280 · FAT: 9G · CARBS: 34G · FIBER: 10G · SUGARS: 12G · ADDED SUGARS: 0G · PROTEIN: 19G

Multi-Fiber Bowl

PREP TIME
5 MINUTES

SERVES
1

Ingredients

½ **cup** berries, fresh or frozen

½ **cup** unsweetened plant milk

2 **tablespoons** slivered almonds or rolled oats

1 **tablespoon** chia or basil seeds

1 **tablespoon** whole roasted hemp seeds

1 **tablespoon** ground flaxseed

1 **teaspoon** Cinnapeel Spicer Power Spice Blend*

Start your day off right and dive into this bowl of vibrant and nourishing goodness. Not only is my multi-fiber bowl a feast for the eyes, but my patients repeatedly appreciate the importance of fiber diversification and this bowl does just that and more. I like to prep a few servings in advance in little jars or for travel. It will keep you feeling satisfied and energized all morning long, wherever you go.

Directions

1. In a serving bowl, mix together all ingredients and enjoy!

 Add to your bowl: ½ teaspoon cacao nibs or cacao powder.

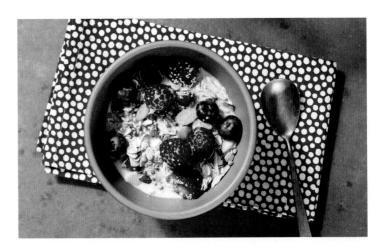

*Substitute spice blend with ¾ teaspoon Ceylon cinnamon, ½ teaspoon granulated orange peel, pinch of ground ginger.

CALORIES: 290 · FAT: 17G · CARBS: 19G · FIBER: 15G · SUGARS: 4G · ADDED SUGARS: 0G · PROTEIN: 15G

Green Power Smoothie

PREP TIME
5 MINUTES

SERVES
1

Ingredients

1½ cups unsweetened plant milk

1 banana, chopped and frozen

½ cup fresh spinach

1 tablespoon watercress or broccoli sprouts

1 tablespoon chia seeds

¼ teaspoon matcha or amla powder, optional

Anyone in the mood for the POWER of greens? Watercress and broccoli sprouts, cruciferous vegetables activated through chewing or blending, are packed with phytochemicals that may help fight cancer! All bananas are great, but use greenish bananas because they offer more resistant starch. Blend up a glass and take on whatever comes your way!

Directions

1. Place all ingredients in a blender. Blend 30 seconds, until smooth.

Add to your smoothie: 1 tablespoon nut or seed protein powder.

CALORIES: 285 · FAT: 10G · CARBS: 24G · FIBER: 12G · SUGARS: 14G · ADDED SUGARS: 0G · PROTEIN: 17G

Warm Apple Crisp

PREP TIME	COOK TIME	SERVES
10 MINUTES	7 MINUTES	1

Ingredients

Avocado oil spray

1 apple, diced

¼ cup rolled oats (sprouted preferred)

2 tablespoons chia seeds or ground flaxseed

½ teaspoon Morning Boost Power Spice Blend*

½ teaspoon maple or date syrup, optional

1 tablespoon plant-based yogurt, optional

If you've ever enjoyed baked fruit, step right in! Let the inviting aroma of the amazing cinnamon and baked apples fill your kitchen as you sit down for this cozy breakfast. This recipe is supercharged with our Morning Boost Power Spice Blend that lends an antioxidant kick and a spicy-sweet depth reminiscent of a baked apple pie. Trust me, it's "a-peeling"! Wake up and smell the apples!

Directions

1. Spray a skillet with avocado oil spray and place over medium heat.

2. Add the diced apples to the skillet and sauté until softened, about 5 minutes.

3. Stir in the oats, chia seeds, and spice blend. Stir in the maple or date syrup for added sweetness, if desired.

4. Sauté 2 minutes before transferring to a serving bowl. Serve topped with a dollop of plant-based yogurt, if desired.

Add to your bowl: lemon or orange zest.

*Substitute spice blend with ½ teaspoon Ceylon cinnamon, pinch of each: ground ginger, nutmeg, allspice, ground cloves.

CALORIES: 285 · FAT: 12G · CARBS: 39G · FIBER: 14G · SUGARS: 11G · ADDED SUGARS: 0G · PROTEIN: 11G

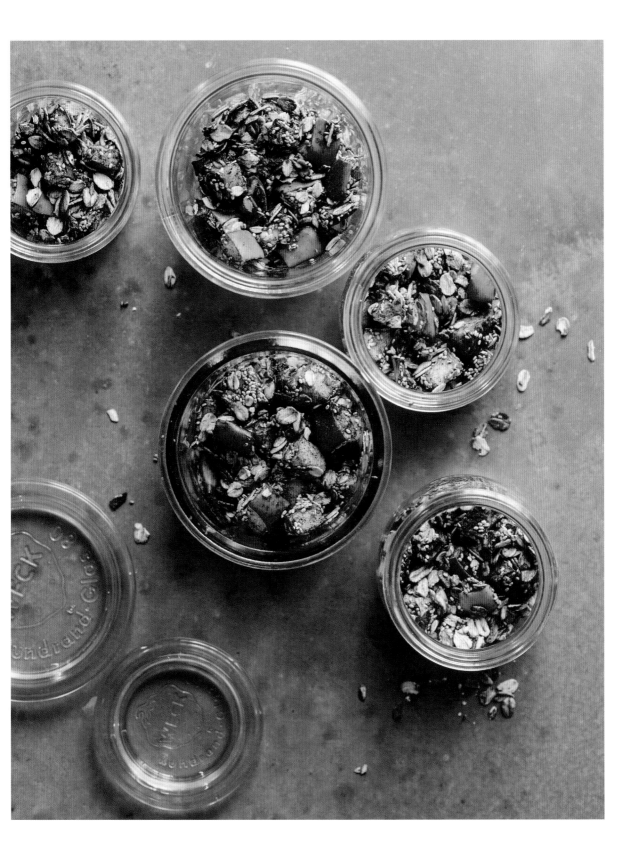

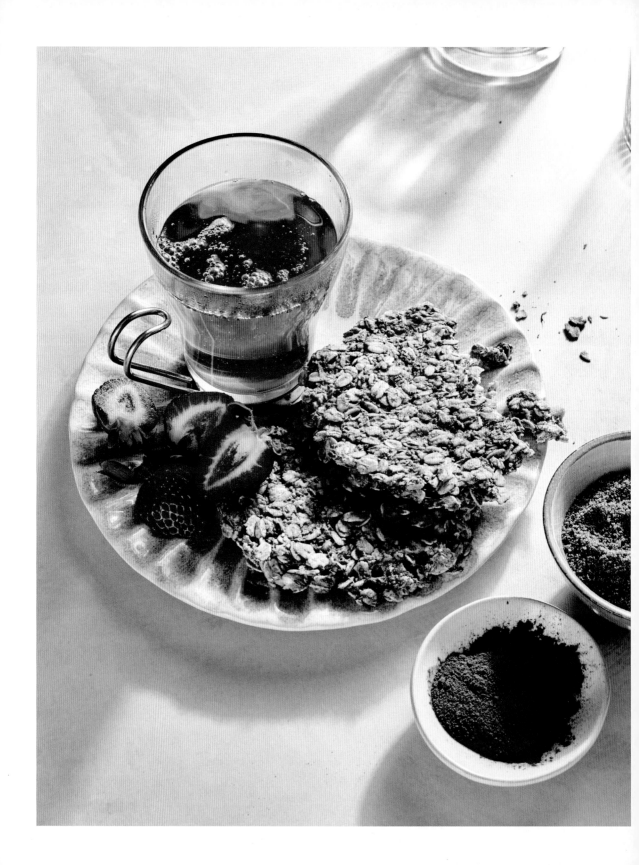

Fiberized Breakfast Cookies

PREP TIME	COOK TIME	SERVING SIZE	SERVES
10 MINUTES	20 MINUTES	2 COOKIES	2

Ingredients

2 bananas, peeled

⅔ cup rolled oats (sprouted preferred)

2 tablespoons chia seeds or ground flaxseed

1 teaspoon avocado oil

1 teaspoon Morning Boost Power Spice Blend*

2 tablespoons protein powder (nut or seed)

Wake up and smell the cookies! You'll definitely want to rise earlier when you have a batch of Rachel Beller's fiber breakfast cookies waiting for you. These tasty treats are a staple of the Beller Method and a favorite among patients looking for a convenient and delicious way to boost their fiber intake. You can make them a million different ways, store them conveniently in the freezer, and take them along for a great travel snack! Preheat your oven and let's get baking! You'll be glad you did.

Directions

1. Preheat oven to 350°F. Line a sheet pan with parchment paper.

2. In a mixing bowl, use the back of a fork to mash the bananas.

3. Fold the remaining ingredients into the mashed bananas and mix well.

4. Using clean hands, create four large cookies. Place on the lined sheet pan.

5. Bake 15–20 minutes, until mostly set.

6. Let cool on the pan 10 minutes before serving.

 Add to batter: 2 teaspoons prebiotic fiber or mushroom powder.

*Substitute ¾ teaspoon Ceylon cinnamon, ⅛ teaspoon ground ginger, ⅛ teaspoon nutmeg, pinch of allspice, pinch of ground cloves.

CALORIES: 309 · FAT: 10G · CARBS: 44G · FIBER: 13G · SUGARS: 10G · ADDED SUGARS: 0G · PROTEIN: 17G

Topped Toasts Three Ways

PREP TIME	COOK TIME	SERVING SIZE	SERVES
5 MINUTES	2 MINUTES	1 SLICE	1

Ingredients

HUMMUS TOAST

1 slice flourless sprouted grain bread

¼ cup hummus

5 cherry tomatoes, halved

¼ teaspoon spices of choice

1 tablespoon hemp, chia, flax, or sunflower seeds

AVOCADO TOAST

1 slice flourless sprouted grain bread

½ avocado, mashed

1 tablespoon nutritional yeast

¼ teaspoon spices of choice

1 tablespoon hemp, chia, flax, or sunflower seeds

PB&J TOAST

1 slice flourless sprouted grain bread

1 tablespoon nut butter

1 tablespoon Rachel's Power Jam (recipe page 176)

1½ teaspoons hemp, chia, flax, or basil seeds

Avo-lutely delicious! Topped Toasts Three Ways is a surefire meal to start your day on the right foot. It may seem like a basic concept, but the secret to success is opting for whole intact, 100% flourless grain bread. It's packed with nutrients and requires more effort for our bodies to digest—a great internal workout that helps your blood sugars stay stable. See for yourself and enjoy this powerful breakfast.

Directions

1. Toast the flourless bread to your liking.

2. Spread the hummus, mashed avocado, or nut butter and jam over top of the toast.

3. Sprinkle with a spice blend and seed of choice.

Add to your toast: sesame seeds.

CALORIES: 290 · FAT: 18G · CARBS: 28G · FIBER: 14G · SUGARS: 2G · ADDED SUGARS: 0G · PROTEIN: 12G

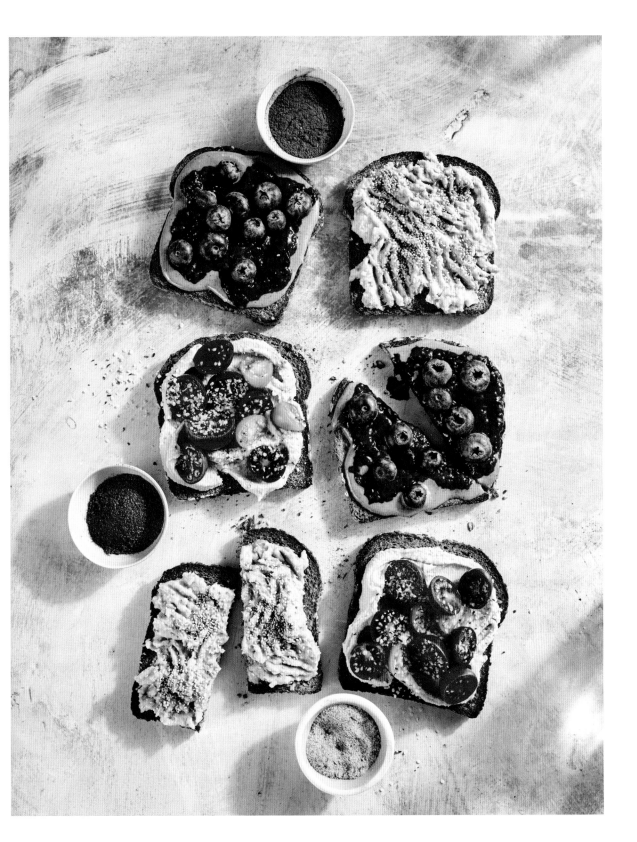

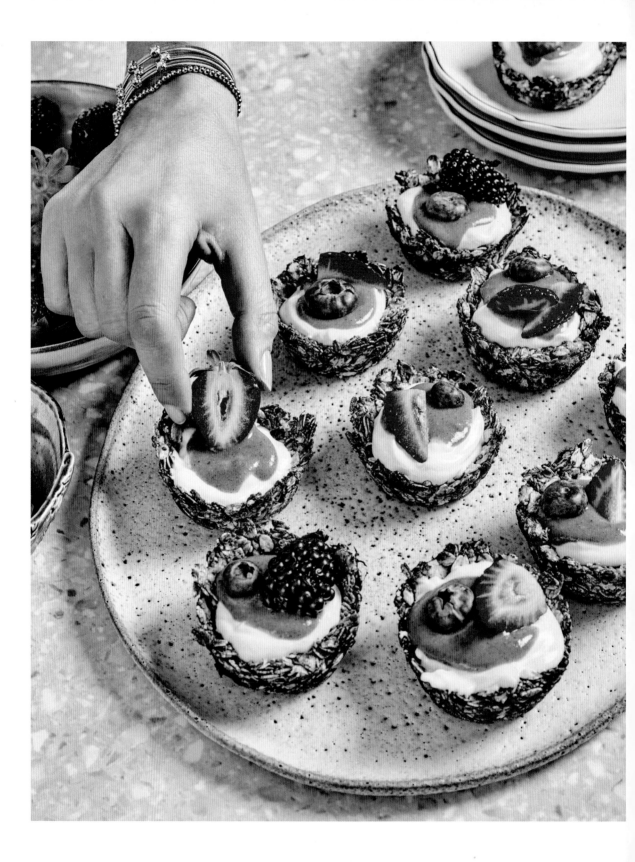

Effortless Oat Cups

PREP TIME	COOK TIME	SERVING SIZE	SERVES
15 MINUTES	2 MINUTES	3 OAT CUPS	4

Ingredients

Avocado oil spray

2 bananas, peeled

2 cups rolled oats (sprouted preferred)

¼ cup chia or basil seeds

1 tablespoon honey, date, or maple syrup

1½ teaspoons vanilla extract

1 teaspoon Morning Boost Power Spice Blend*

Dollops of plant-based yogurt, Rachel's Power Jam (recipe page 176), or nut butter, to top cups

Fresh berries, optional, for garnish

Breakfast, meet your new best friend! Not only are these oat cups fun to dress up, but they are also a quick and convenient on-the-go breakfast when topped with a dollop of nut butter or even my Power Jam. The oats in these fiber powerhouses are a great source of beta-glucans, a special type of soluble fiber that helps support a healthy immune system. So, whether you're hosting a brunch or just looking for a quick breakfast option, give these Effortless Oat Cups a try and see for yourself!

Directions

1. Spray 12 cups of a muffin tin with avocado oil spray.

2. In a mixing bowl, use the back of a fork to mash the bananas. Fold in oats, chia seeds, honey, vanilla extract, and spice blend, until all is combined.

3. Divide the mixture among the 12 cups of the muffin tin and press it up the sides of the muffin cups to create little cups.

4. Preheat oven to 350°F. Bake the oat cups for 15 minutes.

5. Let cool 10 minutes before removing the oat cups from the muffin tin. Fill each with a dollop of your choice of plant-based yogurt, jam, or nut butter. Garnish with fresh berries, if desired.

 Add to the batter:
2 teaspoons acacia prebiotic fiber.

*Substitute spice blend with ¾ teaspoon Ceylon cinnamon, ⅛ teaspoon ground ginger, ⅛ teaspoon nutmeg, pinch of allspice, pinch of ground cloves.

CALORIES: 280 · FAT: 8G · CARBS: 41G · FIBER: 11G · SUGARS: 12G · ADDED SUGARS: 2G · PROTEIN: 10G

Spiced Pour and Go Oats

PREP TIME
5 MINUTES

SERVES
1

Ingredients

⅔ **cup** unsweetened plant milk

⅓ **cup** rolled oats (sprouted preferred)

1 **tablespoon** chia or basil seeds

1 **tablespoon** protein powder (nut or seed)

½ **teaspoon** Cinnapeel Spicer Power Spice Blend*

¼ **cup** berries, fresh or frozen

This breakfast is the perfect solution for those mornings when you're short on time. You can simply pour and go or add all of the ingredients to a jar, give it a shake, and throw it in the fridge before crawling into bed. I like to make a few jars ahead of time for quick grab-and-go breakfasts for the week. And while this recipe is easy to make, it's anything but basic in terms of benefits. Just by adding spices, you've easily transformed an unassuming oatmeal into an antioxidant-supercharged breakfast.

Directions

1. Place plant milk, rolled oats, chia seeds, protein powder, and spice blend in a jar. Seal jar and shake well.

2. The fruit can be added to the jar when preparing or added when ready to serve.

3. Refrigerate overnight or enjoy right after preparing, soaking oat mixture for 10 minutes. Eat warmed up or chilled.

Add to your jar: ½ teaspoon matcha.

---

*Substitute spice blend with ½ teaspoon Ceylon cinnamon, ¼ teaspoon granulated orange peel, pinch of ground ginger.

CALORIES: 288 · FAT: 11G · CARBS: 34G · FIBER: 14G · SUGARS: 4G · ADDED SUGARS: 0G · PROTEIN: 20G

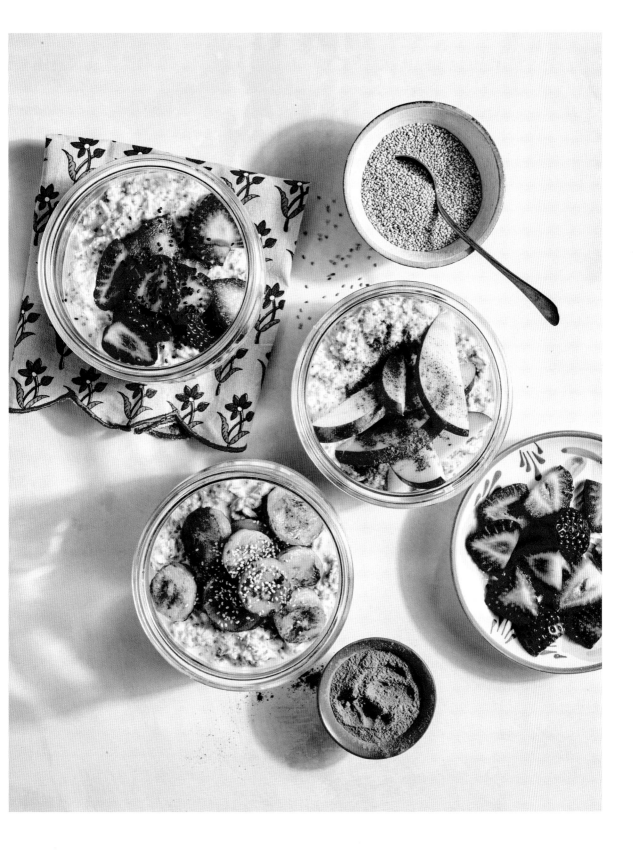

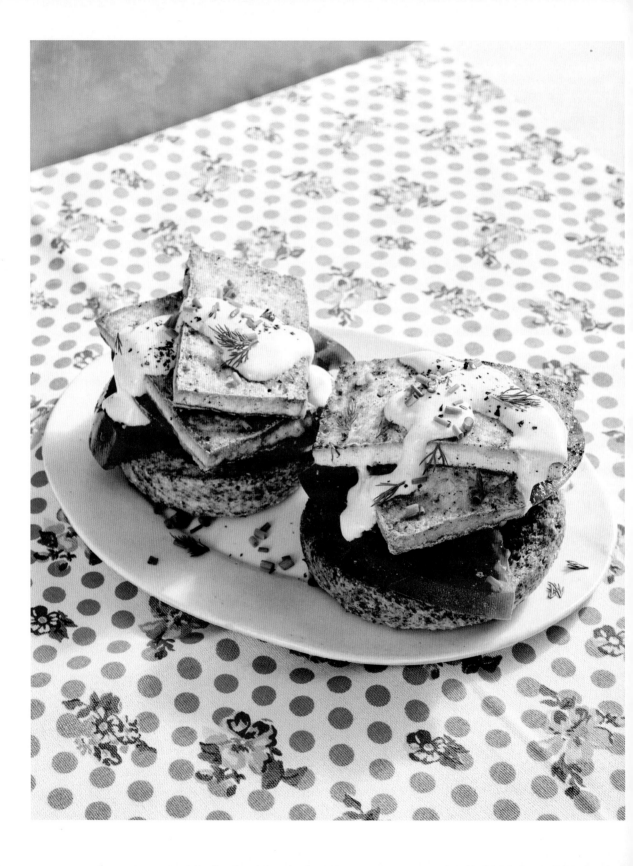

Tofu Benedict

PREP TIME	COOK TIME	SERVES
10 MINUTES	10 MINUTES	2

Ingredients

Avocado oil spray

8 ounces extra-firm tofu, sliced

1 teaspoon Vegitude Power Spice Blend*

Salt and pepper, to taste

2 sprouted flourless English muffins

1 tomato, sliced

PLANT-BASED HOLLANDAISE

½ **cup** plain plant-based yogurt

Juice of ½ lemon

1 tablespoon nutritional yeast

1 teaspoon Dijon mustard

¼ **teaspoon** ground turmeric

Say hello to Tofu Benedict—a playful twist on a classic dish for anyone in the mood for something different. Don't let the tofu scare you off—it's power spiced and contains phytoestrogens, which add a layer of breast cancer protection to the theme of this dish. Flourless muffins give a great texture and are incredibly filling. And let's not forget about the sauce—it's so versatile that you can use it for other meals throughout the week. So what are you waiting for? Whip up a batch at your next brunch and start your weekend off on a delicious note!

Directions

1. Spray a skillet with avocado oil spray and place over medium heat.

2. Place the sliced tofu in the skillet and lightly season with the spice blend, salt, and pepper.

3. Let tofu cook until lightly browned, 4–5 minutes on each side.

4. Meanwhile, toast the English muffins and arrange on 2 serving plates. Top each half of the muffins with an equal amount of sliced tomato.

5. In a small mixing bowl, whisk together all hollandaise ingredients. This can be used as is, or warmed up.

6. Place the cooked tofu over the sliced tomato on the English muffins and top with an equal amount of the hollandaise before serving.

Sprinkle with: fresh parsley or paprika.

*Substitute spice blend with ¼ teaspoon granulated garlic, ¼ teaspoon granulated onion, ¼ teaspoon ground turmeric, ⅛ teaspoon dried parsley, pinch of black pepper.

CALORIES: 320 · FAT: 11G · CARBS: 38G · FIBER: 10G · SUGARS: 4G · ADDED SUGARS: 0G · PROTEIN: 23G

Rachel's Power Jam

PREP TIME	COOK TIME	SERVING SIZE	SERVES
5 MINUTES	15 MINUTES	1 TABLESPOON	30

Ingredients

3 cups berries (any, fresh or frozen)

2 tablespoons lemon juice

2 tablespoons chia or whole hemp seeds

2 tablespoons ground flaxseed

1 teaspoon Cinnapeel Spicer Power Spice Blend*

1 tablespoon honey or date syrup

Sweet and powerful—my favorite combo! This jam is incredibly easy to make, full of crunch, and mildly sweet. The secret is in the power-seed mix that is absolutely jam-packed with good-for-you omega-3 fats, fiber, protein, and anti-inflammatory properties. I love adding this to my oatmeal, yogurt parfaits, or on top of nut butter, spread on my breakfast cookies, or smeared over toast. Make it once and you will be hooked! Truly a hidden "jam"!

Directions

1. Add all ingredients to a saucepan over medium heat.

2. Bring up to a simmer and reduce heat to low.

3. Stirring occasionally, let the jam gently simmer 10–15 minutes, just until it has thickened.

4. Store in a covered jar in the refrigerator for up to 1 week.

 Stir into your jam: 2 tablespoons hemp hearts.

*Substitute spice blend with ¾ teaspoon Ceylon cinnamon, ½ teaspoon granulated orange peel, pinch of ground ginger.

CALORIES: 15 · FAT: 1G · CARBS: 3G · FIBER: 1G · SUGARS: 1G · ADDED SUGARS: 1G · PROTEIN: 1G

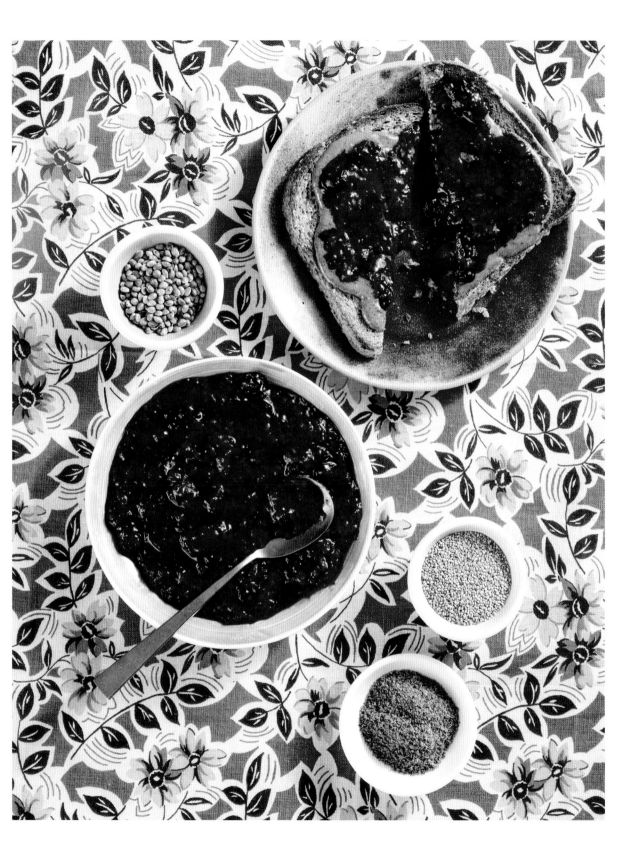

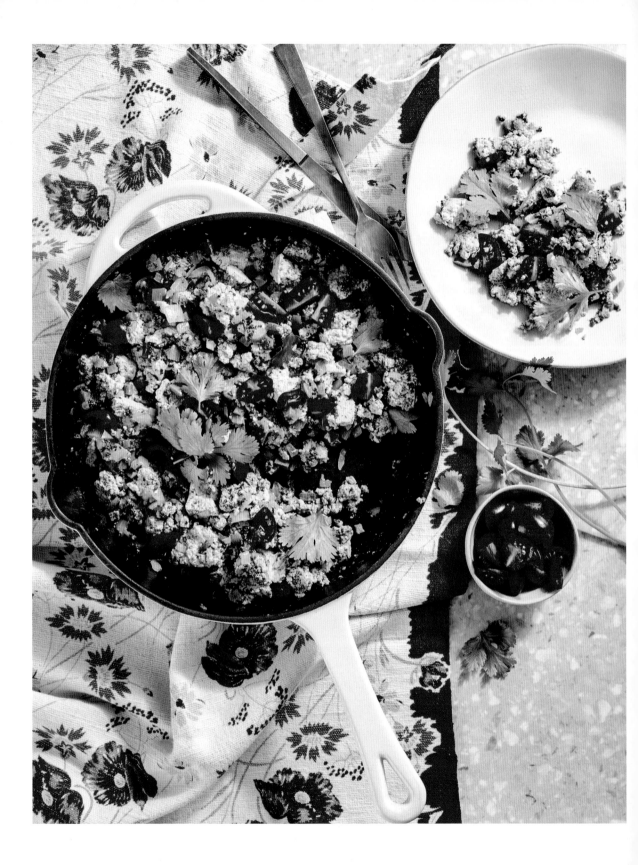

Tex Mex Tofu Scramble

PREP TIME	COOK TIME	SERVES
15 MINUTES	10 MINUTES	2

Ingredients

2 teaspoons avocado oil

1 yellow onion, diced

1 bell pepper, diced

2 Roma tomatoes, diced

2 tablespoons chia seeds

16 ounces medium or soft tofu, drained

2 tablespoons nutritional yeast

2 teaspoons Tex Mex Power Spice Blend*

¼ teaspoon salt

Your morning scramble just got a face-lift! This scramble is creamy, protein-packed, and entirely plant-based thanks to the crumbled tofu; soft tofu is the key to a creamy and "egg-like" consistency. Nutritional yeast adds a savory and almost "cheesy" kick to complement all of the traditional Tex Mex flavors. It makes for great leftovers and probably will not last long; my daughter Keira ate this one up for breakfast AND dinner.

Directions

1. Heat avocado oil in a skillet over medium heat.

2. Add the onion and bell pepper to the skillet and sauté 5 minutes, until the onion is translucent. Add the tomatoes and stir in chia seeds.

3. Meanwhile, in a mixing bowl, use a heavy fork to break up and crumble the tofu into the consistency of scrambled eggs. Fold in nutritional yeast, spice blend, and salt.

4. Stir the tofu mixture into the skillet and sauté 3–5 minutes to heat the tofu throughout.

Top your meal: with fresh cilantro.

*Substitute spice blend with ½ teaspoon chili powder, ¼ teaspoon paprika, ½ teaspoon ground cumin, ¼ teaspoon granulated onion, ¼ teaspoon granulated garlic, ¼ teaspoon dried oregano, ¼ teaspoon crushed red pepper flakes, pinch of each: black pepper, Ceylon cinnamon, ground cloves.

CALORIES: 240 · FAT: 18G · CARBS: 25G · FIBER: 12G · SUGARS: 5G · ADDED SUGARS: 0G · PROTEIN: 22G

Rachel's Cereal Mix

PREP TIME	COOK TIME	SERVING SIZE	SERVES
5 MINUTES	12 MINUTES	1 CUP	6

Ingredients

2 tablespoons avocado oil

1 tablespoon date syrup, pure maple syrup, or honey

1 teaspoon Cinnapeel Spicer Power Spice Blend*

1 teaspoon vanilla extract

⅛ teaspoon salt

1½ cups rolled oats (sprouted preferred)

½ cup sliced almonds

¼ cup whole hemp seeds

2 tablespoons chia or basil seeds

3 cups puffed kamut or millet

It's time to have a little fun! Many of my patients want to bypass traditional boxed cereals loaded with added sugar, refined flours, and a host of other unnecessary ingredients. It's why I created this delicious fiberized cereal mix—so you can **know** exactly what's in your bowl and you can enjoy the kid in you craving the sound, the crunch, the milk being poured. It's versatile and can be taken as an on-the-go snack. So go ahead and let your inner child out with Rachel's Cereal Mix—the perfect way to start your day!

Directions

1. Preheat oven to 325°F. Line a sheet pan with parchment paper.

2. In a large mixing bowl, whisk together avocado oil, date syrup, spice blend, vanilla extract, and salt.

3. Fold in oats, almonds, hemp seeds, and chia seeds, until all is combined. Spread on the prepared sheet pan.

4. Bake 10–12 minutes, stirring halfway through.

5. Let cool 5 minutes before transferring to a food storage container. Add puffed kamut or millet and shake to mix. Serve as a topping, snack, or cereal in plant milk with some fiber-rich berries.

Add to the mix: 2 tablespoons sesame seeds.

*Substitute spice blend with ¾ teaspoon Ceylon cinnamon, ½ teaspoon granulated orange peel, pinch of ground ginger.

CALORIES: 250 · FAT: 13G · CARBS: 26G · FIBER: 7G · SUGARS: 3G · ADDED SUGARS: 2G · PROTEIN: 8G

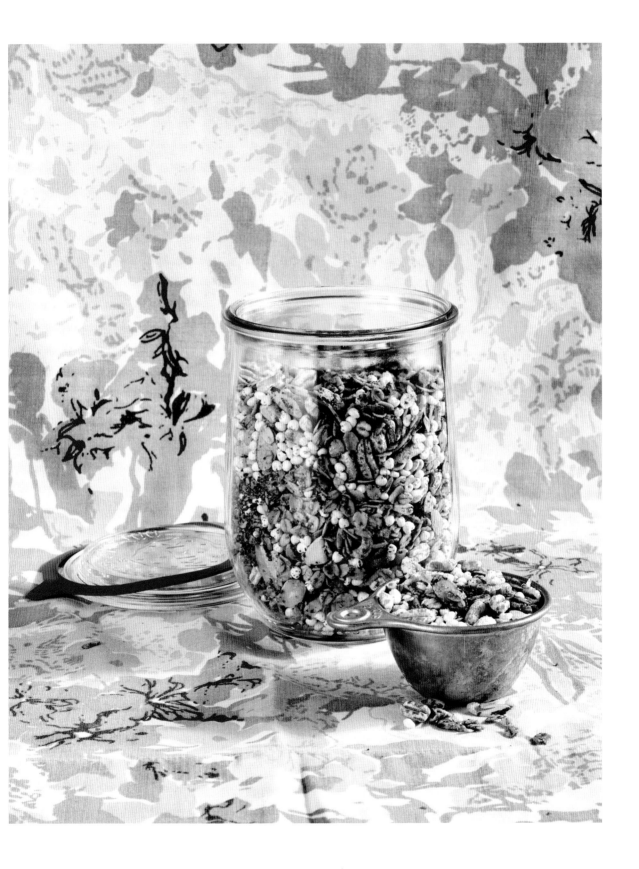

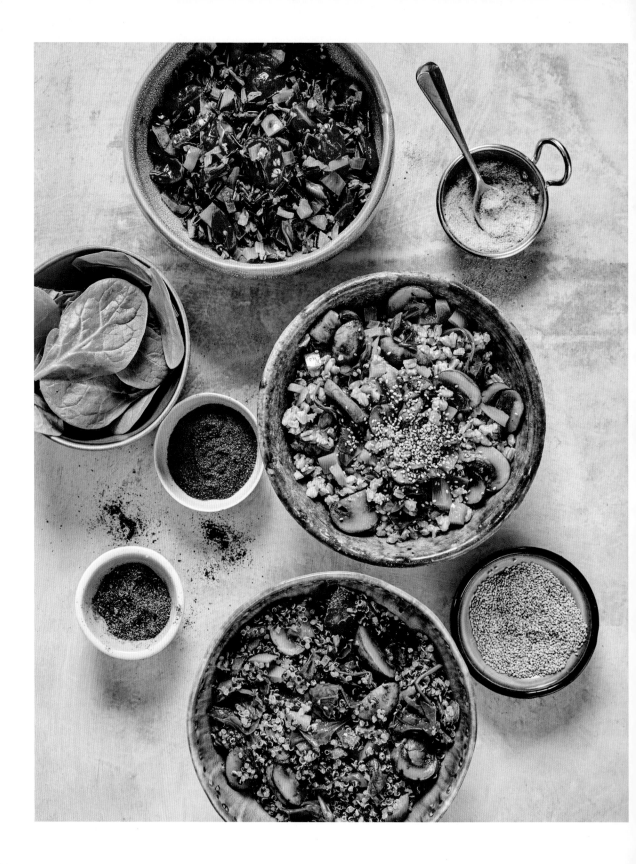

Savory Breakfast Bowl Your Way

PREP TIME	COOK TIME	SERVES
10 MINUTES	10 MINUTES	1

Ingredients

1½ teaspoons avocado oil

2 cups chopped low starch vegetables of choice
or onions, bell peppers, mushrooms, spinach, and tomatoes

¾ cup cooked quinoa, farro, or black rice

1½ teaspoons chia seeds

1 teaspoon Everything Savory Power Spice Blend*

Salt to taste

For those craving something savory to start their day, or anytime really, I've got just the thing. Enjoy a savory breakfast bowl in your own way, the perfect solution for when you want something as easy as a veggie scramble but with the satisfaction of hearty intact whole grains. You can cook up a big batch of any grain or seed of choice and you're set for the week! The best part? You can customize it to your heart's content with your favorite fiber boosters and veggies.

Directions

1. Heat avocado oil in a skillet over medium heat.

2. Add your choice of vegetables to the skillet and sauté until crisp-tender.

3. Stir in your choice of cooked grain, chia seeds, and spice blend. Sauté 2 additional minutes, just until grain is heated through.

4. Season with salt before serving.

Add to bowl: ½ teaspoon mushroom powder.

*Substitute spice blend with ½ teaspoon paprika, ¼ teaspoon granulated garlic, ⅛ teaspoon ground turmeric, ⅛ teaspoon ground cumin, pinch of black pepper, pinch of cayenne pepper.

CALORIES: 330 · FAT: 12G · CARBS: 42G · FIBER: 12G · SUGARS: 5G · ADDED SUGARS: 0G · PROTEIN: 14G

Oat Bran Mini Toasts

PREP TIME	COOK TIME	SERVING SIZE	SERVES
10 MINUTES	20 MINUTES	2 TOASTS	3

Ingredients

2 bananas, peeled

½ teaspoon vanilla extract

1 teaspoon Morning Boost Power Spice Blend*

1 tablespoon protein powder (nut or seed)

1 cup oat bran

2 tablespoons chia or ground flaxseeds

TOPPINGS:

1 tablespoon nut or seed butter

1 tablespoon Rachel's Power Jam (recipe page 176)

These mini oat bran toasts are a fiber-packed way to start your morning. I like to spread a bit of nut or seed butter over top, but they are also delicious all on their own as a grab-n-go snack solution!

Directions

1. Preheat oven to 350°F. Line a sheet pan with parchment paper.

2. In a food processor, process bananas, vanilla, spice blend, and protein powder until creamy and smooth.

3. Add the oat bran and process another 5 seconds, until a dough has formed. Fold in chia or flaxseeds.

4. Using clean hands, press the dough on the parchment paper into 6 round toasts.

5. Bake 15–20 minutes, until golden brown around the edges. Turn oven off and let cool, in the oven with the oven door cracked open, at least 15 minutes, to further crisp up. Feel free to spread nut butter and jam over the top of the toasts.

Add to batter: 1 teaspoon mushroom or prebiotic fiber powder.

Substitute spice blend with ¾ teaspoon Ceylon cinnamon, ⅛ teaspoon ground ginger, ⅛ teaspoon nutmeg, pinch of allspice, pinch of ground cloves.

CALORIES: 260 · FAT: 6G · CARBS: 40G · FIBER: 14G · SUGARS: 7G · ADDED SUGARS: 0G · PROTEIN: 13G

Quinoa Berry Breakfast Squares

PREP TIME	COOK TIME	SERVES
10 MINUTES	60 MINUTES	6

Ingredients

Avocado oil spray

2 medium bananas, peeled

2 cups unsweetened plant milk

1½ cups berries, fresh or frozen

1 cup uncooked quinoa

5 tablespoons chia seeds

2 tablespoons protein powder (nut or seed)

2 tablespoons date syrup

2 teaspoons vanilla extract

2 teaspoons Cinnapeel Spicer Power Spice Blend*

Anyone in need of a super fast and easy breakfast with minimal cleanup and lots of leftovers? Well, these breakfast squares are definitely it. Add all the ingredients into a baking dish, mix it up, throw it in the oven, and boom, you've got a great alternative to muffins or granola bars that ensures you have a high-fiber breakfast on hand for days. The serving size is generous, and each square gets a boost of natural sweetness and flavor complexity from the power combo of Ceylon cinnamon, ginger, and orange peel.

Directions

1. Preheat oven to 350°F. Lightly spray a medium (about 8 x 12-inch) baking dish with avocado oil spray.

2. Place bananas in the baking dish and use a fork to mash.

3. Add the remaining ingredients and stir to combine.

4. Bake for 60 minutes. Let cool at least 15 minutes before slicing to serve. Store covered and refrigerated.

Mix into batter:
2 tablespoons oat fiber.

*Substitute spice blend with 1¼ teaspoon Ceylon cinnamon, ¾ teaspoon granulated orange peel, pinch of ground ginger.

CALORIES: 260 · FAT: 8G · CARBS: 37G · FIBER: 11G · SUGARS: 12G · ADDED SUGARS: 0G · PROTEIN: 13G

Power Breakfast Sweet Potatoes

PREP TIME	COOK TIME	SERVES
5 MINUTES	55 MINUTES	1

Ingredients

1 sweet potato, scrubbed

2 teaspoons nut butter or tahini sauce

2 teaspoons chia seeds

1 tablespoon hemp hearts

1 teaspoon Cinnapeel Spicer Power Spice Blend*

If you've never tried sweet potatoes for breakfast, it's time to start! I love suggesting this filling breakfast to my patients—seeing the light in their eyes of "OH! What a good idea!" before they try it is always so gratifying. Enjoy the wonderful aroma filling your kitchen and make a batch of 3 to 4 and keep it in the fridge for the coming week as a great pre-workout breakfast. Fuel up on these powered up Beller Method sweet potatoes!

Directions

1. Preheat oven to 400°F. Line a sheet pan with parchment paper.

2. Pierce sweet potato in at least 4 places with the tines of a fork and place on the lined sheet pan. You can bake as many potatoes at once as you'd like, as long as there is at least 2 inches of space between each.

3. Bake for 45 minutes– 1 hour, until potatoes are fork-tender.

4. Remove from oven and allow to cool for 5 minutes. Once ready to eat, split the warm sweet potato open with a knife and add the nut butter or tahini, seeds, and spice blend.

 Add to your sweet potato: ½ teaspoon cacao powder.

*Substitute spice blend with ¾ teaspoon Ceylon cinnamon, ½ teaspoon granulated orange peel, pinch of ground ginger.

CALORIES: 311 · FAT: 18G · CARBS: 29G · FIBER: 10G · SUGARS: 10G · ADDED SUGARS: 0G · PROTEIN: 10G

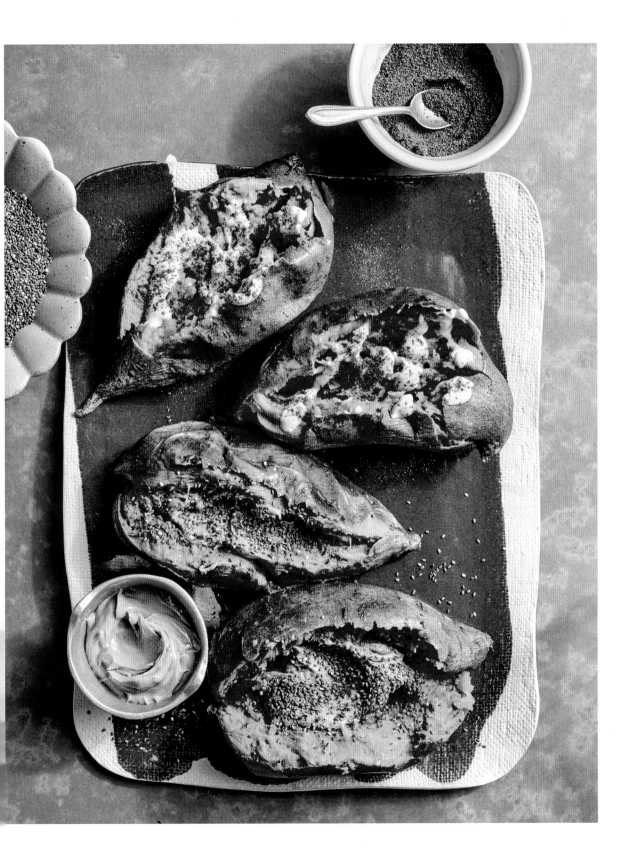

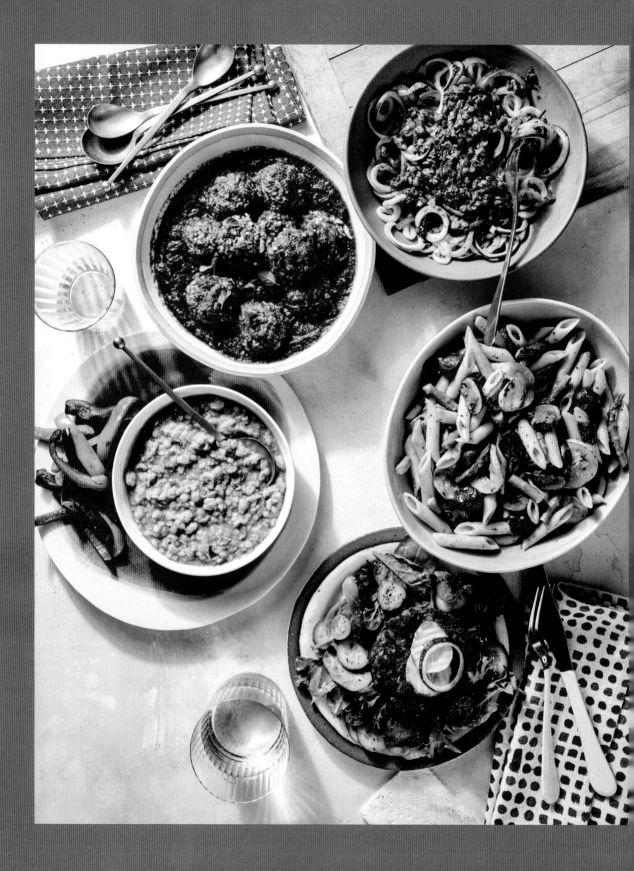

Complete
Meals

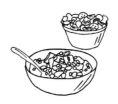

The Beller Method™
Meal Strategy

Meals are the bulk of your food intake for the day! That's why it's essential to have a strategic approach to building them. I've done the hard work for you and have made sure that each of these recipes is packed with anti-cancer foods and spices in appropriate portions to optimize cancer risk reduction and weight management. They have been designed with a key concept in: The Power of 3. Each meal contains three power players that are non-negotiables for every meal. Whether you're following the recipes in this book, cooking on your own, or eating out, make sure that you have The Power of 3 in each meal.

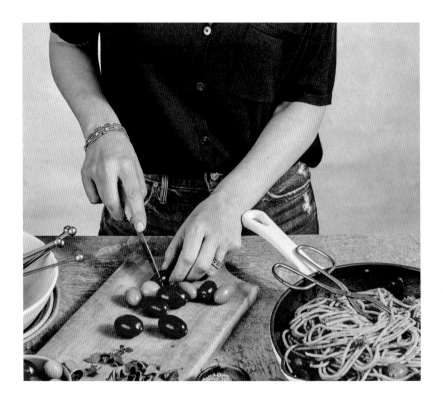

Low Starch Vegetables:
Base of at least 2 cups and more if you like!

They're rich in fiber, antioxidants, cancer-protective phytochemicals, vitamins, and minerals; they also may reduce inflammation, support gut health, and provide volume to assist with weight loss. Veg should be the star of your meal, not a secondary player. Refer to page 66 for a list of low starch veg. We've made sure to include 2 cups or more for each recipe.

Premium Protein:
Generally ¾ cup—1 cup.

Follow my guide in the Go Pro chapter (page 78) to choose premium plant proteins that assist with hormonal balance and are rich in phytochemicals that flood your insides with cancer-protective compounds. All the recipes in this section, of course, use premium protein options.

Beneficial Fats:
About 1 tablespoon oil, 2 tablespoons of dressing/nuts/avocado.

Adding an anti-inflammatory fat keeps you full longer, stabilizes blood sugars, enhances immunity, and increases the absorption of anti-inflammatory and cancer fighting compounds from plant foods and spices. Fats are often incorporated in the cooking method or can be drizzled on top of your meal.

The Power of 3 is a tried and true concept that has helped my patients create easy, simple meals that prioritize cancer protective nutrients, balance blood sugars, and support weight management. Start with this method especially if you are focusing on weight loss, then you may slowly add in appropriate amounts of intact whole grains and high starch veg if desired. See Strike a Sugar Balance Chapter (page 50) and Veg Out Chapter (page 62) for information.

While the Power of 3 is the foundation for each of these meals, I don't stop there. I make sure to include the top-of-the-line Power Up! ingredients. And of course, all the recipes are spiced up to radically transform them into antioxidant and anti-inflammatory powerhouses.

And I've kept things simple. The ingredient lists are short and to the point, and the methods are quick and easy. The recipes are plant-based but are appealing to pescatarians or occasional meat-eaters. They're family friendly (my kids have approved them!) and I can assure you they'll become part of your regular meal rotation in your household.

Shakshuka Your Way

PREP TIME	COOK TIME	SERVES
5 MINUTES	15 MINUTES	2

Ingredients

1 tablespoon extra-virgin olive oil

1 yellow onion, diced

1 bell pepper, chopped

1 teaspoon Everything Savory Power Spice Blend*

1½ cups cooked chickpeas, cannellini, or green peas, drained and rinsed

⅔ cup marinara sauce

3 tablespoons hemp hearts

RECOMMENDED SIDE:

1 cup roasted low starch vegetables per serving

Let's shakshuka things up! This is a dish that is enjoyed worldwide and is delicious, easy to make, and customizable. I like to think of it as an "anything goes" dish. With just a few key ingredients and your choice of protein, you can whip up a meal that's perfect for any time of day. Toss in a teaspoon of my spice blend to make things even simpler while cranking up the flavor and nutritional power!

Directions

1. Heat olive oil in a skillet over medium heat. Add the onion and sauté 5 minutes, just until softened.

2. Stir in bell pepper and sauté an additional 3 minutes. Stir in spice blend.

3. Stir in beans, marinara sauce, and hemp hearts and bring up to a simmer. Let simmer 5 minutes, or until bell pepper is tender.

 Add to the skillet: 1 teaspoon mushroom powder or sumac.

*Substitute spice blend with ½ teaspoon paprika, ¼ teaspoon granulated garlic, ⅛ teaspoon ground turmeric, ⅛ teaspoon ground cumin, pinch of black pepper, pinch of cayenne pepper.

CALORIES: 394 · FAT: 13G · CARBS: 47G · FIBER: 18G · SUGARS: 8G · ADDED SUGARS: 0G · PROTEIN: 23G

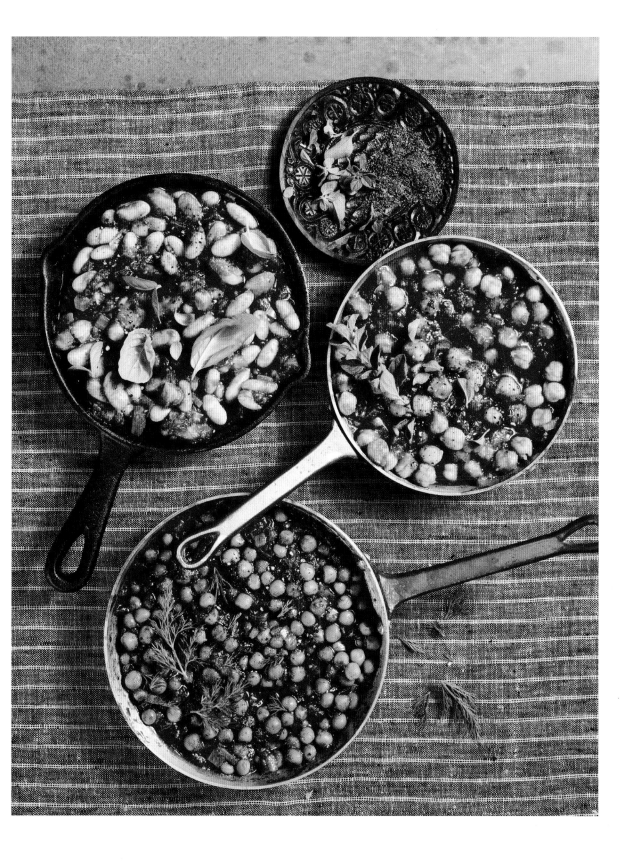

Zucchini Noodle Ramen

PREP TIME	COOK TIME	SERVES
15 MINUTES	10 MINUTES	2

Ingredients

2 teaspoons sesame oil

4 ounces mushrooms, sliced

6 ounces firm tofu, cubed

3 cups vegetable stock

1 tablespoon coconut aminos or tamari

2 teaspoons grated fresh ginger

¼ teaspoon onion powder

2 zucchini, spiralized

¾ cup grated carrots

¾ cup shelled edamame

Get ready for "zoodles" of delicious comfort in a bowl! This recipe for Zucchini Noodle Ramen is the perfect way to enjoy the soothing flavors of ramen without refined starchy noodles. With the addition of tofu and edamame, you'll get a boost of protective phytoestrogens and cancer-fighting compounds, along with a quick and easy solution for a soothing Asian-inspired broth sans the additives.

Directions

1. Heat sesame oil in a pot over medium heat. Add the mushrooms and sauté 5 minutes.

2. Place the cubed tofu in the pot and stir in vegetable stock, coconut aminos, ginger, and onion powder. Bring up to a simmer.

3. Meanwhile, arrange the spiralized zucchini evenly between 2 serving bowls. Top each with an equal amount of the grated carrot and thawed edamame.

4. Once the broth is simmering, pour over the vegetables in each serving bowl. Top each bowl with an equal amount of the simmered mushrooms and tofu.

5. Let rest 2 minutes before serving to allow the hot broth to lightly cook the zucchini and carrot.

TIP: If you don't own a vegetable spiralizer, you can usually buy pre-spiralized zucchini "zoodles" in the refrigerated section of the produce department.

Add to the broth:
1 teaspoon miso paste.

CALORIES: 326 · FAT: 14G · CARBS: 26G · FIBER: 10G · SUGARS: 11G · ADDED SUGARS: 0G · PROTEIN: 28G

Hearty Lentil Stew

PREP TIME	COOK TIME	SERVES
15 MINUTES	30 MINUTES	2

Ingredients

¾ cup dried green lentils, rinsed

2 cups vegetable stock

1 tablespoon extra-virgin olive oil

2 cups sliced mushrooms

2 cups chopped zucchini

2 cups diced tomatoes

1 cup marinara sauce

1 teaspoon Vegitude Power Spice Blend*

Lentils may be small, but they're mighty in this Hearty Lentil Stew! Packed with protein, protective phytochemicals, prebiotic fibers, and more. It's budget friendly, easy to whip up in a rush, and a great option for a quick and satisfying plant-based meal. This recipe will be absolutely "stew-pendous"!

Directions

1. Add lentils and vegetable stock to a pot over high heat. Bring up to a boil. Reduce heat to a simmer and let cook 25 minutes, or until lentils are nearly tender.

2. Meanwhile, heat olive oil in a skillet over medium-high heat. Add mushrooms and sauté 5 minutes.

3. Reduce heat to medium and stir in zucchini and tomatoes. Sauté 5 minutes and remove from heat.

4. Stir the cooked vegetables into the pot of cooked lentils. Stir in marinara sauce and spice blend and bring back up to a simmer. Let simmer 5–10 minutes.

 Add to the pot:
2 teaspoons mushroom powder.

*Substitute spice blend with ¼ teaspoon granulated garlic, ¼ teaspoon granulated onion, ¼ teaspoon ground turmeric, ⅛ teaspoon dried parsley, pinch of black pepper.

CALORIES: 316 · FAT: 7G · CARBS: 49G · FIBER: 11G · SUGARS: 12G · ADDED SUGARS: 0G · PROTEIN: 20G

Pasta Primavera

PREP TIME	COOK TIME	SERVES
15 MINUTES	20 MINUTES	4

Ingredients

6 ounces dry edamame or chickpea pasta

1½ tablespoons extra-virgin olive oil

1 pound mushrooms, sliced

1 pound asparagus, ends discarded, chopped into 1-inch lengths

1 yellow squash, sliced

2 teaspoons minced garlic

Juice of ½ lemon

2 tablespoons nutritional yeast

1 teaspoon Italian seasoning

1 teaspoon Vegitude Power Spice Blend*

1 cup grape tomatoes, halved

Salt and pepper, to taste

There's no springtime bouquet quite as vibrant as my Pasta Primavera! With a strong serving of low starch veggies and protein-packed pasta, this dish is a super "Comfort-me" meal that is rich in protective phytonutrients, protein, and fiber. The addition of nutritional yeast adds a cheesy flavor and a boost of plant-based protein. This dish checks off all the boxes—easy, delicious, and a quick go-to!

Directions

1. Cook pasta according to package directions.

2. Heat olive oil in a large skillet over medium heat. Add the mushrooms and sauté 5 minutes.

3. Add the asparagus, squash, and garlic to the skillet and sauté 7 minutes, just until vegetables are crisp-tender.

4. Reserve at least ½ cup of the pasta boiling water before draining. Add the drained pasta to the skillet with the vegetables and stir in lemon juice, nutritional yeast, Italian seasoning, spice blend, and tomatoes.

5. Pour ½ cup of the reserved pasta boiling water into the skillet and sauté all ingredients together for 2 minutes. Season with salt and pepper to taste before serving.

Add to the skillet:
½ cup chopped fresh basil.

*Substitute spice blend with ¼ teaspoon granulated garlic, ¼ teaspoon granulated onion, ¼ teaspoon ground turmeric, ⅛ teaspoon dried parsley, pinch of black pepper.

CALORIES: 265 · FAT: 8G · CARBS: 27G · FIBER: 15G · SUGARS: 9G · ADDED SUGARS: 0G · PROTEIN: 27G

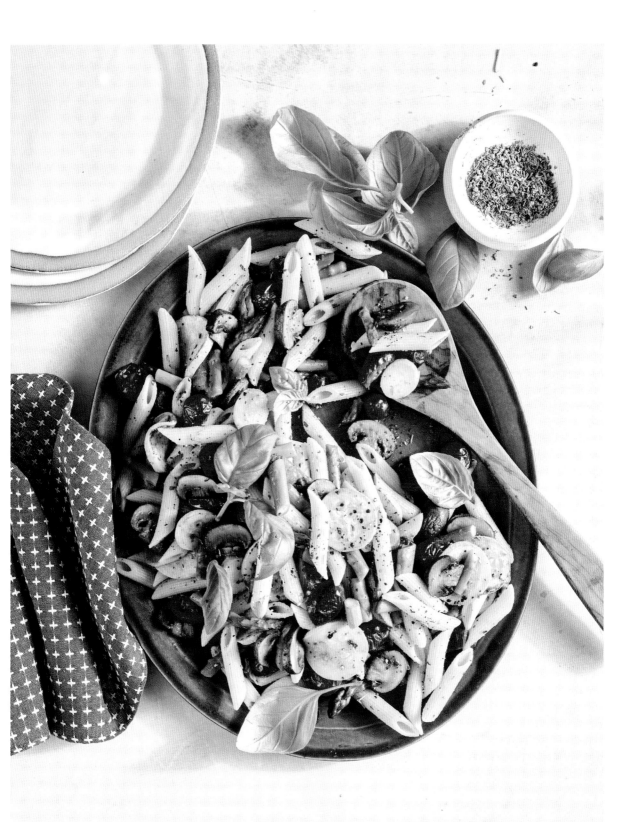

Spiced Tahini Cauliflower and Chickpeas

PREP TIME	COOK TIME	SERVES
10 MINUTES	35 MINUTES	4

Ingredients

1 teaspoon salt

1 head cauliflower, stem removed

2 ½ tablespoons extra-virgin olive oil, divided

2 tablespoons Savory Sizzle Power Spice Blend*, divided

2 tablespoons water

3 cups cooked chickpeas, drained and rinsed

2 tablespoons Golden Tahini Sauce (recipe page 297)

Cauliflower gets a deliciously golden makeover in this spiced and savory recipe. Chickpeas build a strong foundation of protein and every type of fiber that will keep you feeling satisfied. But let's not forget about our star of the show—cauliflower; a cruciferous vegetable packed with glucosinolates makes it a top-tier cancer-fighting veggie. The creamy tahini sauce is infused with Vegitude Power Spice Blend giving it a powerful anti-inflammatory and antioxidant boost. This dish is so good, you'll be "cauliflowering" all your friends to tell them about it!

Directions

1. Preheat oven to 425°F. Bring a large pot of water with 1 teaspoon of salt to a boil.

2. Add the cauliflower to the boiling water and cook for 5 minutes, just until soft on the outside but crisp on the inside, as it will continue to cook in the oven.

3. Drain and transfer the cauliflower to a parchment-lined baking dish.

4. In a small bowl, whisk together 1½ tablespoons of the olive oil, 1 tablespoon of the spice blend, and 2 tablespoons water.

Brush this mixture over the cauliflower. Bake 5 minutes.

5. Meanwhile, toss the chickpeas in the remaining 1 tablespoon of olive oil and remaining 1 tablespoon of spice blend.

6. Place chickpeas in a single layer around the cauliflower in the baking dish and bake 20 minutes, until both cauliflower and chickpeas are golden brown.

7. Transfer the cauliflower and chickpeas to a serving platter. Serve drizzled with the tahini sauce.

*Substitute spice blend with 1 tablespoon paprika, 1½ teaspoons granulated garlic, 1 teaspoon ground turmeric, ½ teaspoon ground cumin, ¼ teaspoon cayenne pepper, dash of black pepper.

CALORIES: 345 · FAT: 12G · CARBS: 40G · FIBER: 12G · SUGARS: 6G · ADDED SUGARS: 0G · PROTEIN: 15G

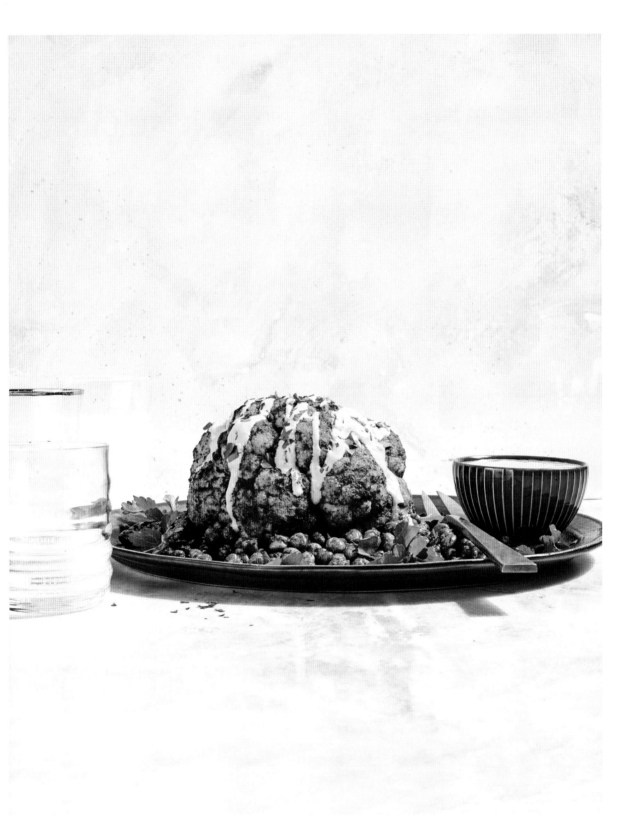

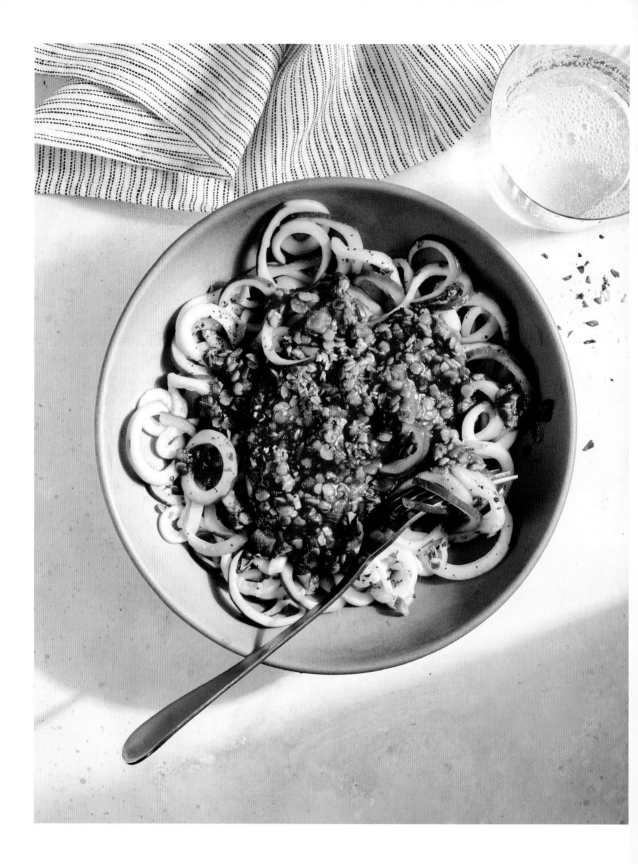

Red Lentil Bolognese

PREP TIME	COOK TIME	SERVES
10 MINUTES	35 MINUTES	4

Ingredients

1 tablespoon extra-virgin olive oil

1 yellow onion, diced

1 pound baby bella mushrooms, diced

3 cloves garlic, minced

1 cup dried red lentils, rinsed

2 tablespoons tomato paste

2 tablespoons balsamic vinegar, divided

3 cups vegetable stock

1 cup marinara sauce

3 tablespoons hemp hearts

¾ teaspoon Italian seasoning

RECOMMENDED SIDE:

1 cup cooked zucchini noodles or broccoli per serving

Lentil-tastic! This red lentil bolognese recipe will be a tasty way to nourish your body. It's not only rich, robust, and delicious but also filled with nourishing ingredients. These little filling lentils provide fiber, protein, and a whole host of essential vitamins to keep your body in tip-top shape.

Directions

1. Heat olive oil in a pot over medium heat.

2. Add the onion to the pot and sauté 3 minutes, just until the onion begins to sweat. Add mushrooms and garlic and sauté 2 additional minutes.

3. Stir in lentils, tomato paste, and 1 tablespoon of the balsamic vinegar. Stir just to help break up the tomato paste before stirring in the vegetable stock, marinara sauce, hemp hearts, and Italian seasoning.

4. Bring up to a gentle boil, reduce heat to low, and let simmer 30 minutes, or until lentils are tender.

5. Stir in the remaining tablespoon of balsamic vinegar and let simmer an additional 2 minutes.

6. Serve over 1 cup of cooked broccoli or zucchini noodles per serving.

 Sprinkle over top: crushed red pepper or nutritional yeast.

CALORIES: 335 · FAT: 9G · CARBS: 48G · FIBER: 13G · SUGARS: 13G · ADDED SUGARS: 0G · PROTEIN: 21G

Quinoa Quiches

PREP TIME	COOK TIME	SERVING SIZE	SERVES
10 MINUTES	30 MINUTES	2 QUICHES	3

Ingredients

1 cup unsweetened plant milk

⅓ cup almond flour

2 tablespoons nutritional yeast

1½ tablespoons avocado oil

1 teaspoon Vegitude Power Spice Blend*

½ teaspoon salt

1½ cups cooked quinoa

¼ cup chopped chives, scallions, or parsley

RECOMMENDED SIDE:

2 cups cooked low starch vegetables per serving

Move over omelets and muffins, there's a new hybrid in town—my Quinoa Quiches! These little poppers are soft, moist, and full of flavor—they make a great alternative to traditional veggie burgers and are a favorite among my patients. The combination of nutritional yeast and Vegitude Power enhances the yellow hue, allowing the vibrancy and power to shine through. Enjoy them on top of a salad, alongside roasted veggies, or simply as a satisfying snack. It's time to put these Quinoa Quiches into your life!

Directions

1. Preheat oven to 350°F. Line a muffin tin with 6 paper muffin cups.

2. In a mixing bowl, whisk together the plant milk, flour, nutritional yeast, avocado oil, spice blend, and salt.

3. Fold the cooked quinoa and chopped chives into the wet ingredients to create a batter. Divide the batter evenly among the 6 muffin cups.

Use a spoon to press down on the top of the batter in each cup, compressing it.

4. Bake 30 minutes. Let cool at least 5 minutes before serving warm, or cover and refrigerate to serve chilled.

5. Serve alongside 2 cups of cooked low starch vegetables of choice per serving.

Mix in before baking: 1 teaspoon prebiotic fiber powder.

*Substitute spice blend with ¼ teaspoon granulated garlic, ¼ teaspoon granulated onion, ¼ teaspoon ground turmeric, ⅛ teaspoon dried parsley, pinch of black pepper.

CALORIES: 355 · FAT: 16G · CARBS: 42G · FIBER: 10G · SUGARS: 4G · ADDED SUGARS: 0G · PROTEIN: 17G

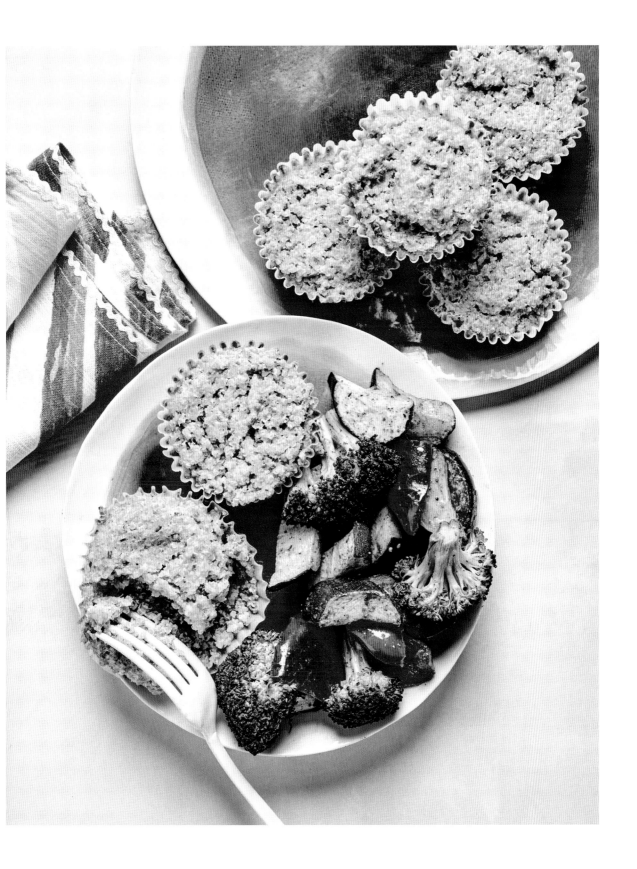

Tomato, White Bean, and Pasta Soup

PREP TIME	COOK TIME	SERVES
15 MINUTES	15 MINUTES	6

Ingredients

6 ounces edamame or chickpea pasta

1 tablespoon extra-virgin olive oil

1 yellow onion, diced

2 carrots, peeled and chopped

1 tablespoon minced garlic

3 cups cooked cannellini white beans, drained and rinsed

1½ cups diced tomatoes, with liquid

1½ teaspoons dried basil

1 teaspoon Vegitude Power Spice Blend*

8 cups vegetable stock, divided

4 cups baby spinach, chopped

"Soup"ercharge your taste buds with this comforting and filling Tomato, White Bean, and Pasta Soup! The creamy broth, made with blended white beans and carrots, is the perfect complement to protein-packed pasta and fresh baby spinach, which adds a pop of color and nutrition. Fun fact: spinach is a great source of glutathione, one of the most powerful antioxidants in the body that may help fight cancer, heart disease, and dementia. Go ahead and enjoy this soup with gusto—you'll thank me later!

Directions

1. Boil pasta according to the package directions and drain.

2. Meanwhile, heat olive oil in a pot over medium heat. Add the onion, carrots, and garlic and sauté 5 minutes, just until the onion has softened.

3. Stir in beans, tomatoes, basil, and spice blend and continue cooking for 5 minutes.

4. Transfer half of the bean, vegetable, and tomato mixture to a blender. Add half of the vegetable stock and blend until smooth. Return blended mixture to the pot with the unblended vegetables and stir in the remaining vegetable stock.

5. Stir in cooked pasta and bring up to a simmer. Let cook for 3 minutes. Remove from heat and stir in chopped spinach to let the residual heat wilt it.

Add to your bowl: chopped parsley.

*Substitute spice blend with ¼ teaspoon granulated garlic, ¼ teaspoon granulated onion, ¼ teaspoon ground turmeric, ⅛ teaspoon dried parsley, pinch of black pepper.

CALORIES: 265 · FAT: 4G · CARBS: 41G · FIBER: 17G · SUGARS: 6G · ADDED SUGARS: 0G · PROTEIN: 22G

"Chickpea of the Sea" Salad

PREP TIME
15 MINUTES

SERVES
4

Ingredients

3 cups cooked chickpeas, drained and rinsed

2 stalks celery, diced

½ cup diced red onion

1 dill pickle, diced

Juice of 1 lemon

1 large avocado, mashed, or **3 tablespoons** tahini sauce

1 teaspoon Vegitude Power Spice Blend*

3 tablespoons nutritional yeast

RECOMMENDED SIDE:

2 cups of lettuce leaves, mixed greens, kale, or baby spinach per serving

(V) (GF)

Let's take a dive into my fiber-fueled, Chickpea of the Sea Salad! With lightly mashed chickpeas taking center stage, it's a plant-based delight that's both creamy and satisfying. This salad is perfect as a main protein over a bed of greens or even as a snack with some cut-up veggies. For an added boost of special marine prebiotic fiber, roll it up with some nori and lettuce for a fun, nutrient-packed sushi-esque hand roll!

Directions

1. Place chickpeas in a mixing bowl and use a heavy fork to mash and break them up into smaller pieces.

2. Add all remaining ingredients to the chickpeas and fold together until all is combined. Season with salt and pepper to taste.

3. Cover and refrigerate until ready to serve.

4. Serve in lettuce wraps or over 2 cups of mixed greens, kale, or baby spinach per serving.

Roll it up: in a sheet of nori.

*Substitute spice blend with ¼ teaspoon granulated garlic, ¼ teaspoon granulated onion, ¼ teaspoon ground turmeric, ⅛ teaspoon dried parsley, pinch of black pepper.

CALORIES: 355 · FAT: 14G · CARBS: 46G · FIBER: 15G · SUGARS: 3G · ADDED SUGARS: 0G · PROTEIN: 18G

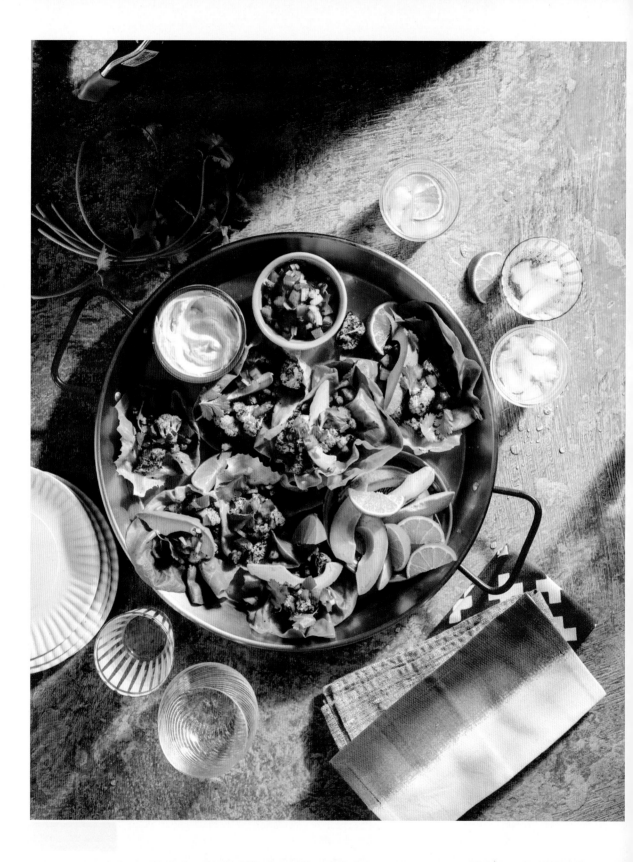

Cauliflower Chickpea Lettuce Cup Tacos

PREP TIME	COOK TIME	SERVES
15 MINUTES	30 MINUTES	2

Ingredients

1 medium cauliflower, cut into florets

1½ cups cooked chickpeas, drained and rinsed

1 tablespoon avocado oil

1 tablespoon Tex Mex Power Spice Blend*

Juice of 1 small lime

8 large lettuce leaves

4 tablespoons salsa

2 tablespoons nutritional yeast

¼ cup plant-based sour cream or plant-based plain yogurt, optional

(V) (GF)

Your Taco Tuesdays just got a major upgrade in flavor, function, and ease! These Cauliflower Chickpea Lettuce Cup Tacos are the perfect solution when you're in need of something quick after a long day and are a great alternative to ordering takeout. Cauliflower contains a compound called indole-3-carbinol that makes this dish a cancer-fighting cruciferous superhero. Paired with fiber and protein-fueled chickpeas and my Tex Mex Spice Blend, that brings a South-of-the-Border, antioxidant-rich flair and you easily have a meal that will go to great lengths to protect your health.

Directions

1. Preheat the oven to 400°F. Line a sheet pan with parchment paper.

2. In a mixing bowl, toss cauliflower florets and chickpeas in the avocado oil, spice blend, and lime juice. Transfer to the prepared sheet pan.

3. Bake 30 minutes, using a spatula to flip the cauliflower and chickpeas halfway through.

4. Assemble the lettuce cup tacos by spooning the cauliflower and chickpea filling into large lettuce leaves. Top with salsa, nutritional yeast, and a dollop of plant-based sour cream or yogurt, if desired, before serving.

Top with: micro broccoli.

---

*Substitute spice blend with 1 teaspoon chili powder, ½ teaspoon paprika, ½ teaspoon ground cumin, ¼ teaspoon granulated onion, ¼ teaspoon granulated garlic, ¼ teaspoon dried oregano, ⅛ teaspoon crushed red pepper flakes, and ⅛ teaspoon black pepper, pinch of Ceylon cinnamon and pinch of ground cloves.

CALORIES: 355 · FAT: 9G · CARBS: 48G · FIBER: 16G · SUGARS: 8G · ADDED SUGARS: 0G · PROTEIN: 18G

Plant-Based Lasagna

PREP TIME	COOK TIME	SERVES
30 MINUTES	60 MINUTES	6

Ingredients

1 tablespoon extra-virgin olive oil

1 yellow onion, sliced

2 zucchini, chopped

8 ounces mushrooms, sliced

2 teaspoons dried oregano

Salt and pepper, to taste

14–16 ounces (1 package) firm tofu, drained and patted dry

1 teaspoon Vegitude Power Spice Blend*

1 tablespoon lemon juice

2 tablespoons nutritional yeast

½ cup fresh basil, chopped

3½ cups marinara sauce

8 ounces lentil-based lasagna noodles (oven ready)

4 cups frozen spinach, thawed and drained

Rejoice! This plant-based lasagna packs a flavorful punch. This recipe is a favorite among my patients. Sure, it may take a bit of extra effort compared to your average recipe, but it's worth it. The secret? A dairy-free ricotta made from protein-packed tofu, antioxidant-packed Italian herbs, and nutritional yeast for that "cheesy" flavor. Loaded with nutrient-rich vegetables, this lasagna makes for a tasty plant-based option and incredible leftovers all week long.

Directions

1. Preheat oven to 400°F. Heat olive oil in a large skillet over medium heat.

2. Add the onion to the skillet and sauté 5 minutes. Stir in zucchini, mushrooms, and oregano and sauté an additional 5 minutes, just until mushrooms begin to cook down. Drain any excess liquid. Lightly season with salt and pepper to taste.

3. In a separate bowl, squeeze tofu until all liquid is released and has the consistency of ricotta cheese. Add spice blend, lemon juice, nutritional yeast, and basil until fully combined.

4. Assemble the lasagna in a 13 x 9-inch casserole dish. Start by spreading 1 cup of the marinara sauce at the bottom of the dish and arrange a layer of the noodles over the sauce. Top the noodles with ⅓ of the tofu ricotta and then ½ of the thawed spinach.

5. Make a second layer of 1 cup sauce, noodles, ⅓ tofu ricotta, and the remaining spinach.

6. Make a third layer of 1 cup sauce, noodles, and the remaining tofu ricotta. Then top the lasagna with all of the cooked onion, zucchini, and mushroom mixture. Top the vegetables with the remaining ½ cup of marinara sauce.

7. Cover with parchment paper followed by aluminum foil and bake 30 minutes. Remove foil and bake uncovered for an additional 20 minutes. Let rest 10 minutes before serving.

*Substitute spice blend with ¼ teaspoon granulated garlic, ¼ teaspoon granulated onion, ¼ teaspoon ground turmeric, ⅛ teaspoon dried parsley, pinch of black pepper.

CALORIES: 335 · FAT: 8G · CARBS: 43G · FIBER: 10G · SUGARS: 7G · ADDED SUGARS: 0G · PROTEIN: 27G

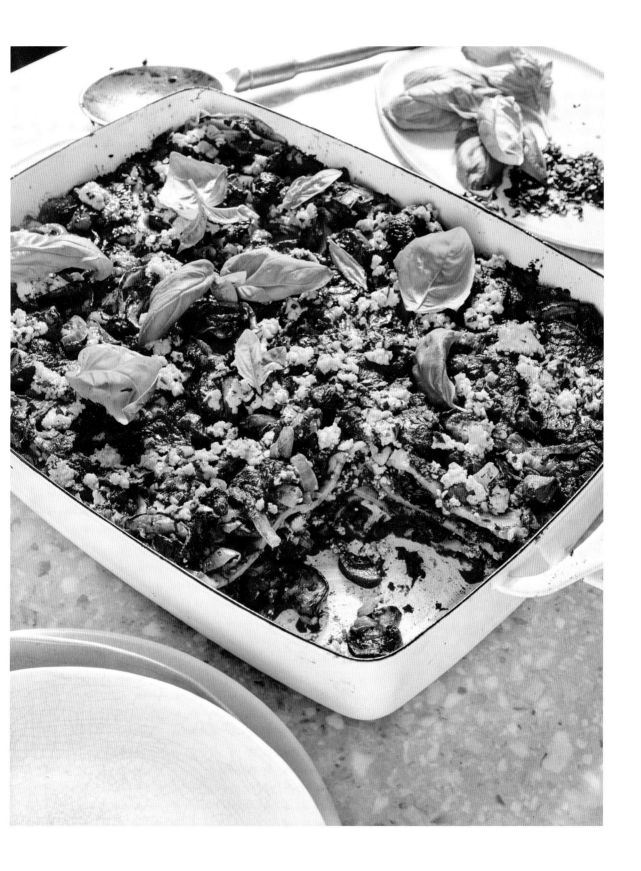

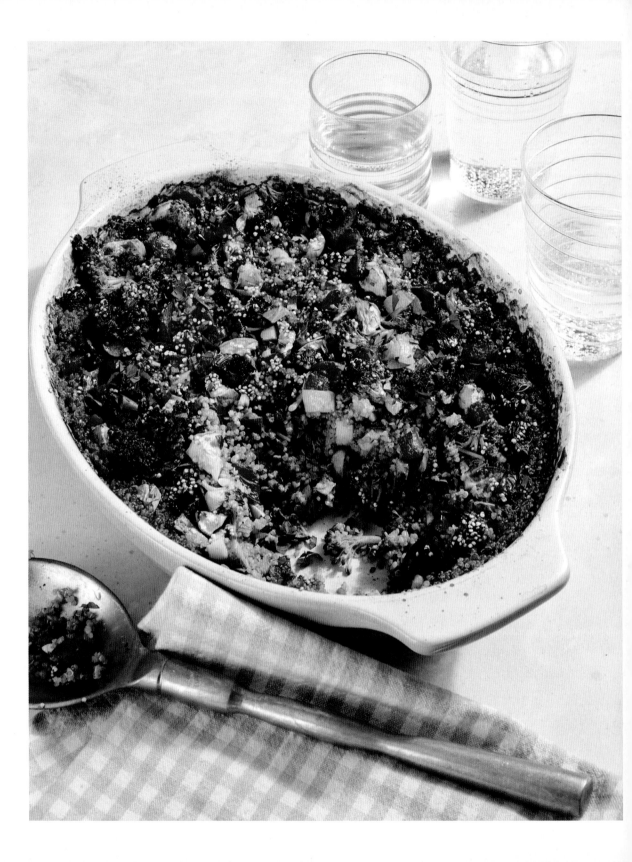

Veggie Quinoa Casserole

PREP TIME	COOK TIME	SERVES
10 MINUTES	60 MINUTES	4

Ingredients

Olive oil spray

6 cups chopped vegetables (any combination of broccoli, zucchini, yellow squash, mushrooms, tomatoes, or shredded carrots)

2 cups vegetable stock

1 cup uncooked quinoa

¼ cup hemp hearts or chopped walnuts

3 tablespoons nutritional yeast

2 teaspoons Everything Savory Spice Blend*

½ teaspoon salt

This dish is tasty and super quick to make; I love making it on Sunday to have easy to pack or reheat leftovers. The best part is, you can effortlessly change up the veggies depending on what you have on hand or what's in season. It's not only delicious, but packed with protein-rich quinoa and a variety of nutrient-dense low starch vegetables. It's the perfect meal to fuel your body and keep you feeling satisfied. Don't settle for a boring dinner when you can have these convenient yummy squares.

Directions

1. Preheat the oven to 350°F. Lightly spray an 8 x 12-inch baking dish with olive oil spray.

2. Add all ingredients to the prepared baking dish and stir to mix the spice blend into the stock. Ensure the vegetables and quinoa are evenly dispersed.

3. Bake 60 minutes, until the center is firm. Let cool for at least 5 minutes before slicing to serve. Store covered and refrigerated.

Top with: chopped cilantro.

*Substitute spice blend with 1 teaspoon paprika, ½ teaspoon granulated garlic, ¼ teaspoon ground turmeric, ¼ teaspoon ground cumin, dash of black pepper, dash of cayenne pepper.

CALORIES: 339 · FAT: 11G · CARBS: 42G · FIBER: 7G · SUGARS: 3G · ADDED SUGARS: 0G · PROTEIN: 18G

Curry Lentil and Chickpea Stew

PREP TIME	COOK TIME	SERVES
10 MINUTES	40 MINUTES	8

Ingredients

1 tablespoon extra-virgin olive oil

1 yellow onion, chopped

4 cloves garlic, chopped

1½ tablespoons grated fresh ginger

1½ tablespoons curry powder

1 teaspoon ground cumin

6 cups vegetable stock

2 cups dry red lentils

1½ cups cooked chickpeas, drained and rinsed

1 cup diced tomatoes, fresh or packaged

RECOMMENDED SIDE:

1½ cups cauliflower rice or **2 cups** roasted low starch vegetables per serving

Ready for a protein and fiber powerhouse? My program participants can't get enough of this Curry Lentil and Chickpea Stew! And the best part? It's quick and easy to make! Just pair it with some low starch veggies like riced cauliflower or riced broccoli and you've got a complete meal that will leave you satisfied and energized. It's curry-licious!

Directions

1. Heat olive oil in a pot over medium heat. Add the onion and sauté 3 minutes.

2. Stir in garlic, ginger, curry powder, and cumin and sauté an additional 2 minutes.

3. Stir in vegetable stock, lentils, chickpeas, and tomatoes and bring up to a simmer. Cover, reduce heat to low, and let simmer 30 minutes, or until lentils are tender.

4. Serve alongside 1½ cups of cauliflower rice or 2 cups roasted low starch vegetables of choice per serving.

Top with: grated ginger.

CALORIES: 255 · FAT: 5G · CARBS: 46G · FIBER: 16G · SUGARS: 5G · ADDED SUGARS: 0G · PROTEIN: 17G

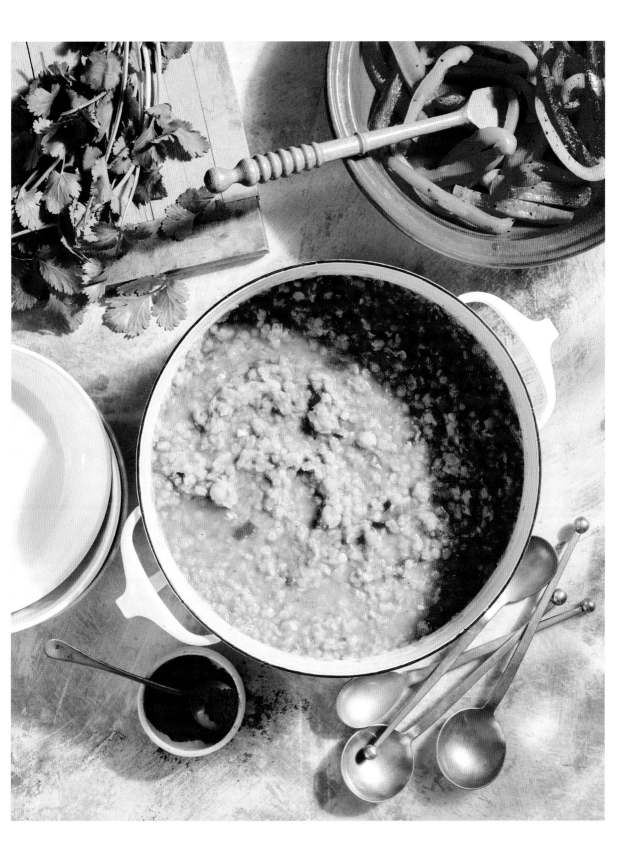

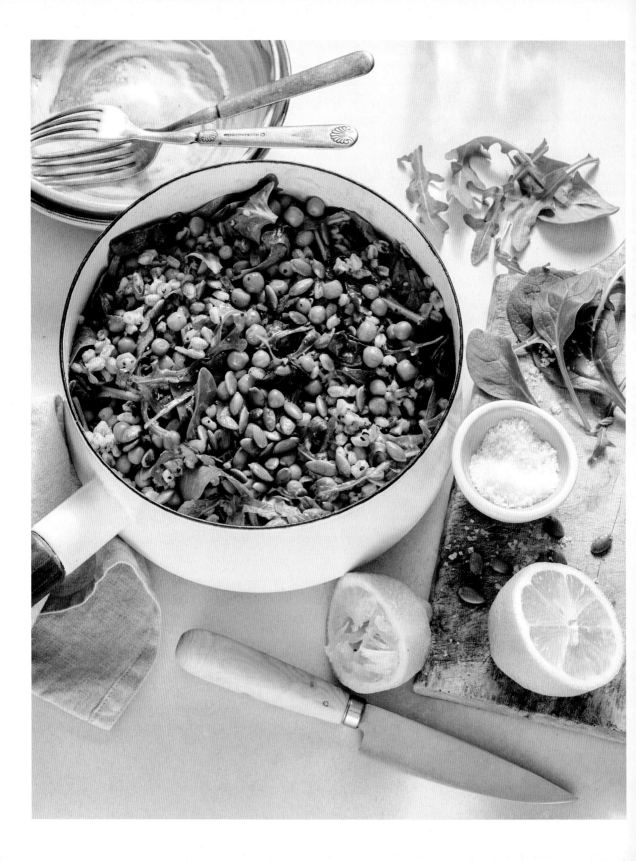

Green Goodness Farro Bowls

PREP TIME	COOK TIME	SERVES
5 MINUTES	25 MINUTES	4

Ingredients

1 tablespoon extra-virgin olive oil

1 cup uncooked pearled farro, rinsed

3 cups vegetable stock

½ teaspoon Italian seasoning

½ teaspoon onion powder

8 cups fresh arugula or spinach

2 ½ cups frozen peas

Juice of ½ lemon

½ cup pepitas

The ultimate green team—packed with all the nutritious goodness you need to power through your day! My Green Goodness Farro Bowls are just the ticket to shake up your plant-based meal routine. The nutty, toothsome intact whole grain is semi-rich in protein, adds a unique texture and flavor, and is a great option for those looking to incorporate more plant-based meals but are feeling bored with the usual suspects like beans and tofu. Unlike rice, farro is hard to overcook. Come back here when you're craving some variety!

Directions

1. Heat olive oil in a pot over medium-high heat. Add farro and sauté 1 minute.

2. Stir in vegetable stock, Italian seasoning, and onion powder.

3. Bring up to a simmer, cover, and reduce heat to low. Let simmer 20–30 minutes.

4. Stir in arugula, frozen peas, and lemon juice and sauté until arugula has wilted and peas are heated through, 4–5 minutes.

5. Top with pepitas.

 Top with: chopped watercress.

CALORIES: 380 · FAT: 11G · CARBS: 54G · FIBER: 12G · SUGARS: 7G · ADDED SUGARS: 0G · PROTEIN: 18G

Easiest Black Bean Chili

PREP TIME	COOK TIME	SERVES
10 MINUTES	15 MINUTES	2

Ingredients

1 tablespoon avocado or extra-virgin olive oil

1 yellow onion, chopped

2 bell peppers, chopped

1 tablespoon Tex Mex Power Spice Blend*

1½ cups cooked black beans, drained and rinsed

¾ cup tomato sauce

3 tablespoons hemp hearts

Salt and pepper, to taste

2 tablespoons plant-based sour cream, optional

RECOMMENDED SIDE:

1 cup cooked low starch vegetables per serving

A chili that's so easy, it's practically on autopilot. This recipe is an all-star recipe among my patients and was so popular it was featured on *Good Morning America*! The Tex Mex Spice Blend adds an antioxidant-rich flavor fiesta to any dish. Not only that, but all the spices in this dish have an additive effect that may help decrease cholesterol. Come see what all the hype is about!

Directions

1. Heat avocado oil in a saucepan over medium-high heat.

2. Add onion to the pot and sauté 3 minutes. Stir in bell peppers and sauté 3 minutes.

3. Stir in spice blend and sauté 1 minute to toast the spices.

4. Stir in black beans, tomato sauce, and hemp hearts. Bring up to a simmer, reduce heat to low, and let simmer 8 minutes, or until peppers are tender.

5. Season with salt and pepper to taste before serving. Top with a dollop of plant-based sour cream, if desired.

Top with: chopped cilantro and/or crushed red pepper flakes.

*Substitute spice blend with 1 teaspoon chili powder, ½ teaspoon paprika, ½ teaspoon ground cumin, ¼ teaspoon granulated onion, ¼ teaspoon granulated garlic, ¼ teaspoon dried oregano, ⅛ teaspoon crushed red pepper flakes, and ⅛ teaspoon black pepper, pinch of Ceylon cinnamon and pinch of ground cloves.

CALORIES: 408 · FAT: 16G · CARBS: 47G · FIBER: 15G · SUGARS: 8G · ADDED SUGARS: 0G · PROTEIN: 20G

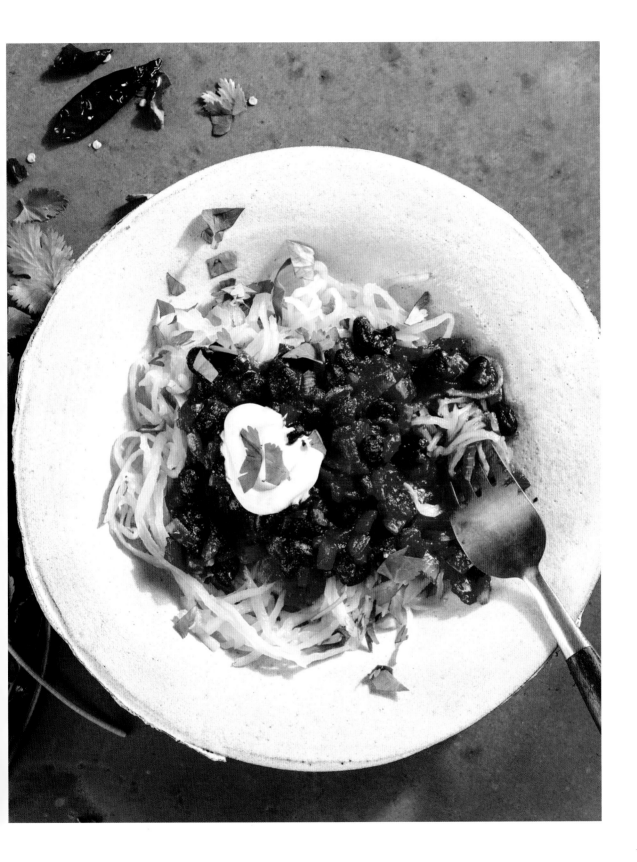

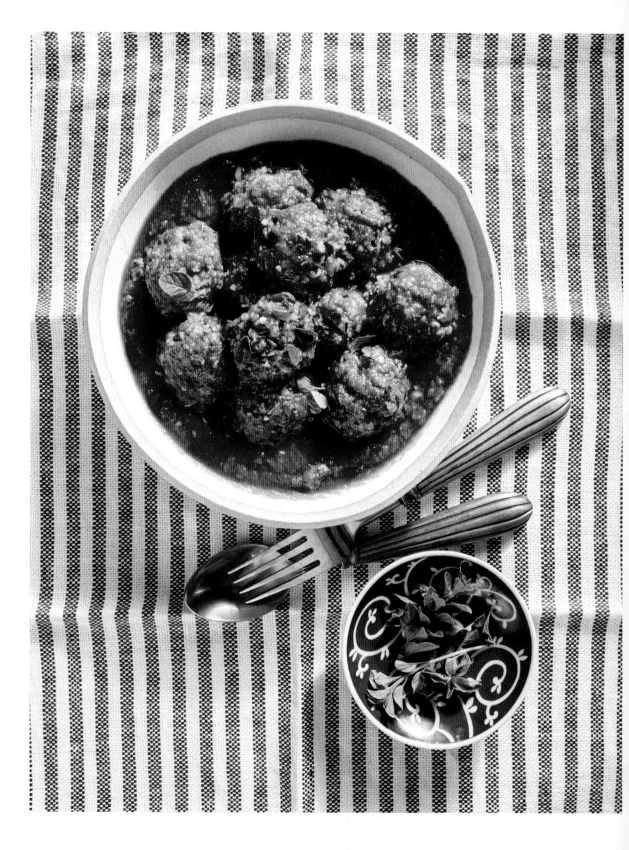

Simple Lentil Meatballs

PREP TIME	COOK TIME	SERVES
15 MINUTES	30 MINUTES	2

Ingredients

1½ cups cooked lentils

½ cup rolled oats (sprouted preferred)

1 tablespoon lemon juice

1 teaspoon Vegitude Power Spice Blend*

1 teaspoon Italian seasoning

½ teaspoon salt

1 cup shredded zucchini

1 cup marinara sauce

RECOMMENDED SIDE:

1 cup cooked zucchini noodles or low starch vegetables per serving

A meatball alternative that won't have you rolling around in the kitchen for hours. Often when I tell people about this, they think it's a lot of work; this recipe is such a breeze to whip up it has even some of my busiest patients astonished. Feel free to purchase pre-steamed lentils, which are usually sold in the refrigerated case in the grocer's produce section. You'll feel amazed nourishing your body and giving confidence to your empowered self!

Directions

1. Preheat oven to 375°F. Line a sheet pan with parchment paper.

2. Place lentils, oats, lemon juice, spice blend, Italian seasoning, and salt in a food processor and pulse 10 seconds, or until the mixture will hold together when pressed between your fingers.

3. Transfer the lentil mixture to a mixing bowl and fold in zucchini.

4. Using clean hands, form the lentil and zucchini mixture into 12 meatballs and transfer to the prepared sheet pan.

5. Bake 25 minutes, until golden brown.

6. Heat marinara sauce in a saucepan over medium heat. Add the baked meatballs and bring up to a simmer. Cover, reduce heat to low, and let simmer 5 minutes before serving.

7. Serve alongside 1 cup of cooked zucchini noodles or low starch vegetables of choice per serving.

 Top with: 1 tablespoon nutritional yeast.

*Substitute spice blend with ¼ teaspoon granulated garlic, ¼ teaspoon granulated onion, ¼ teaspoon ground turmeric, ⅛ teaspoon dried parsley, pinch of black pepper.

CALORIES: 333 · FAT: 2G · CARBS: 49G · FIBER: 16G · SUGARS: 7G · ADDED SUGARS: 0G · PROTEIN: 20G

Warm Caesar Salad

PREP TIME	COOK TIME	SERVES
15 MINUTES	25 MINUTES	4

Ingredients

14–16 ounces (1 package) extra-firm tofu, cut into 1-inch cubes

1 tablespoon extra-virgin olive oil, divided

1 pound Brussels sprouts, quartered

1 teaspoon Everything Savory Spice Blend*

¼ teaspoon salt

8 cups chopped romaine lettuce

1 tomato, diced

¼ cup sliced almonds, raw or toasted

½ cup (4 servings) Plant-Based Caesar Dressing (recipe page 302)

This Warm Caesar Salad with tofu and Brussels sprouts is a delightful twist on the classic dish. The tofu adds a rich source of protective phytoestrogens and is the perfect canvas for the Everything Savory Spice Blend, which cranks up the antioxidant and anti-inflammatory properties to another level. The warm tofu and Brussels sprouts blend perfectly with the Caesar dressing, creating a deliciously satisfying meal. If you're looking for a new way to incorporate tofu, this recipe is a must-try!

Directions

1. Preheat oven to 400°F. Line a sheet pan with parchment paper.

2. Place tofu on the prepared sheet pan and brush with ½ of the olive oil.

3. Toss the Brussels sprouts in the remaining ½ tablespoon of olive oil and arrange around the tofu. Season all with the spice blend and salt.

4. Bake 20–25 minutes, flipping all halfway through, until tofu is beginning to brown and sprouts are crisp.

5. Arrange the salads by splitting the lettuce among 4 serving bowls. Top each with an equal amount of the tofu and Brussels sprouts.

6. Sprinkle each salad with diced tomato and sliced almonds. Drizzle with dressing before serving.

 Top with: broccoli sprouts.

*Substitute spice blend with ½ teaspoon paprika, ¼ teaspoon granulated garlic, ⅛ teaspoon ground turmeric, ⅛ teaspoon ground cumin, dash of black pepper, dash of cayenne pepper.

CALORIES: 280 · FAT: 14G · CARBS: 20 G · FIBER: 10G · SUGARS: 6G · ADDED SUGARS: 0G · PROTEIN: 23G

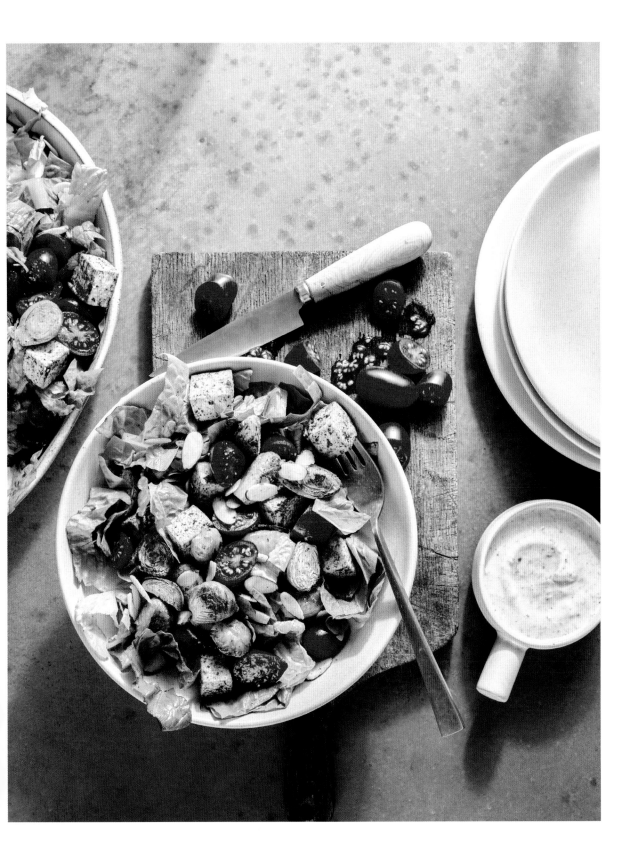

Spicy Asian Noodles

PREP TIME
2 MINUTES

SERVES
2

Ingredients

12 ounces kelp noodles

3 cups shredded purple cabbage

1 cup grated carrots

2 cups shelled edamame

1 tablespoon rice wine vinegar

1 tablespoon baking soda

¼ cup (2 servings) Spicy Nut Sauce (recipe page 299)

2 scallions, sliced

1 teaspoon toasted sesame seeds

Inspired by some LA poke spots, I often get excited to share this recipe when my patients crave a spicy nut sauce. This recipe features cancer-protective edamame and kelp noodles—a gut-friendly low starch marine vegetable that contains prebiotic fibers and calcium and is oh-so satisfying. These noodles are so tasty, you'll be "shore" to want seconds!

Directions

1. Place dry kelp noodles, shredded cabbage, grated carrots, and edamame in a large mixing bowl.

2. Drizzle with vinegar, sprinkle with baking soda, and then cover all with hot tap water.

3. Let sit 10 minutes to soften the noodles. Meanwhile, prepare the spicy nut sauce.

4. Drain and rinse the noodles and vegetables under cold water.

5. Fold the spicy nut sauce into the noodles and vegetables. For best flavor and temperature, cover and refrigerate 15–30 minutes.

6. Serve topped with sliced scallions and toasted sesame seeds.

Top with: nori shreds.

CALORIES: 360 · FAT: 13G · CARBS: 37G · FIBER: 14G · SUGARS: 15G · ADDED SUGARS: 1G · PROTEIN: 24G

Buffalo Tempeh with Slaw

PREP TIME	COOK TIME	SERVES
15 MINUTES	25 MINUTES	2

Ingredients

6 ounces tempeh, sliced

2 tablespoons hot sauce

1 tablespoon extra-virgin olive oil, divided

6 stalks celery, cut into 2-inch lengths

1 teaspoon Vegitude Power Spice Blend*

1 batch (2 servings) Barbecue Braised Slaw (recipe page 262)

Introducing the punk rock of plant-based meals—my Buffalo Tempeh with Slaw. If you're not familiar with tempeh, don't be scared—think of it as an upgraded version of tofu that's been fermented. Once you try it, you'll wonder why you ever feared it! The slaw adds a crunchy twist to this dish, and the buffalo sauce is so delicious, you'll want to put it on everything. Trust us, this tempeh dish will have you saying "oh my tempeh" with every bite!

Directions

1. Preheat oven to 400°F. Line a sheet pan with parchment paper.

2. In a mixing bowl, toss tempeh in hot sauce and ½ tablespoon of the olive oil. Transfer to the prepared sheet pan.

3. Toss celery with the spice blend, and the remaining ½ tablespoon of olive oil. Transfer to the prepared sheet pan.

4. Bake 20–25 minutes, flipping tempeh and celery halfway through. Cook until the hot sauce and celery begin to brown.

5. Meanwhile, prepare the braised slaw to serve alongside the cooked tempeh and celery.

 Top with: chopped parsley.

*Substitute spice blend with ¼ teaspoon granulated garlic, ¼ teaspoon granulated onion, ¼ teaspoon ground turmeric, ⅛ teaspoon dried parsley, pinch of black pepper.

CALORIES: 330 · FAT: 16G · CARBS: 27G · FIBER: 12G · SUGARS: 11G · ADDED SUGARS: 3G · PROTEIN: 21G

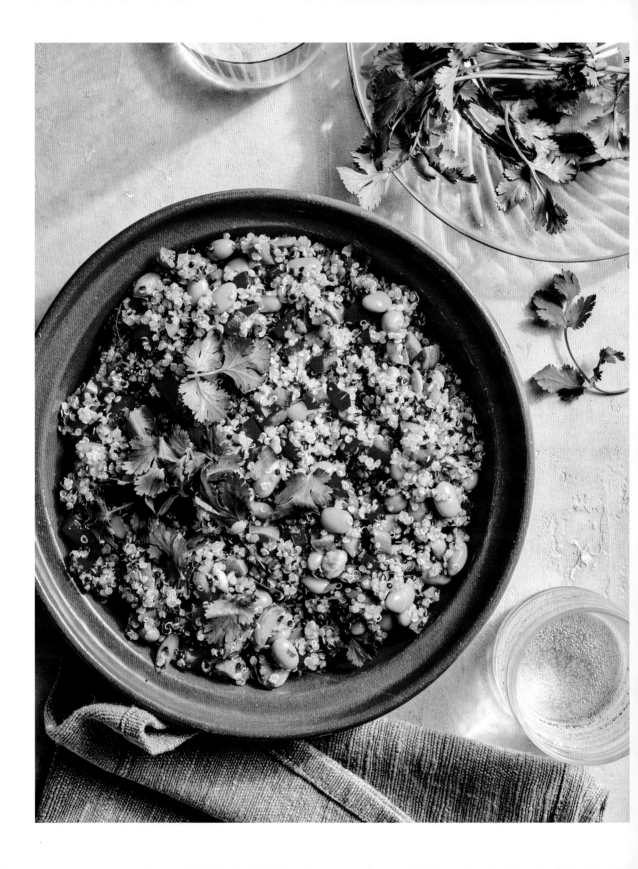

Quinoa and Edamame Salad

PREP TIME	COOK TIME	SERVES
10 MINUTES	5 MINUTES	2

Ingredients

1 cup cooked quinoa

1 cup shelled edamame

1 bell pepper, chopped

½ cup cilantro, chopped

1 scallion, sliced

2 tablespoons (2 servings) Sesame Dressing (recipe page 304)

RECOMMENDED SIDE:

2 cups chopped cucumber, kale, cabbage, broccoli, or carrots

(V) (GF)

From potlucks to packed lunches, my Quinoa and Edamame Salad is a crowd-pleaser and loved by my patients across the globe! This recipe was once tucked in the back of my recipe library before resurfacing and has now become a fan favorite. It's no wonder—the combination of quinoa and edamame provides a perfect balance of plant-based protein and delicious flavor.

Directions

1. In a mixing bowl, fold together all ingredients.

2. For the best flavor, cover and refrigerate at least 15 minutes before serving.

3. Serve alongside 2 cups of cooked low starch vegetables of choice per serving.

Top with : 1 teaspoon sesame seeds.

CALORIES: 400 · FAT: 12G · CARBS: 44G · FIBER: 13G · SUGARS: 10G · ADDED SUGARS: 2G · PROTEIN: 20G

Quinoa Spanish "Rice"

PREP TIME	COOK TIME	SERVES
10 MINUTES	45 MINUTES	6

Ingredients

1½ tablespoons extra-virgin olive oil

1 onion, chopped

2 bell peppers, chopped

2 cups dry quinoa

2 teaspoons Vegitude Power Spice Blend*

4 cups vegetable stock

2 cups diced tomatoes, from package, drained

Salt, to taste

RECOMMENDED SIDE:

2 cups cooked low starch vegetables per serving

If you're looking for a hearty and comforting recipe that packs a nutritional punch, then try this flavorful twist on a traditional Spanish dish. I wasn't planning on including this recipe in my book (my editor said we are maxed out!), but since my daughter Keira asks me to make it at least once a week and my niece Karin begs me to make it every time we have a family dinner, I figured, I'll make it happen! It's easy to make and super delish! Pair with some roasted multicolored peppers or any low starch veg for an instant power meal.

Directions

1. Heat olive oil in a pot over medium heat. Add the onion and bell pepper and sauté 5 minutes.

2. Stir in quinoa and spice blend and sauté 3 minutes to lightly toast the quinoa.

3. Stir in vegetable stock, tomatoes, and bring up to a simmer. Cover, reduce heat to low, and let simmer 30–35 minutes.

4. Remove from heat, uncover, and let rest 5 minutes, until all liquid has been absorbed. Season with salt to taste and fluff with a fork before serving.

5. Serve alongside 2 cups of cooked low starch vegetables of choice per serving.

Top with: ¼ cup chopped fresh cilantro and 1 tablespoon nutritional yeast.

*Substitute spice blend with ½ teaspoon granulated garlic, ½ teaspoon granulated onion, teaspoon ground turmeric, ¼ teaspoon dried parsley, pinch of black pepper.

CALORIES: 328 · FAT: 8G · CARBS: 52G · FIBER: 9G · SUGARS: 8G · ADDED SUGARS: 0G · PROTEIN: 15G

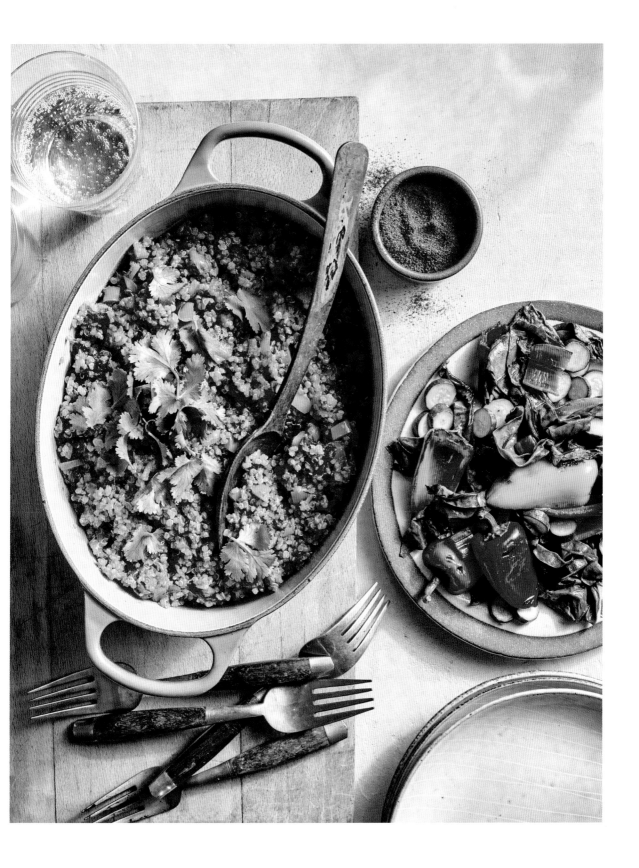

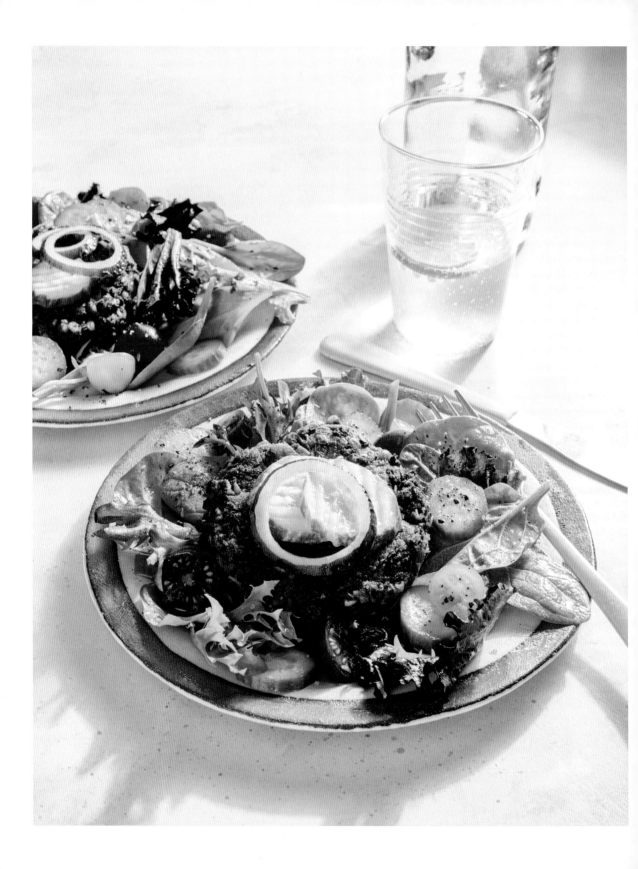

Black Bean Burgers

PREP TIME	COOK TIME	SERVING SIZE	SERVES
20 MINUTES	15 MINUTES	1 BURGER	4

Ingredients

1 tablespoon extra-virgin olive oil

1 yellow onion, diced

2 carrots, peeled and shredded

3 cloves garlic, minced

1 teaspoon Everything Savory Power Spice Blend*

3 cups cooked black beans, drained and rinsed

½ cup rolled oats (sprouted preferred)

2 tablespoons coconut aminos or tamari

Olive oil spray

RECOMMENDED SIDE:

2 cups mixed greens or cooked low starch vegetables per serving

Black Bean Burgers are the MVP of meatless meals. This tasteful twist on a classic store-bought veggie burger is overflowing with cancer-protective ingredients and surprisingly simple to prep. They're a great foundation for a "burger bowl" or wrapped in lettuce with additional vegetables for a complete meal. I love fixings like probiotic-rich kraut, pickles, or even a smear of hummus on top. The protein and fiber from the black beans will have you fueled up and ready to tackle the day. It's always fun when a recipe that seems like a ton of work is actually easy to make, delicious, and great for meals all week long.

Directions

1. Heat olive oil in a skillet over medium heat. Add the onion and sauté 3 minutes.

2. Stir in carrots, garlic, and spice blend and sauté 5 minutes, or until carrots are tender.

3. In a mixing bowl, use a potato masher or heavy fork to mash the cooked black beans. Add the oats, coconut aminos (or tamari if using), and cooked vegetables from the skillet and fold together to form a burger mixture.

4. Form the burger mixture into 4 patties and place on plates lined with parchment paper to prevent sticking. Place in freezer for 20 minutes to set.

5. To cook the patties: Spray a skillet with olive oil spray and place over medium heat. Add burger patties and cook for 4–5 minutes on each side.

6. Serve over mixed greens or alongside 2 cups of cooked low starch vegetables of choice per serving.

*Substitute spice blend with ½ teaspoon paprika, ¼ teaspoon granulated garlic, ⅛ teaspoon ground turmeric, ⅛ teaspoon ground cumin, pinch of black pepper, pinch of cayenne pepper.

CALORIES: 315 · FAT: 5G · CARBS: 39G · FIBER: 10G · SUGARS: 5G · ADDED SUGARS: 0G · PROTEIN: 15G

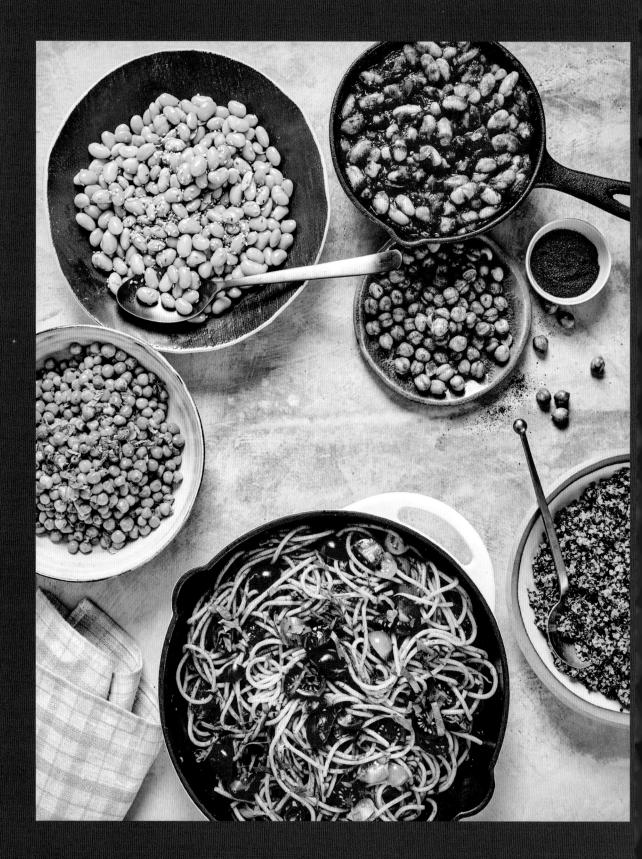

Mix & Match Meals

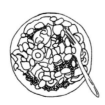

The Beller Method™ Easy Meal Combos

Sometimes you want to cook off the cuff—in those cases, it's helpful to have some simple yet flavorful recipes to mix and match. Here are some of my go-to premium protein and low starch veg recipes that you can incorporate into your regular routine. Pick a protein and pair with some of our veg recipes (the fat is included in the cooking method) to make your own combination meal using the Power of 3. As a timesaver, I often whip up a batch of protein (lentils or zesty edamame, for example) to keep on hand for the week and serve with any veg recipe.

RACHEL'S 5 FAVORITE DINNER COMBOS:

- Miso Glazed Tempeh with Soy Ginger Broccolini
- Everyday Immune-Support Quinoa with Simple Roasted Vegetables
- Lemon Mint Peas with Fried Cauliflower Rice
- Protein Pasta with Sautéed Mushrooms
- Zesty Edamame with Snow Peas and Greens

Quinoa or Tofu Taco "Meat"

PREP TIME	COOK TIME	SERVES
10 MINUTES	30 MINUTES	4

Ingredients

3 cups cooked quinoa or
14–16 ounces (1 package)
extra-firm tofu

3 tablespoons hemp hearts

1 tablespoon avocado oil

1 tablespoon Tex Mex Power
Spice Blend*

¾ cup salsa

Salt, to taste

These tasty tacos fall right in line with the concept of quick and easy, making them the perfect go-to meal for when you're trying to cut back on ordering takeout and short on time. With a side of roasted veggies, this meal is sure to leave you feeling satisfied and energized!

Directions

1. Preheat oven to 375°F. Line a sheet pan with parchment paper. If using tofu, crumble it into small pieces using two forks.

2. In a mixing bowl, fold together cooked quinoa or crumbled tofu, hemp hearts, avocado oil, and spice blend.

3. Spread the seasoned quinoa or tofu out evenly on the prepared sheet pan.

4. Bake 25–30 minutes, until quinoa or tofu is golden brown.

5. Transfer the quinoa or tofu back to a mixing bowl and stir in salsa before seasoning with salt to taste. Serve in place of traditional taco meat.

*Substitute spice blend with 1 teaspoon chili powder, ½ teaspoon paprika, ½ teaspoon ground cumin, ¼ teaspoon granulated onion, ¼ teaspoon granulated garlic, ¼ teaspoon dried oregano, ⅛ teaspoon crushed red pepper flakes, and ¼ teaspoon black pepper, pinch of Ceylon cinnamon and pinch of ground cloves.

TOFU CALORIES: 206 · FAT: 13G · CARBS: 5G · FIBER: 3G · SUGARS: 2G · ADDED SUGARS: 0G · PROTEIN: 15G
QUINOA CALORIES: 266 · FAT: 10G · CARBS: 32G · FIBER: 4G · SUGARS: 1G · ADDED SUGARS: 0G · PROTEIN: 10G

Miso Glazed Tempeh

PREP TIME	COOK TIME	SERVES
10 MINUTES	25 MINUTES	2

Ingredients

2 teaspoons sesame oil

2 teaspoons white miso paste

1 teaspoon honey

1 teaspoon coconut aminos or tamari

¼ teaspoon ground ginger

6 ounces tempeh, cut into triangles or cube

RECOMMENDED TOPPING:

2 tablespoons hemp hearts

Marinated in a savory probiotic-rich miso paste, a touch of sweet honey glaze and baked to perfection, this fermented and nutrient-rich protein source is a tasty way to support your health and add some variety to your meals. Don't be tempeh-ted to skip this one!

Directions

1. Preheat oven to 400°F. Line a sheet pan with parchment paper.

2. In a mixing bowl, whisk together all ingredients except tempeh to create a marinade. Add tempeh and toss to coat. Let sit 5 minutes to marinate.

3. Transfer marinated tempeh to sheet pan and drizzle with any remaining marinade.

4. Bake 20–25 minutes, flipping halfway through, until the tempeh begins to brown.

CALORIES: 223 · FAT: 11G · CARBS: 14G · FIBER: 9G · SUGARS: 4G · ADDED SUGARS: 3G · PROTEIN: 18G

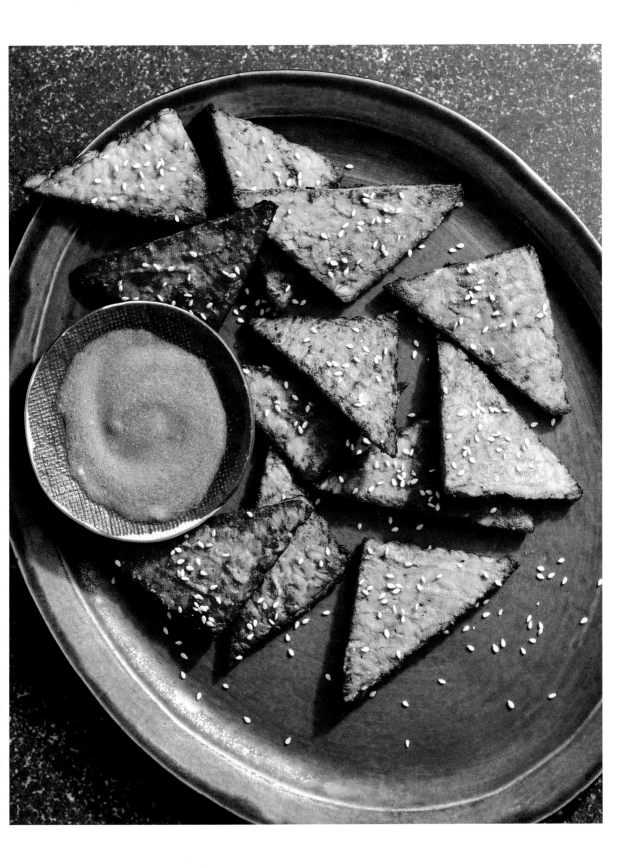

Everyday Immune-Support Quinoa

PREP TIME	COOK TIME	SERVES
5 MINUTES	20 MINUTES	4

Ingredients

1 cup dry quinoa

2 cups vegetable stock

1 teaspoon Vegitude Power Spice Blend*

RECOMMENDED TOPPING:

2 tablespoons hemp hearts

Quin-wow! Most of my patients have this one on autopilot when they need a quick and easy batch of a plant-based protein to keep them fueled. With a beautiful yellow hue coming from the Vegitude Power Spice Blend, which contains garlic, onion, turmeric, pepper, and parsley, it's a delicious way to support your immune system. A huge plus—it's quicker and easier to cook than rice, a real win-win!

Directions

1. Stir the quinoa, vegetable stock, and spice blend into a pot over medium-high heat.

2. Bring to a boil, cover, and reduce heat to low.

3. Let simmer 15–20 minutes, until all the broth has absorbed.

4. Remove from heat and let sit for 3 minutes before fluffing with a fork. Top with hemp hearts.

*Substitute spice blend with ¼ teaspoon granulated garlic, ¼ teaspoon granulated onion, ¼ teaspoon ground turmeric, ⅛ teaspoon dried parsley, pinch of black pepper.

CALORIES: 210 · FAT: 6G · CARBS: 29G · FIBER: 5G · SUGARS: 3G · ADDED SUGARS: 0G · PROTEIN: 10G

Baja Black Beans

PREP TIME	COOK TIME	SERVES
5 MINUTES	10 MINUTES	2

Ingredients

2 teaspoons avocado oil

½ onion, chopped

1 ½ cups cooked black beans, drained and rinsed

2 tablespoons salsa

1 teaspoon Tex Mex Power Spice Blend*

Salt, to taste

RECOMMENDED TOPPING:

1 tablespoon nutritional yeast

Whether you're a fan of Mexican cuisine or just looking for a simple and flavorful way to diversify your plant-based protein rotation, this recipe will bring you one step closer to incorporating black beans into your regular meal prep routine. Get ready to enjoy restaurant quality Baja Black Beans in the comfort of your own home!

Directions

1. Heat avocado oil in a skillet over medium heat.

2. Add the onion and sauté 5 minutes.

3. Stir in black beans, salsa, and spice blend and sauté 5 minutes, just until beans are heated through.

4. Season with nutritional yeast and salt to taste before serving.

*Substitute spice blend with ¼ teaspoon chili powder, ⅛ teaspoon paprika, ¼ teaspoon ground cumin, ⅛ teaspoon granulated onion, ⅛ teaspoon granulated garlic, ⅛ teaspoon dried oregano, ⅛ teaspoon crushed red pepper flakes, pinch of each: black pepper, Ceylon cinnamon, ground cloves.

CALORIES: 250 · FAT: 5G · CARBS: 27G · FIBER: 8G · SUGARS: 3.5G · ADDED SUGARS: 0G · PROTEIN: 12G

Teriyaki Tofu

PREP TIME	COOK TIME	SERVES
10 MINUTES	10 MINUTES	3

Ingredients

1 tablespoon coconut aminos or tamari

Juice of ½ orange

2 teaspoons sesame oil

1 teaspoon honey

¼ teaspoon onion powder

1 teaspoon avocado oil

14-16 ounces (1 package) extra-firm tofu, drained and sliced 1-inch thick

Tofu is the all-star of proteins, and when it comes to teriyaki, it's no exception! If you're craving teriyaki and trying to bypass a lot of added sugars—this is a nice way to make it happen.

Directions

1. In a wide bowl, whisk together coconut aminos, orange juice, sesame oil, honey, and onion powder to create a teriyaki marinade. Flip tofu in the marinade and let sit at least 10 minutes to marinate.

2. Heat avocado oil in a skillet over medium heat.

3. Add the tofu and any marinade from the bowl to the skillet in a single layer and cook for 4–5 minutes on each side, just until it begins to lightly brown.

CALORIES: 225 · FAT: 12G · CARBS: 6G · FIBER: 0G · SUGARS: 4G · ADDED SUGARS: 2G · PROTEIN: 21G

Pesto White Beans

PREP TIME	COOK TIME	SERVES
5 MINUTES	6 MINUTES	2

Ingredients

1 tablespoon extra-virgin olive oil

1½ cups cooked cannellini white beans, drained and rinsed

2 cloves garlic, minced

1 tablespoon nutritional yeast

¼ cup chopped fresh basil

Salt to taste

Creamy and satisfying cannellini beans pair perfectly with the bold and fresh flavors of homemade pesto, making for a dish that's both comforting and full of bright, zesty flavor. It's a match made in culinary heaven that you won't want to miss!

Directions

1. Heat olive oil in a skillet over medium heat.

2. Add the white beans, garlic, and nutritional yeast to the skillet and sauté 5 minutes.

3. Stir in basil and sauté 1 additional minute, just until basil wilts and beans are heated through.

4. Season with salt to taste.

CALORIES: 245 · FAT: 7G · CARBS: 29G · FIBER: 10G · SUGARS: 0G · ADDED SUGARS: 0G · PROTEIN: 15G

Lemon Mint Peas

PREP TIME	COOK TIME	SERVES
5 MINUTES	8 MINUTES	2

Ingredients

2 teaspoons extra-virgin olive oil

3 cups frozen peas

Juice and zest of ½ lemon

1 tablespoon chopped fresh mint

Salt and pepper, to taste

With the zesty combo of lemon and mint, these peas are an underrated plant protein-packed dish that comes right out of the freezer and onto the plate in no time flat. Plus, they're easy on the wallet and add a refreshing plant-based protein to any salad or cooked vegetables. It's time we give peas some well deserved PR!

Directions

1. Heat olive oil in a skillet over medium heat.

2. Add the peas, lemon juice and zest, and mint and sauté 7–8 minutes, just until peas are heated through.

3. Season with salt and pepper to taste before serving.

CALORIES: 179 · FAT: 6G · CARBS: 26G · FIBER: 9G · SUGARS: 13G · ADDED SUGARS: 0G · PROTEIN: 12G

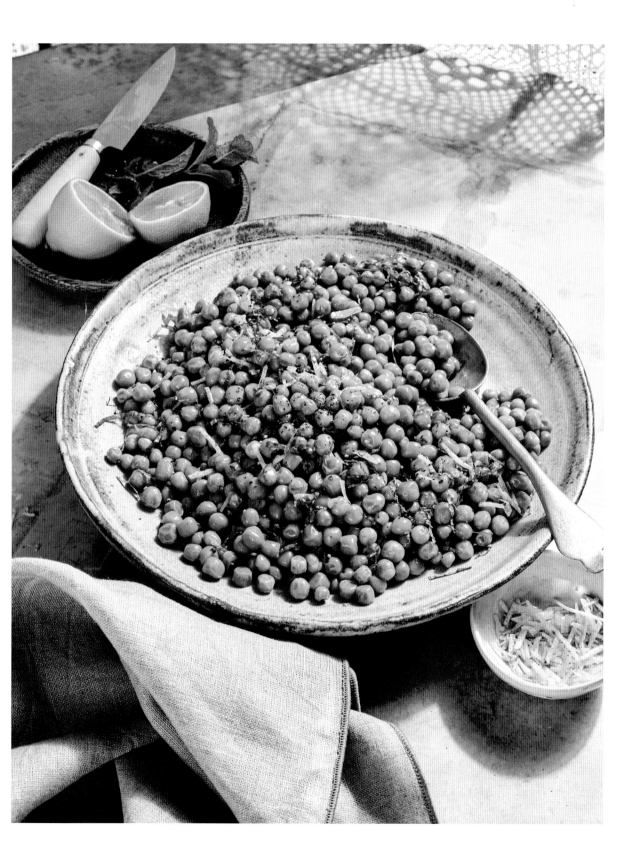

Yummy Beans Your Way

PREP TIME	COOK TIME	SERVES
10 MINUTES	10 MINUTES	2

Ingredients

2 teaspoons extra-virgin olive oil

½ red onion, chopped

1½ cups cooked lentils, garbanzo, black, or cannellini beans, drained and rinsed

1 teaspoon Savory Sizzle, Tex Mex, or Vegitude Power Spice Blend*

Salt, to taste

Choose your own adventure with your favorite plant-based protein. It's an easy, go-to meal staple that's as quick and simple as scrambling a couple eggs. So let your imagination run wild with the flavor and enjoy feeling empowered having this one on autopilot!

Directions

1. Heat olive oil in a skillet over medium heat.

2. Add the onion and sauté 5 minutes.

3. Stir in your choice of beans and spice blend and sauté 5 minutes, just until beans are heated through.

4. Season with salt to taste before serving.

*Savory Sizzle: Substitute spice blend with ½ teaspoon paprika, ¼ teaspoon granulated garlic, ⅛ teaspoon ground turmeric, ⅛ teaspoon ground cumin, ⅛ teaspoon cayenne pepper, pinch of black pepper.

*Tex Mex: Substitute spice blend with ¼ teaspoon chili powder, ⅛ teaspoon paprika, ¼ teaspoon ground cumin, ⅛ teaspoon granulated onion, ⅛ teaspoon granulated garlic, ⅛ teaspoon dried oregano, ⅛ teaspoon crushed red pepper flakes, pinch of each: black pepper, Ceylon cinnamon, ground cloves.

*Vegitude: Substitute spice blend with ¼ teaspoon granulated garlic, ¼ teaspoon granulated onion, ¼ teaspoon ground turmeric, ⅛ teaspoon dried parsley, pinch of black pepper.

CALORIES: 230 · FAT: 5G · CARBS: 33G · FIBER: 11G · SUGARS: 3G · ADDED SUGARS: 0G · PROTEIN: 16G

Red Curry Chickpeas

PREP TIME	COOK TIME	SERVES
5 MINUTES	10 MINUTES	2

Ingredients

2 teaspoons avocado oil

½ yellow onion, chopped

1½ cups cooked chickpeas, drained and rinsed

1 tablespoon Thai red curry paste

2 tablespoons unsweetened plant milk

Salt, to taste

Skip the takeout and try these easy peasy chickpeas! Chickpeas are sautéed with onion in Thai red curry paste for a delicious and different protein that goes great with riced cauliflower or any roasted veg side dish.

Directions

1. Heat avocado oil in a skillet over medium heat.

2. Add the onion and sauté 5 minutes.

3. Stir in chickpeas, curry paste, and plant-based milk and sauté 5 minutes, just until chickpeas are heated through.

4. Season with salt to taste before serving.

CALORIES: 240 · FAT: 6G · CARBS: 33G · FIBER: 9G · SUGARS: 4G · ADDED SUGARS: 0G · PROTEIN: 11G

Simple Power Spiced Lentils

PREP TIME	COOK TIME	SERVES
5 MINUTES	20 MINUTES	4

Ingredients

1 cup dried brown lentils, rinsed

2 ¼ cups vegetable stock, divided

2 cups water

1 teaspoon extra-virgin olive oil

2 cloves garlic, minced

½ cup tomato sauce

1 tablespoon lemon juice

1 teaspoon Everything Savory Power Spice Blend*

Salt, to taste

Every week, I'll whip up a batch of these little legumes as my secret weapon for a powerful week ahead. They become my go-to protein source for quick and nutritious meals, whether I'm tossing them into a vibrant salad, warming them up on a pan, or mixing them into quinoa for a great protein combo. Having these lentils on autopilot in your routine is a shortcut to mealtime victory. Get ready to "lentil" a world of deliciousness and simplicity!

Directions

1. Place the lentils, 2 cups of the vegetable broth, and 2 cups water in a medium pot over medium-high heat.

2. Bring up to a boil, reduce heat to low, and let simmer 20 minutes, or until lentils are tender.

3. Drain any excess water.

4. Heat the olive oil in a saucepan over medium heat. Add the garlic and sauté 1 minute, until fragrant.

5. Stir in cooked lentils, tomato sauce, lemon juice, spice blend, and remaining ¼ cup vegetable broth. Bring up to a simmer. Remove from heat and season with salt to taste.

*Substitute spice blend with ½ teaspoon paprika, ¼ teaspoon granulated garlic, ⅛ teaspoon ground turmeric, ⅛ teaspoon ground cumin, pinch of black pepper, pinch of cayenne pepper.

CALORIES: 185 · FAT: 1G · CARBS: 29G · FIBER: 15G · SUGARS: 2G · ADDED SUGARS: 0G · PROTEIN: 14G

Zesty Edamame

PREP TIME	SERVES
5 MINUTES	2

Ingredients

2 cups shelled edamame

1 tablespoon coconut aminos or tamari

1½ teaspoons rice vinegar

1½ teaspoons avocado oil

1 teaspoon toasted sesame seeds

½ teaspoon sesame oil

Edamame might sound like a mouthful, but these will definitely be gone before you know it! This recipe is a favorite among my patients and perfect for meal prepping and snacking throughout the week. The longer they marinate, the better the flavor gets; so be sure to make enough to enjoy!

Directions

1. Place edamame in a mixing bowl or food storage container.

2. Add the remaining ingredients and toss to evenly coat.

3. Cover and refrigerate at least 15 minutes before serving.

TIP: Serve over a bed of greens for a complete salad meal. Dressing is included!

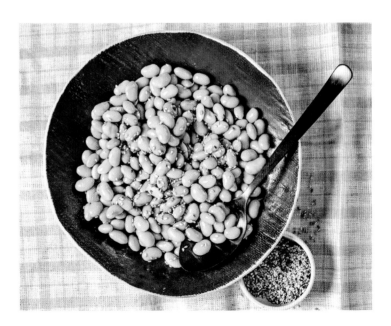

CALORIES: 220 · FAT: 13G · CARBS: 15G · FIBER: 8G · SUGARS: 6G · ADDED SUGARS: 0G · PROTEIN: 18G

Protein Pasta Three Ways

PREP TIME	COOK TIME	SERVES
5 MINUTES	15 MINUTES	4

Ingredients

8 ounces chickpea or lentil pasta

ALFREDO PASTA

1 cup Vegan Alfredo Sauce (recipe page 298)

PESTO PASTA

1 cup Vegan Pesto Sauce (recipe page 303)

MARINARA PASTA

1½ cups marinara sauce

With its neutral flavor, protein-packed goodness, and myriad preparation options, protein pasta is like a blank canvas for your culinary creativity. Whether you like it spicy, savory, or creamy, you can have it any way you'd like. So why not let your imagination run wild and create a pasta dish that's uniquely you?

Directions

1. Cook pasta according to the package directions.

2. Mix pasta with your choice of sauce.

ALFREDO: CALORIES: 330 · FAT: 12G · CARBS: 39G · FIBER: 7G · SUGARS: 2G · PROTEIN: 18G
PESTO: CALORIES: 290 · FAT: 11G · CARBS: 36G · FIBER: 6G · SUGARS: 1G · PROTEIN: 15G
MARINARA: CALORIES: 240 · FAT: 3G · CARBS: 39G · FIBER: 7G · SUGARS: 5G · PROTEIN: 15G

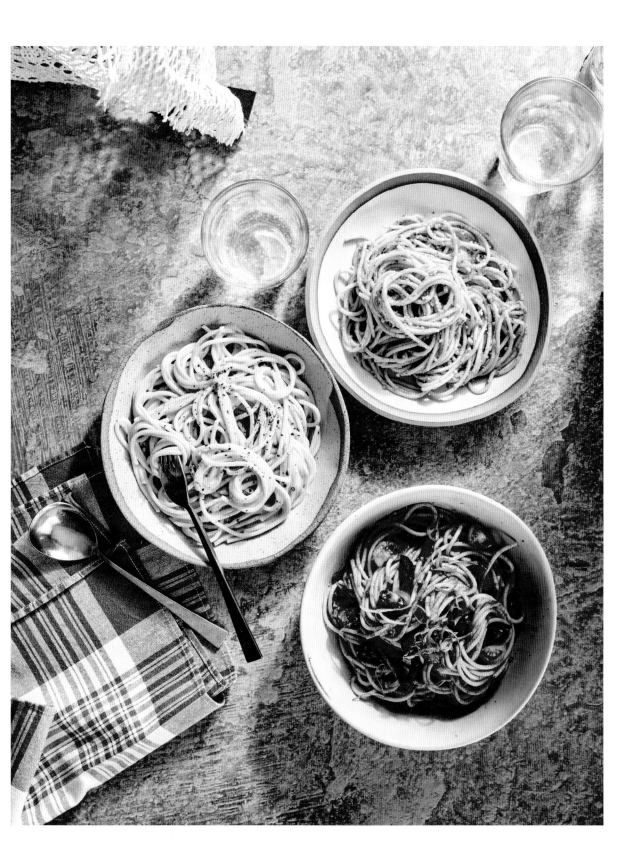

Roasted Veggies Your Way

PREP TIME	COOK TIME	SERVES
15 MINUTES	30 MINUTES	6

Ingredients

1 eggplant, chopped

2 zucchini, chopped

2 cups broccoli florets

1 bell pepper, cored and chopped

1½ tablespoons extra-virgin olive oil

2 teaspoons Vegitude Power Spice Blend*

Salt to taste

Get ready to power up your veggie game with this recipe for Roasted Veggies Your Way! It's a no-brainer dish that you can make on autopilot. Just grab your favorite veggies (eggplant, zucchini, broccoli, bell pepper, you name it!), toss them in one of our Power Spice Blends with some oil, and roast them on a baking sheet. It's the perfect way to level up the antioxidant value of your veg with delicious flavors.

Directions

1. Preheat oven to 400°F. Line a sheet pan with parchment paper.

2. In a mixing bowl, toss all vegetables with olive oil and spice blend. Lightly season with salt and pepper. Transfer to sheet pan.

3. Bake 20–30 minutes, flipping at least twice, until veggies are golden brown. Season with salt, to taste.

*Substitute spice blend with ½ teaspoon granulated garlic, ½ teaspoon granulated onion, ½ teaspoon ground turmeric, ¼ teaspoon dried parsley, dash of black pepper.

CALORIES: 60 · FAT: 3G · CARBS: 7G · FIBER: 5G · SUGARS: 2G · ADDED SUGARS: 0G · PROTEIN: 3G

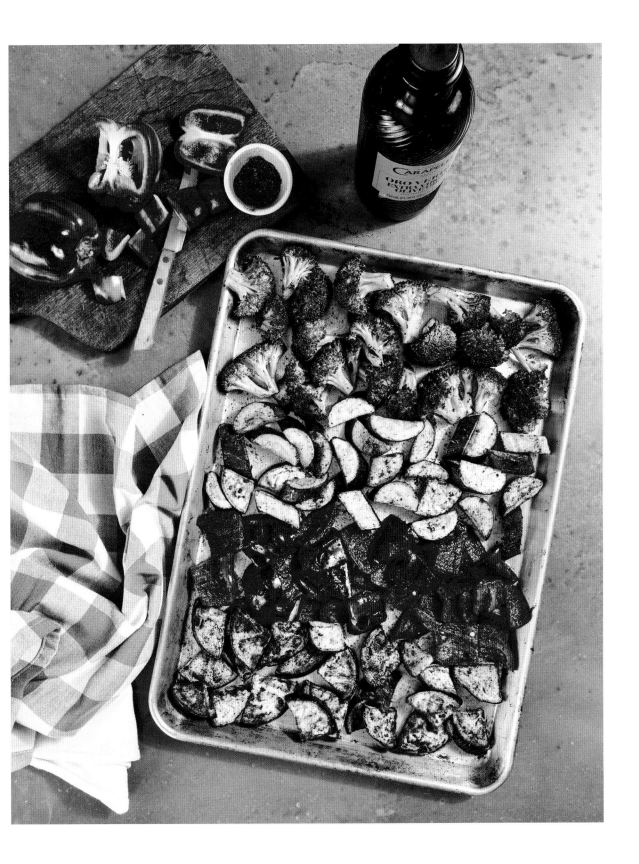

Easy Eggplant Ratatouille

PREP TIME	COOK TIME	SERVES
10 MINUTES	30 MINUTES	4

Ingredients

1 large eggplant, chopped

4 Roma tomatoes, chopped

1 tablespoon extra-virgin olive oil

2 cloves garlic, minced

1 teaspoon Italian seasoning

Salt and pepper, to taste

Eggplants are truly "eggcellent," especially when roasted alongside Roma tomatoes and paired with the bold flavor of garlic. This fiber-filled side dish will leave you feeling full and satisfied.

Directions

1. Preheat oven to 400°F. Line a sheet pan with parchment paper.

2. In a mixing bowl, toss eggplant and tomatoes in olive oil, minced garlic, and Italian seasoning. Lightly season with salt and pepper. Transfer to sheet pan.

3. Bake 20–30 minutes, flipping halfway through, just until eggplant is roasted and tender.

CALORIES: 82 · FAT: 5G · CARBS: 8G · FIBER: 5G · SUGARS: 3G · ADDED SUGARS: 0G · PROTEIN: 3G

Snow Peas or Asparagus with Lemon

PREP TIME	COOK TIME	SERVES
5 MINUTES	5 MINUTES	4

Ingredients

12 ounces snow peas, or
1 pound asparagus, stalks trimmed

¼ cup water

2 cloves garlic, minced

2 teaspoons extra-virgin olive oil

1 teaspoon Vegitude Power Spice Blend*

2 teaspoons lemon zest

Salt and pepper, to taste

Whether you go with the crisp snow peas or the speary asparagus, this simple skillet preparation with lemon is sure to please. Starting with just a little bit of water, these veggies are lightly steamed to perfection before the liquid evaporates for a richer flavor. Plus, it pairs perfectly with just about any of our protein selections.

Directions

1. Place snow peas or asparagus, water, garlic, olive oil, Vegitude Power spice blend, and lemon zest in a skillet over medium heat.

2. Bring up to a simmer and sauté 3–5 minutes, just until the water has evaporated and vegetables are crisp-tender.

3. Season with salt and pepper to taste before serving.

*Substitute ¼ teaspoon granulated garlic, ¼ teaspoon granulated onion, ¼ teaspoon ground turmeric, ⅛ teaspoon dried parsley, pinch of black pepper.

CALORIES: 45 · FAT: 2G · CARBS: 4G · FIBER: 2.5G · SUGARS: 2G · ADDED SUGARS: 0G · PROTEIN: 3G

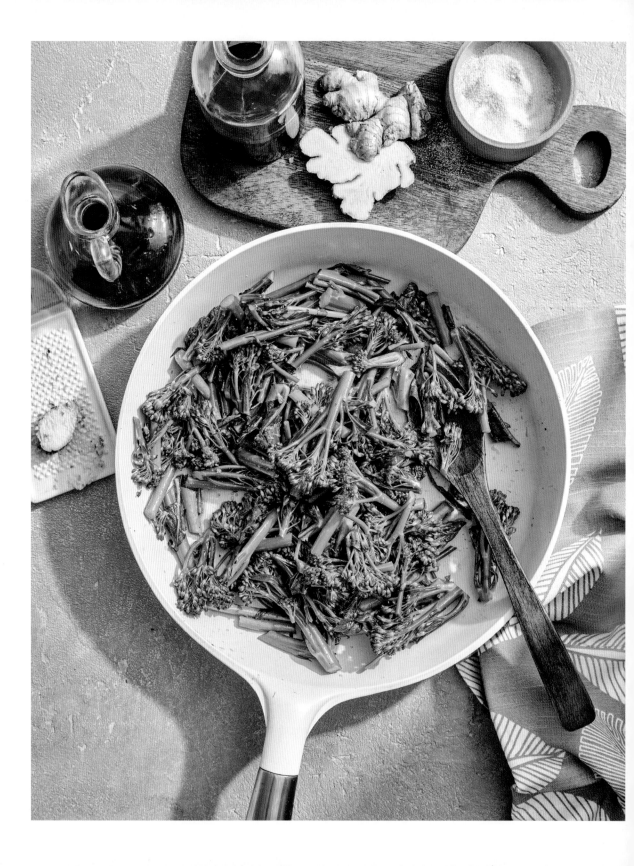

Soy Ginger Broccolini

PREP TIME	COOK TIME	SERVES
5 MINUTES	8 MINUTES	4

Ingredients

2 bunches (about 1 pound) Broccolini

3 tablespoons water

1 tablespoon coconut aminos or tamari

2 teaspoons sesame oil

1½ teaspoons fresh grated ginger

¼ teaspoon onion powder

Pick your favorite green, and with just a few simple ingredients, you'll feel like you're indulging in takeout without all the extra refined oils and additives. It's a delicious way to enjoy a top-tier cancer-fighting cruciferous veg. Go ahead, give Broccolini a nod and whip up this fancy but actually super simple dish!

Directions

1. Place Broccolini, water, coconut aminos, sesame oil, ginger, and onion powder in a skillet over medium heat.

2. Cover, bring up to a simmer, and let cook 3 minutes.

3. Uncover and sauté an additional 5 minutes, just until the water has evaporated and vegetables are crisp-tender.

CALORIES: 45 · FAT: 2.5G · CARBS: 4G · FIBER: 3G · SUGARS: 1G · ADDED SUGARS: 0G · PROTEIN: 3G

Tex Mex Cauliflower Rice

PREP TIME	COOK TIME	SERVES
10 MINUTES	10 MINUTES	4

Ingredients

2 teaspoons avocado oil

½ onion, chopped

1 bell pepper, chopped

3 cups riced cauliflower

1 clove garlic, minced

1 teaspoon Tex Mex Power Spice Blend*

2 tablespoons salsa

Salt, to taste

"Rice" to the occasion with this Southwestern cauliflower rice dish! Grated cauliflower is a perfect, nutrient-rich base alongside your favorite dishes; the Tex Mex Power Spice Blend flavors pair perfectly with black beans for a hearty cancer protective meal.

Directions

1. Heat avocado oil in a skillet over medium heat.

2. Add the onion and bell pepper and sauté 3 minutes.

3. Stir in the cauliflower rice, garlic, and spice blend and sauté 3–5 minutes, just until cauliflower is translucent and beginning to lightly brown.

4. Stir in salsa and season with salt to taste before serving.

*Substitute spice blend with ¼ teaspoon chili powder, ⅛ teaspoon paprika, ¼ teaspoon ground cumin, ⅛ teaspoon granulated onion, ⅛ teaspoon granulated garlic, ⅛ teaspoon dried oregano, ⅛ teaspoon crushed red pepper flakes, pinch of each: black pepper, Ceylon cinnamon, ground cloves.

CALORIES: 55 · FAT: 2.5G · CARBS: 7G · FIBER: 3G · SUGARS: 2G · ADDED SUGARS: 0G · PROTEIN: 2G

Spiced Up Green Beans

PREP TIME	COOK TIME	SERVES
5 MINUTES	8 MINUTES	4

Ingredients

1 pound green beans, ends trimmed

¼ cup water

2 teaspoons extra-virgin olive oil

1 teaspoon Savory Sizzle Power Spice Blend*

Salt, to taste

Add some sizzle to your side dish game with these skillet green beans! These green beauties are jazzed up with my Savory Sizzle spice blend, so you know they're packed with flavor and antioxidant power. It's a tasty way to get your greens in and keep you feeling your best. Plus, they're so easy to make—just a few minutes in a hot skillet and you're done!

Directions

1. Place green beans, water, olive oil, and spice blend in a skillet over medium heat.

2. Bring up to a simmer and sauté 4–6 minutes, just until the water has evaporated and green beans are crisp-tender.

3. Season with salt to taste before serving.

*Substitute spice blend with ½ teaspoon paprika, ¼ teaspoon granulated garlic, ⅛ teaspoon ground turmeric, ⅛ teaspoon ground cumin, ⅛ teaspoon cayenne pepper, pinch of black pepper.

CALORIES: 48 · FAT: 2.5G · CARBS: 5G · FIBER: 3.5G · SUGARS: 1G · ADDED SUGARS: 0G · PROTEIN: 2G

Golden Brussels Sprouts

PREP TIME	COOK TIME	SERVES
10 MINUTES	25 MINUTES	4

Ingredients

1 pound Brussels sprouts, halved

1 tablespoon extra-virgin olive oil

2 teaspoons apple cider vinegar

1 teaspoon honey

1 teaspoon Vegitude Power Spice Blend*

Salt and pepper, to taste

Top-tier Brussels sprouts are roasted to crispy, golden brown perfection in this delicious side dish! These little guys may look unassuming, but they pack a punch when it comes to their cancer protective value. When roasted with a splash of apple cider vinegar and our Vegitude Power blend, they receive a major anticancer upgrade that's sure to steal the show at any meal.

Directions

1. Preheat oven to 400°F. Line a sheet pan with parchment paper.

2. In a mixing bowl, toss Brussels sprouts in olive oil, vinegar, honey, and spice blend. Lightly season with salt and pepper. Transfer to sheet pan.

3. Bake 20–25 minutes, flipping halfway through, until sprouts are golden brown and crisp-tender.

*Substitute spice blend with ¼ teaspoon granulated garlic, ¼ teaspoon granulated onion, ¼ teaspoon ground turmeric, ⅛ teaspoon dried parsley, pinch of black pepper.

CALORIES: 85 · FAT: 3.5G · CARBS: 11G · FIBER: 4.5G · SUGARS: 4G · ADDED SUGARS: 1.5G · PROTEIN: 4G

Sautéed Balsamic Mushrooms

PREP TIME	COOK TIME	SERVES
10 MINUTES	10 MINUTES	2

Ingredients

8 ounces baby bella mushrooms, halved

1 clove garlic, minced

1 tablespoon balsamic vinegar

2 teaspoons coconut aminos or tamari

2 teaspoons avocado oil

These Sautéed Balsamic Mushrooms are sure to steal the spotlight! Packed with flavor and a surprising source of protein, they're the perfect addition to any meal. The aromatase inhibitors in mushrooms help reduce estrogen levels and support breast cancer risk reduction—a top-tier rec at Beller Nutrition!

Directions

1. In a mixing bowl, toss mushrooms with garlic, balsamic vinegar, and coconut aminos. Let sit at least 10 minutes to marinate.

2. Heat avocado oil in a skillet over medium-high heat.

3. Add the marinated mushrooms to the skillet and sauté until tender and beginning to brown, 8–10 minutes.

CALORIES: 70 · FAT: 5G · CARBS: 5G · FIBER: 2G · SUGARS: 3G · ADDED SUGARS: 0G · PROTEIN: 4G

Everything Savory Cauliflower

PREP TIME	COOK TIME	SERVES
10 MINUTES	25 MINUTES	4

Ingredients

1 head cauliflower, cut into florets

1 ½ tablespoons extra-virgin olive oil

Juice of ½ lime

1 tablespoon Everything Savory Power Spice Blend*

Salt and pepper, to taste

Cauliflower, with my Everything Savory Power Spice Blend, is a flavor-packed side dish that becomes so easy to prepare you'll have this one on autopilot. It's both of my daughters' favorite veggie dish that I serve at least twice a week and I love knowing that by power spicing it, I have dramatically elevated the anti-inflammatory and antioxidant value of this cruciferous veg every time it's served!

Directions

1. Preheat oven to 400°F. Line a sheet pan with parchment paper.

2. In a mixing bowl, toss cauliflower in olive oil, lime juice, and spice blend. Lightly season with salt and pepper. Transfer to sheet pan.

3. Bake 20–25 minutes, flipping halfway through, until cauliflower is tender and beginning to brown.

*Substitute 1½ teaspoons paprika, ¾ teaspoon granulated garlic, ½ teaspoon ground turmeric, ¼ teaspoon ground cumin, ⅛ teaspoon cayenne pepper, pinch of black pepper.

CALORIES: 75 · FAT: 5G · CARBS: 6G · FIBER: 4G · SUGARS: 2.5G · ADDED SUGARS: 0G · PROTEIN: 3G

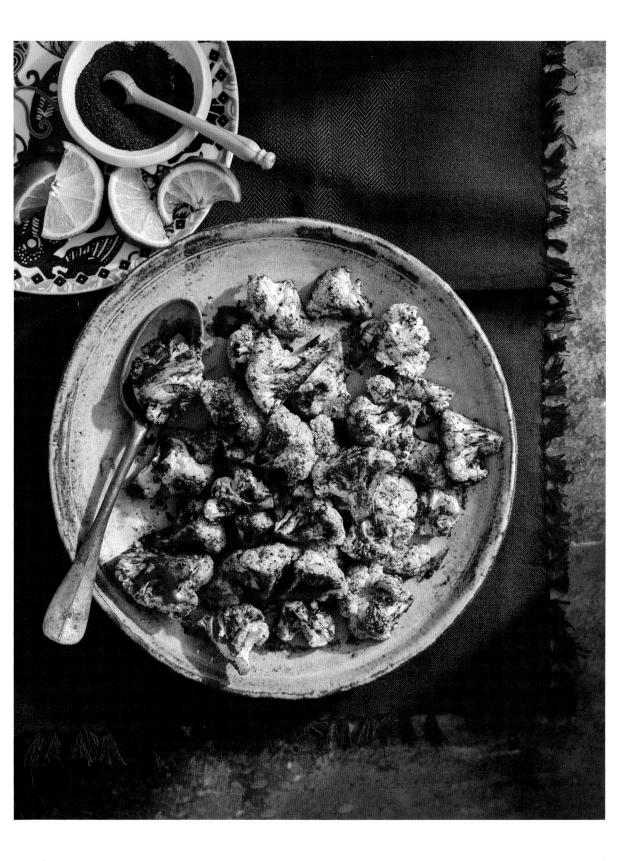

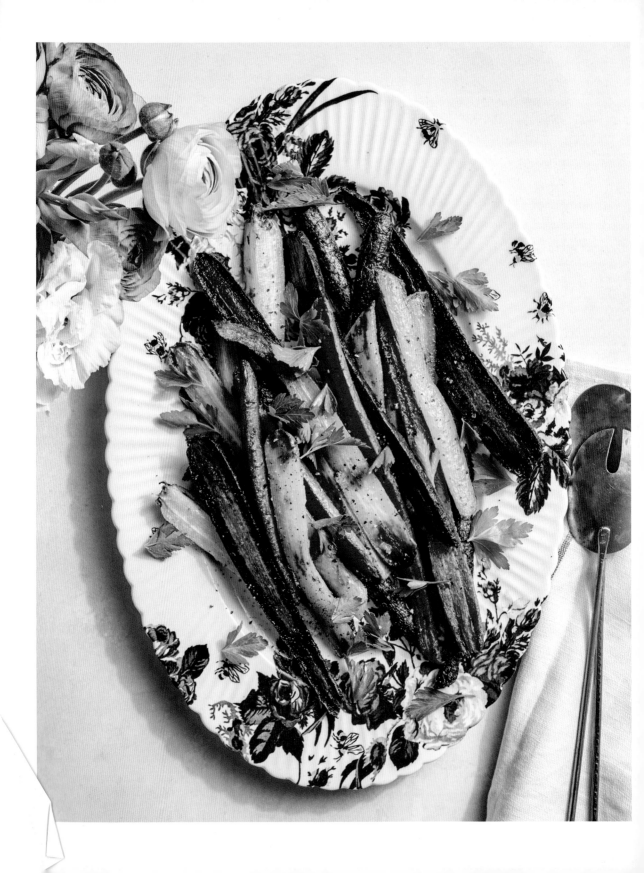

Dijon Glazed Carrots

PREP TIME	COOK TIME	SERVES
10 MINUTES	30 MINUTES	8

Ingredients

1½ tablespoons avocado oil

1 tablespoon pure maple syrup

2 teaspoons Dijon mustard

1 teaspoon Vegitude Power Spice Blend*

2 pounds carrots, peeled and halved lengthwise

Salt, to taste

This nourishing and satisfying side dish is a real crowd-pleaser at my Thanksgiving dinner table, glazed with the perfect balance of flavors. A tiny bit of maple syrup, along with Dijon and my Vegitude Power Spice Blend go a long way in making these carrots a standout in both presentation and flavor. A must-try!

Directions

1. Preheat oven to 425°F. Line a sheet pan with parchment paper.

2. In a mixing bowl, whisk together oil, maple syrup, Dijon mustard, and spice blend to create a glaze.

3. Place the carrots on the lined sheet pan and pour the glaze over top, brushing to ensure an even coat. Lightly season with salt and pepper.

4. Bake 20–30 minutes, until the carrots are fully roasted and fork-tender.

*Substitute spice blend with ¼ teaspoon granulated garlic, ¼ teaspoon granulated onion, ¼ teaspoon ground turmeric, ⅛ teaspoon dried parsley, pinch of black pepper.

CALORIES: 70 · FAT: 3G · CARBS: 11G · FIBER: 4G · SUGARS: 6.5G · ADDED SUGARS: 1.5G · PROTEIN: 2G

Barbecue Braised Slaw

PREP TIME	COOK TIME	SERVES
5 MINUTES	15 MINUTES	4

Ingredients

2 teaspoons avocado oil

4 cups shredded purple cabbage, coleslaw cabbage mix, or broccoli slaw mix

1 tablespoon apple cider vinegar

2 teaspoons smoked paprika or Everything Savory Power Spice Blend*

1 teaspoon honey

½ teaspoon onion powder

Salt, to taste

Traditional coleslaw with a barbecue braised twist! This warm and comforting slaw is the perfect addition to any meal, from backyard barbecues to cozy dinners at home. It's made with easy-to-find ingredients and can be whipped up in no time.

Directions

1. Heat avocado oil in skillet.

2. Stir in the shredded cabbage, cider vinegar, paprika or power spice blend, honey, and onion powder and sauté 10–13 minutes, just until cabbage is tender and beginning to brown.

3. Season with salt to taste before serving.

*Substitute spice blend with 1 teaspoon paprika, ½ teaspoon granulated garlic, ¼ teaspoon ground turmeric, ¼ teaspoon ground cumin, pinch of black pepper, pinch of cayenne pepper.

CALORIES: 45 · FAT: 2.55G · CARBS: 5.5G · FIBER: 2G · SUGARS: 4G · ADDED SUGARS: 1.6G · PROTEIN: 2G

Fried Cauliflower Rice

PREP TIME	COOK TIME	SERVES
10 MINUTES	7 MINUTES	4

Ingredients

2 teaspoons sesame oil

3 cups riced cauliflower

½ cup shredded carrots

½ teaspoon ground ginger

½ teaspoon onion powder

1 tablespoon coconut aminos or tamari

From the cauliflower patch to the frying pan, this savory and comforting fried cauliflower rice is sure to satisfy any craving. Packed with fiber and essential nutrients, this top-tier anticancer vegetable pairs perfectly with peas for an easy, plant protein-packed meal.

Directions

1. Heat sesame oil in a skillet over medium heat.

2. Add the riced cauliflower, carrots, ground ginger, and onion powder and sauté 5–7 minutes, just until riced cauliflower is translucent and beginning to lightly brown.

3. Stir in coconut aminos and remove from heat to serve.

CALORIES: 50 · FAT: 2.5G · CARBS: 6G · FIBER: 2.5G · SUGARS: 4G · ADDED SUGARS: 0G · PROTEIN: 2G

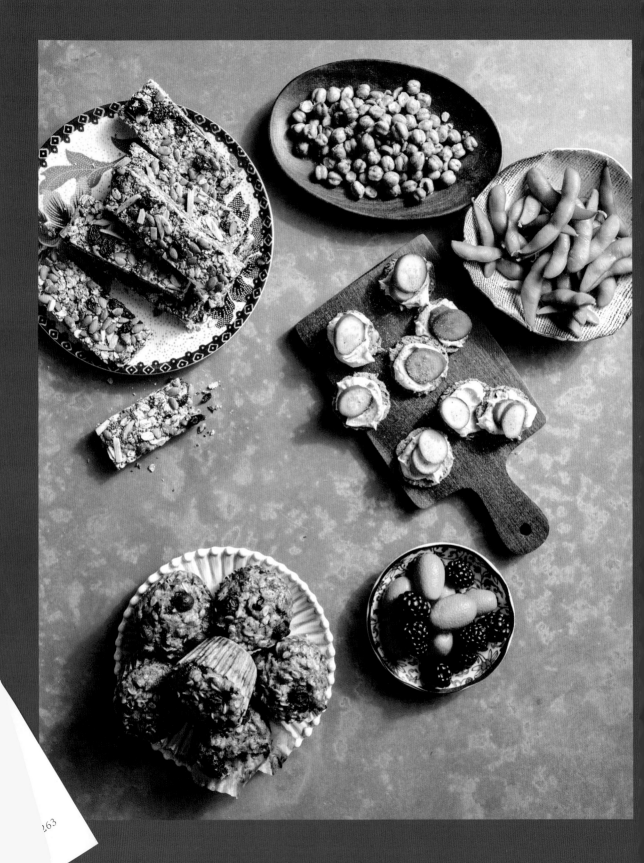

Snacks

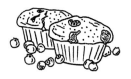

The Beller Method™
Power Snacks

If you're hungry between meals or need an extra boost, feel
free to enjoy 1–2 snacks per day. I don't need you to be counting
calories, but it's easy to go overboard on snacks, so mindfully
keep snacks to 150–200 wholesome calories. Choose from any
of my snack recipes in this section.

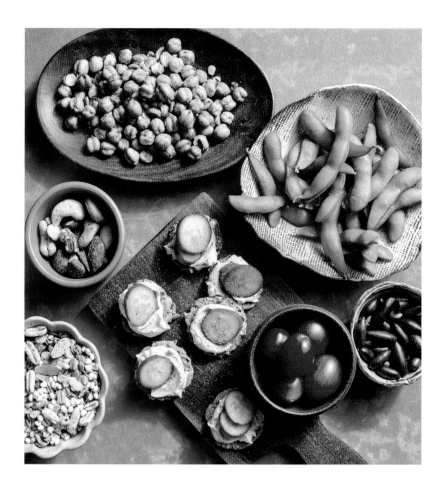

A Beller Method snack supports weight management and breast cancer risk reduction by:

- Preventing overeating
- Satiating your appetite
- Stabilizing blood sugars
- Burning more energy during digestion
- Reducing inflammation

You can include a snack between each meal if you're hungry, but most people feel that an afternoon snack is the most helpful to have due to the long stretch of time between lunch and dinner. If you skip it, you are more likely to overeat before or during mealtimes.

And of course, if you find yourself hungry at any point during the day, feel free to munch on some low starch vegetables as an anytime snack. They'll provide protective phytochemicals and fiber, but aren't high in calories and won't spike your blood sugar. Go for low starch veg any way—raw, cooked, or even in a vegetable soup!

We have some easy recipes that follow, but here are my Top 10 Pantry Grab and Go Favorites.

TOP 10 EASY BELLER SNACK FAVORITES

- ¾ cup shelled edamame sprinkled with 1 teaspoon sesame seeds
- 30 pistachios with mandarin orange or ½ cup berries
- 1+ cups raw veggies (peppers, snap peas, cucumbers, carrots) with 2 tablespoons hummus)
- 1 cup celery sticks with 1 tablespoon nut or seed butter
- 1 apple with 2 teaspoons nut butter or 10 nuts
- 3 cups popcorn with 1 tablespoon nutritional yeast
- 2 tablespoons slivered almonds + ½ cup puffed kamut + ½ cup freeze dried berries
- 2 dates stuffed with 3 almonds each.
- 1 brown rice cake with ½ small avocado, smashed
- 8 multi-seed crackers with 1 tablespoon tahini sauce with cucumber slices

Oat Seed Energy Bars

PREP TIME	COOK TIME	SERVES
15 MINUTES	25 MINUTES	12

Ingredients

3 bananas, peeled

2 cups rolled oats (sprouted preferred)

½ cup no sugar added dried fruit

½ cup shelled pumpkin seeds

⅓ cup sliced almonds

¼ cup chia seeds

1 teaspoon vanilla extract

1 teaspoon Cinnapeel Spicer Power Spice Blend*

Oat Seed Energy Bars are one of my all-time favorite, on-the-go energy snacks—they're perfect for travel and are a great alternative to store-bought snack bars. The recipe is flexible—whether you like a seedy vs nutty texture, a touch more sweetness from specific fruit, or changing up those powerful spice blends, you can easily enjoy a different flavor with each bite.

Directions

1. Preheat oven to 350°F. Line a 13 x 9-inch baking dish with parchment paper.

2. In a large mixing bowl, mash bananas until smooth.

3. Fold in all remaining ingredients, until thoroughly mixed.

4. Transfer mixture to the parchment-lined dish and press down to smooth the top and firmly pack the ingredients.

5. Bake 25 minutes, until firm and lightly browned around the edges.

6. Remove from oven and slice into bars. Store in an airtight container for up to 7 days. Bars can also be stored in the freezer for up to 2 months. Thaw for 20–30 minutes before serving.

TIP: Any no sugar added dried fruit can be used such as chopped apricots, prunes, or raisins.

*Substitute spice blend with ¾ teaspoon Ceylon cinnamon, ½ teaspoon granulated orange peel, pinch of ground ginger.

CALORIES: 160 · FAT: 6G · CARBS: 21G · FIBER: 5G · SUGARS: 4G · ADDED SUGARS: 0G · PROTEIN: 5G

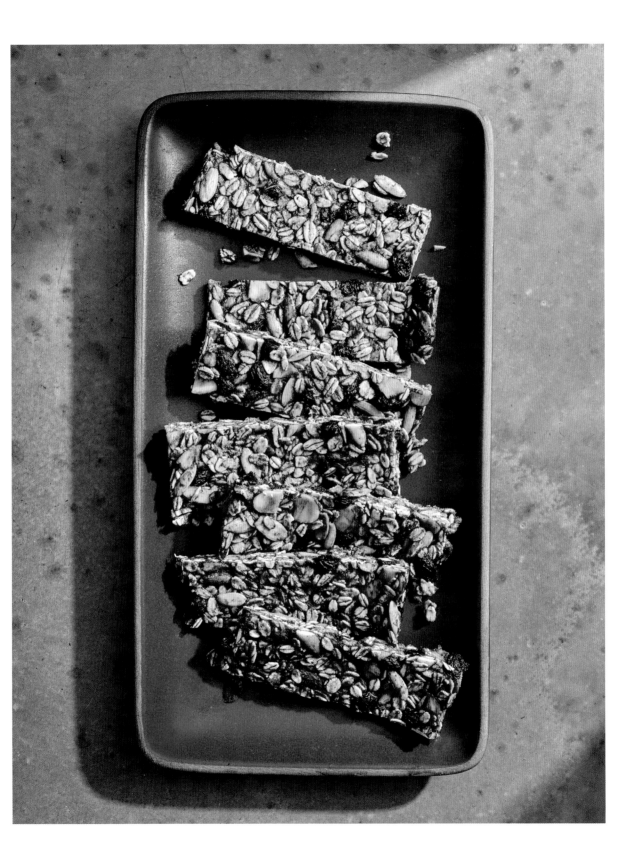

No-Hassle Snack Mix

PREP TIME
5 MINUTES

SERVES
6

Ingredients

12 cups plain or lightly salted popcorn

1 cup freeze dried fruit

⅓ cup shelled pumpkin seeds

⅓ cup sliced almonds

Snack time is the best time, and with this easy no-hassle snack mix, you can satisfy your cravings anytime, anywhere. This crunchy and wholesome snack offers fiber, protein, and essential fats and is perfect for on-the-go munching. Just grab a handful and enjoy the crunch!

Directions

1. Place all ingredients in a large food storage container and toss to combine. Store in an airtight container for up to 5 days.

TIP: 6 cups of puffed millet, quinoa, or kamut can be used in place of the popcorn.

CALORIES: 150 · FAT: 7G · CARBS: 15G · FIBER: 4G · SUGARS: 3G · ADDED SUGARS: 0G · PROTEIN: 5G

Bell Pepper Nachos

PREP TIME	COOKING TIME	SERVES
10 MINUTES	12 MINUTES	4

Ingredients

4 bell peppers, cut into triangles or strips

1½ cups cooked black beans, drained and rinsed

½ cup diced red onion

2 teaspoons Tex Mex Power Spice Blend*

¼ teaspoon salt

1 tomato, diced

¼ cup chopped fresh cilantro

¼ cup Creamy Avocado Lime Dressing (recipe page 301)

These are "nacho" ordinary nachos! This filling snack built on multi-colored bell peppers is decorated with fiber, protein, and antioxidant rich ingredients that make this a phytonutrient rich plate. The creaminess of the Avocado Lime Dressing adds the texture and flavor reminiscent of traditional nacho ingredients. Get ready to pepper those taste buds with some bold flavors!

Directions

1. Preheat oven to 425°F and line a sheet pan with parchment paper.

2. Cut tops off bell peppers and discard. Remove and discard seeds. Cut each bell pepper into triangular pieces or strips and arrange on the prepared sheet pan.

3. Sprinkle black beans and onion over the cut bell peppers and then season with spice blend and salt.

4. Bake 10–12 minutes, just until peppers begin to brown around the edges. Center of peppers should still be crisp.

5. Sprinkle the cooked peppers with diced tomato and chopped cilantro before drizzling with the dressing. Serve immediately.

TIP: This can also be made with mini multi-colored peppers in place of full-sized bell peppers. Simply cut the mini peppers in half and scoop out the seeds.

*Substitute spice blend with ½ teaspoon chili powder, ¼ teaspoon paprika, ½ teaspoon ground cumin, ¼ teaspoon granulated onion, ¼ teaspoon granulated garlic, ¼ teaspoon dried oregano, ¼ teaspoon crushed red pepper flakes, dash of each: black pepper, Ceylon cinnamon, ground cloves.

CALORIES: 155 · FAT: 2G · CARBS: 22G · FIBER: 6G · SUGARS: 5G · ADDED SUGARS: 1G · PROTEIN: 6G

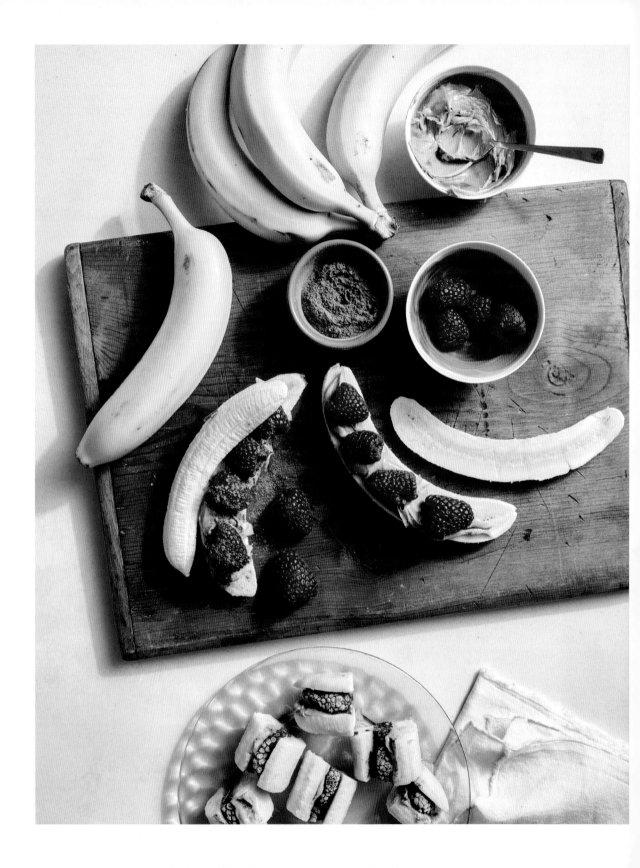

Frozen 'Nana "Sandwich"

PREP TIME	FREEZING TIME	SERVES
5 MINUTES	1 HOUR	1

Ingredients

2 teaspoons nut or seed butter

1 banana, peeled and halved lengthwise

½ teaspoon Golden Breakfast Power Spice Blend*

4–5 raspberries, optional

Frozen 'nana sandwich! A hands-down favorite among my teen and adult patients; it's filling, satisfying, and the perfect anytime snack. If you'd like to make a larger batch all at once, these will keep in the freezer for up to 3 months.

Directions

1. Spread half of the nut butter on each ½ of the banana.

2. Sprinkle lightly with spice blend. Add raspberries, if desired.

3. Place the second half of the banana over top the first to create a sandwich.

4. Wrap the banana sandwich with parchment paper and then place in a storage bag or airtight container. Freeze at least 1 hour.

5. Serve the banana sandwich as is, or sliced into bite-sized pieces.

*Substitute spice blend with ¼ teaspoon Ceylon cinnamon, ¼ teaspoon cacao powder, ⅛ teaspoon ground turmeric, pinch of ground ginger.

CALORIES: 155 · FAT: 5G · CARBS: 25G · FIBER: 4G · SUGARS: 12G · ADDED SUGARS: 0G · PROTEIN: 4G

Green Pea Hummus

PREP TIME	SERVING SIZE	SERVES
5 MINUTES	¼ CUP	10

Ingredients

1½ cups cooked chickpeas, drained and rinsed

1½ cups frozen peas, thawed

3 tablespoons tahini paste

2 tablespoons extra-virgin olive oil

Juice of 1 lemon

1 teaspoon Vegitude Power Spice Blend*

Salt and pepper, to taste

Hummus where the heart is, and my heart is in this green pea hummus! This hybrid dip is made with a duo of plant-based proteins for extra flavor and nutrient value. I get rave reviews with this one, pairing perfectly with freshly cut cucumbers, celery, carrots, or even my Super Seed Crackers (page 287).

Directions

1. Place all ingredients in a food processor and process until smooth and creamy. If mixture is too thick, add warm water, 1 tablespoon at a time, until it loosens up.

2. Season with salt and pepper to taste before serving. Store in an airtight container in the fridge for up to 5 days.

*Substitute spice blend with ¼ teaspoon granulated garlic, ¼ teaspoon granulated onion, ¼ teaspoon ground turmeric, ⅛ teaspoon dried parsley, pinch of black pepper.

CALORIES: 110 · FAT: 6G · CARBS: 9G · FIBER: 3G · SUGARS: 1G · ADDED SUGARS: 0G · PROTEIN: 5G

Spinach and Artichoke Dip

PREP TIME	SERVING SIZE	SERVES
10 MINUTES	½ CUP	6

Ingredients

2 cups plain plant-based yogurt

12 ounces jarred artichoke hearts, drained and chopped

2 cups frozen chopped spinach, thawed

½ bell pepper, diced

2 teaspoons minced garlic

3 tablespoons nutritional yeast

1 teaspoon Italian seasoning

Salt and pepper, to taste

Here's a dip that's sure to leave you feeling "artichoked" up with joy! We skipped all the junk and left you with a fiber-filled, protein-packed snack solution you'll love dipping into again and again. Serve warm or chilled, it's great as leftovers and makes for a satisfying party dish!

Directions

1. Preheat oven to 350°F.

2. In a baking dish, stir together all ingredients to create a thick dip.

3. Bake 20–25 minutes, just until bubbly hot. Serve immediately. Leftovers are also great chilled.

CALORIES: 85 · FAT: 4G · CARBS: 10G · FIBER: 6G · SUGARS: 2G · ADDED SUGARS: 0G · PROTEIN: 7G

Banana Berry Oat Muffins

PREP TIME	COOK TIME	SERVES
10 MINUTES	35 MINUTES	12

Ingredients

1¼ cups oat flour

1¼ cups rolled oats (sprouted preferred)

⅓ cup coconut sugar

2 tablespoons baking powder

½ teaspoon baking soda

3 small bananas, peeled

¼ cup unsweetened plant milk

¼ cup avocado oil

1 teaspoon vanilla extract

1 teaspoon Cinnapeel Spicer Power Spice Blend*

1 cup fresh berries

These Banana Berry Oat Muffins are a treat that can't be "battered"! They're the perfect hybrid between a snack and a sweet treat, making them a great on-the-go snack or a satiating dessert. The Cinnapeel Power Spice Blend adds natural sweetness and a unique fragrance that really shines through. These muffins will have you going bananas!

Directions

1. Preheat oven to 350°F. Line a muffin tin with 12 paper liners.

2. In a mixing bowl, stir together oat flour, oats, coconut sugar, baking powder, and baking soda.

3. In a separate mixing bowl, mash bananas using a heavy fork. Stir in plant milk, avocado oil, vanilla extract, and spice blend.

4. Stir the dry ingredients into the wet ingredients, until all is combined. Fold in berries.

5. Scoop the batter into the lined muffin cups using a measuring cup or ice cream scoop.

6. Bake 30–35 minutes, until a toothpick inserted into the center of a muffin comes out mostly clean. Let rest at least 5 minutes before serving.

*Substitute spice blend with ¾ teaspoon Ceylon cinnamon, ½ teaspoon granulated orange peel, pinch of ground ginger.

CALORIES: 155 · FAT: 6G · CARBS: 23G · FIBER: 4G · SUGARS: 7G · ADDED SUGARS: 4G · PROTEIN: 3G

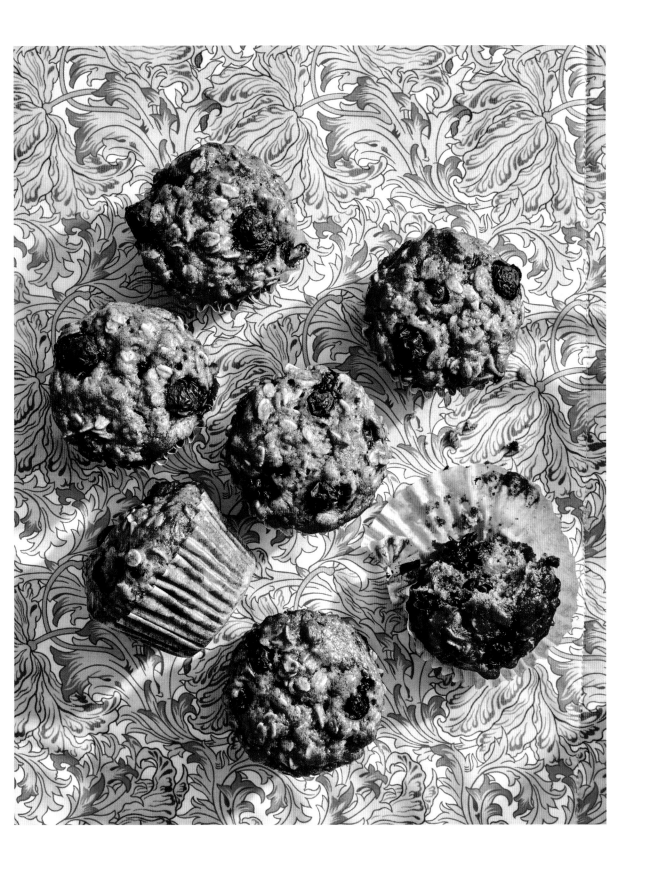

Falafel Snack Wraps

PREP TIME	COOK TIME	SERVES
10 MINUTES	5 MINUTES	4

Ingredients

2 cups cooked chickpeas, drained and rinsed

½ small yellow onion, chopped

½ cup fresh cilantro

2 cloves garlic

1 teaspoon Savory Sizzle Power Spice Blend*

½ teaspoon salt

1 tablespoon extra-virgin olive oil

8 large lettuce leaves

These Falafel Snack Wraps hit the spot! The wonderful smells of onion, cilantro, and smashed chickpeas are so fragrant and especially enjoyable because they're so quick and easy to make. They make for great leftovers for a flavorful plant-based protein I can enjoy during mealtime. Enjoy them wrapped in lettuce or on their own with a drizzle of hummus or tahini sauce. No regrets!

Directions

1. Place chickpeas, onion, cilantro, garlic, spice blend, and salt in a food processor and process until smooth.

2. Heat olive oil in a skillet over medium-high heat.

3. Transfer the chickpea mixture to the skillet and sauté 5 minutes, or until golden brown.

4. Fill lettuce leaves with the browned chickpea mixture before serving.

*Substitute spice blend with ½ teaspoon paprika, ¼ teaspoon granulated garlic, ⅛ teaspoon ground turmeric, ⅛ teaspoon ground cumin, ⅛ teaspoon cayenne pepper, pinch of black pepper.

CALORIES: 160 · FAT: 4G · CARBS: 22G · FIBER: 6G · SUGARS: 1G · ADDED SUGARS: 0G · PROTEIN: 7G

Multi-Fiber Protein Bites

PREP TIME	SERVING SIZE	SERVES
15 MINUTES	2 PROTEIN BITES	12

Ingredients

2 cups hemp hearts

⅓ cup rolled oats (sprouted preferred)

¼ cup almond flour

¼ cup ground flaxseed

3 tablespoons nut or seed butter

2 tablespoons date syrup or honey

2 tablespoons chia seeds

1 teaspoon Golden Breakfast Power Spice Blend*

Unsweetened plant milk, if needed

These little bites are like rolled up mini-energy bars, with all the ingredients you'd want for a pre or post-workout boost. If I were shopping for an energy bar at a health food store, these are the ingredients I would love to see listed. I keep mine in the freezer for a chewier, longer lasting bite. The best part is these bites are budget-friendly and can be adjusted to your liking. So go ahead—indulge with each delicious bite of energy!

Directions

1. In a large mixing bowl, fold together all ingredients, except the plant milk.

2. If the mixture is too thick to work with, add plant milk a few teaspoons at a time until a dough has formed.

3. Use a tablespoon to scoop out dough and roll into 1-inch balls. Transfer to a parchment paper-lined dish.

4. Cover and refrigerate at least 20 minutes before serving.

*Substitute ½ teaspoon Ceylon cinnamon, ½ teaspoon cacao powder, ¼ teaspoon ground turmeric, pinch of ground ginger.

CALORIES: 160 · FAT: 11G · CARBS: 7G · FIBER: 4G · SUGARS: 3G · ADDED SUGARS: 2G · PROTEIN: 8G

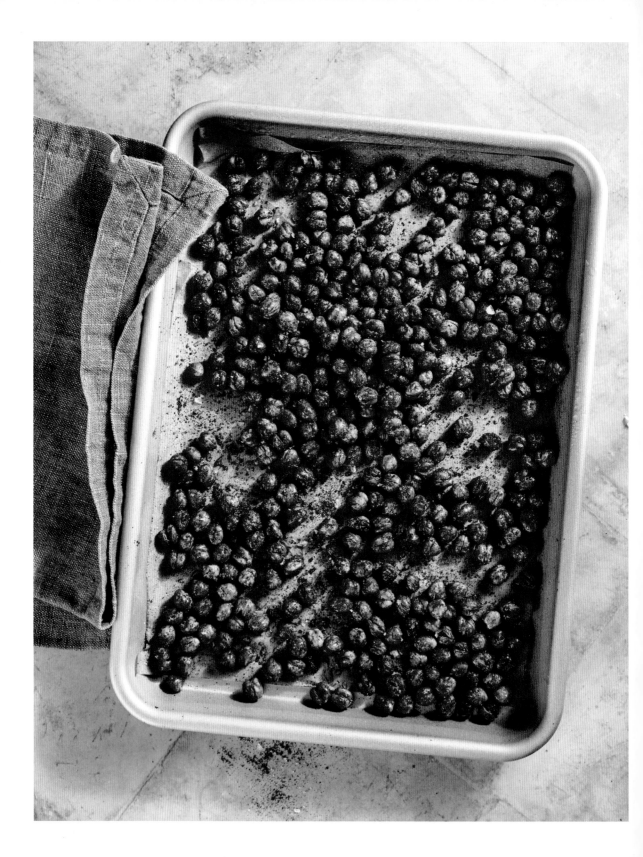

Savory Chickpea Snacks

PREP TIME	COOK TIME	SERVING SIZE	SERVES
5 MINUTES	45 MINUTES	1 TABLESPOON	4 PEOPLE

Ingredients

1½ cups cooked chickpeas, drained and rinsed

2 teaspoons extra-virgin olive oil

1 tablespoon Everything Savory Power Spice Blend*

¼ teaspoon salt

Chickpeas take it to the next level being high in fiber, protein, and tossed in a perfect blend of spices that pack a punch of cancer protective nutrients and flavor. I love how versatile they are—not only do they make for a great snack, but they can also be used as a plant-based protein topper for salads or bowls. It's like getting two in one!

Directions

1. Preheat oven to 375°F. Line a sheet pan with parchment paper.

2. In a mixing bowl, toss chickpeas with olive oil, spice blend, and salt.

3. Arrange seasoned chickpeas in a single layer on the prepared sheet pan.

4. Bake 25–35 minutes, shaking the pan twice during cooking to rotate the chickpeas.

5. Let cool 5 minutes before serving. Store in an airtight container for up to 3 days.

*Substitute spice blend with 1½ teaspoons paprika, ¾ teaspoon granulated garlic, ½ teaspoon ground turmeric, ¼ teaspoon ground cumin, ⅛ teaspoon cayenne pepper, pinch of black pepper.

CALORIES: 115 · FAT: 3G · CARBS: 16G · FIBER: 5G · SUGARS: 1G · ADDED SUGARS: 0G · PROTEIN: 5G

English Muffin Pizzas

PREP TIME	COOK TIME	SERVES
10 MINUTES	7 MINUTES	4

Ingredients

2 sprouted flourless English muffins

½ cup marinara sauce

¼ cup plain plant-based yogurt

3 tablespoons nutritional yeast

½ teaspoon Italian seasoning

Pinch salt

½ cup sliced mushrooms

¼ cup diced bell pepper

Who doesn't like toaster oven pizza? These English Muffin Pizzas are a perfect midday pick-me-up when you're craving something savory and satisfying. You can indulge in a pizza party any day of the week! They're a fun and easy snack to make with kids; get creative with toppings and stack on the veggies for a tower of deliciousness! Truly a slice above the rest!

Directions

1. Preheat oven to 425°F. Split English muffins and place on a sheet pan.

2. Spread 2 tablespoons of marinara sauce across each half of muffin.

3. In a small mixing bowl, stir together yogurt, nutritional yeast, Italian seasoning, and salt. Spread ¼ of this mixture over the marinara on each half of muffin.

4. Top all with an equal amount of the mushrooms and bell pepper. Sprinkle with additional Italian seasoning, if desired.

5. Bake 8–10 minutes, just until the edges of English muffin begin to brown. Serve immediately.

CALORIES: 115 · FAT: 1G · CARBS: 19G · FIBER: 5G · SUGARS: 1G · ADDED SUGARS: 0G · PROTEIN: 7G

Buffalo Cauliflower Bites

PREP TIME	COOK TIME	SERVES
10 MINUTES	20 MINUTES	4

Ingredients

1 head cauliflower, cut into small florets

3 tablespoons hot sauce

2 tablespoons almond flour

2 tablespoons ground flaxseed

1 tablespoon extra-virgin olive oil

1 teaspoon Savory Sizzle Power Spice Blend*

Salt, to taste

Buffalo Cauliflower Bites are a tasty twist on a classic appetizer! These bites are a plant-based alternative to traditional restaurant wings that are often loaded with ingredients that are not so ideal for our health. Using cauliflower instead of wings and some added ground flax, you can level up your snack game and pump more fiber goodness into your midday routine.

Directions

1. Preheat oven to 400°F. Line a sheet pan with parchment paper.

2. In a mixing bowl, toss all ingredients to evenly coat the cauliflower florets. Transfer to the prepared sheet pan.

3. Bake 20 minutes, flipping halfway through. Cauliflower should be lightly browned around the edges, but still crisp in the center.

TIP: For something cooling to dip these into, try my Plant-Based Caesar Dressing (recipe page 302), Creamy Avocado Lime Dressing (recipe page:301), or Golden Tahini Sauce (recipe page 297).

*Substitute spice blend with ½ teaspoon paprika, ¼ teaspoon granulated garlic, ⅛ teaspoon ground turmeric, ⅛ teaspoon ground cumin, ⅛ teaspoon cayenne pepper, pinch of black pepper.

CALORIES: 115 · FAT: 7G · CARBS: 9G · FIBER: 6G · SUGARS: 4G · ADDED SUGARS: 0G · PROTEIN: 5G

Cacao Muffins

PREP TIME	COOK TIME	SERVES
10 MINUTES	40 MINUTES	12

Ingredients

2 cups unsweetened plant-based milk

⅓ cup date syrup or pure maple syrup

¼ cup nut or sunflower seed butter

1 teaspoon vanilla extract

2 cups rolled oats (sprouted preferred)

⅓ cup raw cacao powder

⅓ cup chia seeds

1 teaspoon Golden Breakfast Power Spice Blend*

1 teaspoon baking powder

¼ cup cacao nibs or dark chocolate chips

These Cacao Muffins are a mildly sweet snack to really sink that chocolate craving! With a sizable amount of protein and fiber, they make for a great snack or even weekend breakfast. Cacao, rich in protective polyphenols, paired with the turmeric in my Golden Breakfast Blend synergizes to add even more cancer-fighting properties to this delicious treat. Occasional sweets with benefits? Sign me up!

Directions

1. Preheat oven to 350°F. Line a muffin tin with 12 paper liners.

2. In a mixing bowl, whisk together plant milk, date syrup, nut butter, and vanilla extract.

3. In a separate mixing bowl, fold together rolled oats, cacao powder, chia seeds, spice blend, and baking powder.

4. Stir the dry ingredients into the wet ingredients, until all is combined. Fold in chocolate chips or cacao nibs.

5. Scoop the batter into lined muffin cups using a measuring cup or ice cream scoop.

6. Bake 35–40 minutes, until a toothpick inserted into the center of a muffin comes out mostly clean. Let rest at least 5 minutes before serving.

*Substitute spice blend with ½ teaspoon Ceylon cinnamon, ½ teaspoon cacao powder, ¼ teaspoon ground turmeric.

CALORIES: 175 · FAT: 6G · CARBS: 23G · FIBER: 6G · SUGARS: 7G · ADDED SUGARS: 5G · PROTEIN: 7G

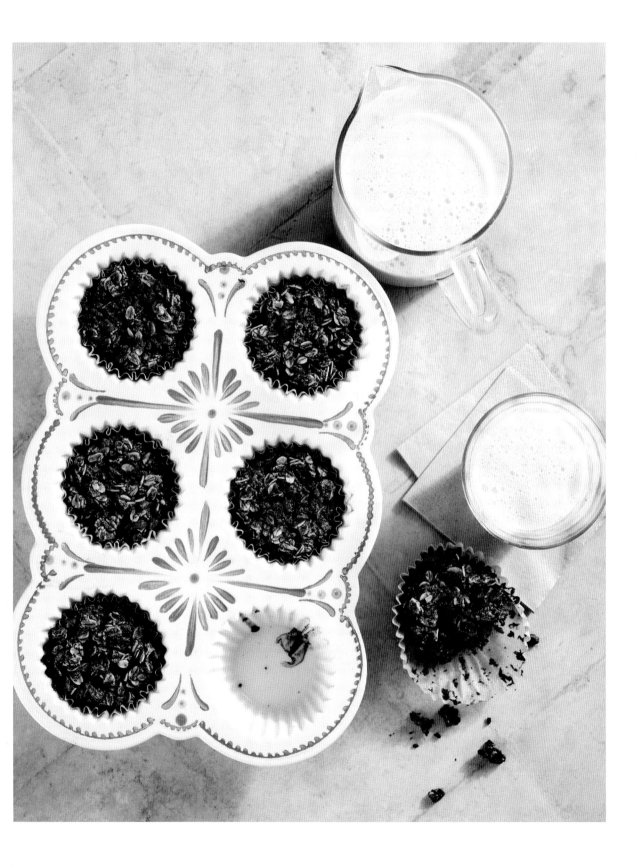

Banana Chia Crisps

PREP TIME	COOK TIME	SERVES
10 MINUTES	30 MINUTES	4

Ingredients

2 bananas, peeled

¼ **cup** chia seeds

2 **tablespoons** sliced almonds

1½ **tablespoons** cacao powder

1 **teaspoon** Cinnapeel Spicer Power Spice Blend*

1 **teaspoon** vanilla extract

These slightly sweet Banana Chia Crisps are the perfect chewy and portable snack to toss in a bag for a busy day on your feet. A generous dose of chia, with its extra fiber and omega-3s, and a few pinches of my flavorful warming Power Spices, you're on your way to a powerful day. Simplicity at its best!

Directions

1. Preheat oven to 350°F. Line a sheet pan with parchment paper.

2. In a mixing bowl, mash bananas with a fork. Fold in all remaining ingredients to create a dough.

3. Transfer small dollops of the dough to the prepared sheet pan and press down to flatten with the back of a fork.

4. Bake 25–30 minutes, until crisp around the edges. Let cool at least 10 minutes as they will crisp further as they cool.

TIP: Store covered and refrigerated for up to 5 days. To re-crisp, place in a toaster oven for 3 minutes.

*Substitute spice blend with ¾ teaspoon Ceylon cinnamon, ½ teaspoon granulated orange peel, pinch of ground ginger.

CALORIES: 165 · FAT: 8G · CARBS: 21G · FIBER: 9G · SUGARS: 6G · ADDED SUGARS: 0G · PROTEIN: 6G

Super Seed Crackers

PREP TIME	COOK TIME	SERVING SIZE	SERVES
10 MINUTES	60 MINUTES	6 CRACKERS	20

Ingredients

1½ cups almond flour

1 cup water

¾ cup sesame seeds

3 tablespoons extra-virgin olive oil

3 tablespoons tahini paste

4 tablespoons chia or ground flaxseeds

1 teaspoon Vegitude Power Spice Blend*

⅛ teaspoon salt

On one of my culinary adventures in Israel, my good friend Diti served my family and me these crackers that were perfect alongside some homemade hummus. This recipe was so delicious and nutrient-packed that I offered her a jar of my Vegitude Power Spice Blend in exchange for the recipe; I now proudly serve these crackers to my guests, who can't help but ask where I buy them. Now, it's your turn to enjoy these super powered-up, great-for-you flavors right in the comfort of your own home!

Directions

1. Preheat oven to 275°F.

2. In a mixing bowl, combine all ingredients. Set aside and let dough rest 30 minutes. If it feels dry, add a little water.

3. Split the dough in half, and place each half of the dough onto a piece of parchment paper. Cover the top of the dough with another piece of parchment paper and use a rolling pin to spread until dough is about ⅛-inch thick. Remove and discard the top sheet of the parchment. Transfer the rolled dough, with the bottom sheets of parchment, onto 2 sheet pans.

4. Bake 60 minutes, until golden and dry. Break into cracker-sized pieces before serving.

*Substitute spice blend with ¼ teaspoon granulated garlic, ¼ teaspoon granulated onion, ¼ teaspoon ground turmeric, ⅛ teaspoon dried parsley, pinch of black pepper.

CALORIES: 110 · FAT: 8G · CARBS: 5G · FIBER: 3G · SUGARS: 1G · ADDED SUGARS: 0G · PROTEIN: 3G

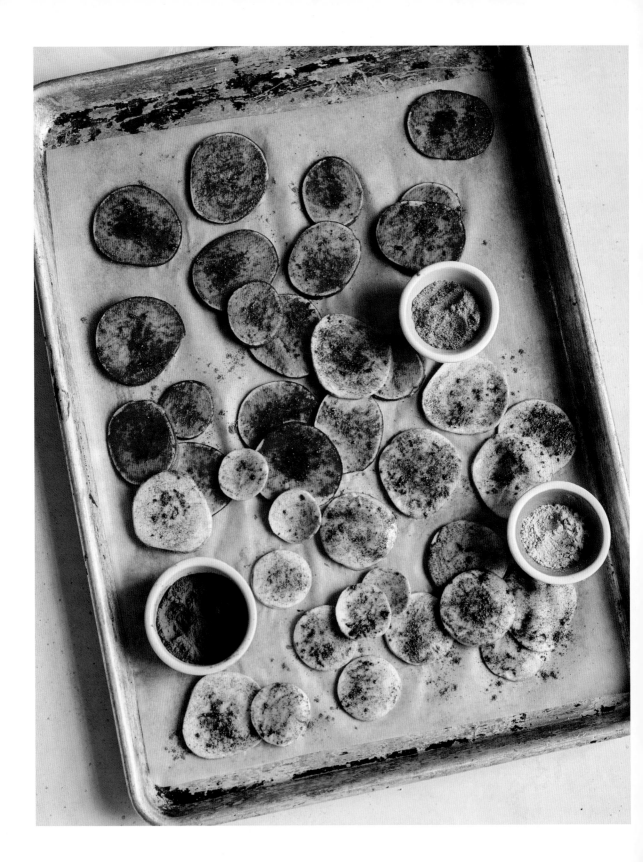

Spiced Sweet Potato and Parsnip Chips

PREP TIME	COOK TIME	SERVES
15 MINUTES	35 MINUTES	4

Ingredients

2 medium sweet potatoes

2 parsnips

1 tablespoon avocado oil

1 teaspoon Morning Boost Power Spice Blend*

Salt, to taste

These simple and savory crisps make a warm treat as an afternoon snack or even a great appetizer for a holiday event! The spice blend adds a warm, spicy-sweet depth (think apple pie!) with Ceylon cinnamon, allspice, nutmeg, ginger, and cloves—dramatically cranking up the antioxidant and anti-inflammatory punch of these coins. Here are some fun facts—clove has ranked as the #1 food in terms of antioxidant content. Ceylon cinnamon imbues a warm sweetness and— along with allspice, nutmeg, and ginger—may help balance blood sugars. A pinch of flavor and protection goes a long way!

Directions

1. Preheat oven to 400°F. Line a sheet pan with parchment paper.

2. Thinly slice the sweet potatoes and parsnips into chips.

3. In a mixing bowl, toss the sweet potatoes and parsnips in oil and spice blend.

4. Arrange in a single layer on the prepared sheet pan.

5. Bake 30–35 minutes, until crispy and browned around the edges. Lightly season with salt to taste as soon as they are removed from the oven.

*Substitute spice blend with ¾ teaspoon Ceylon cinnamon, pinch of each: ground ginger, nutmeg, allspice, ground cloves.

CALORIES: 135 · FAT: 4G · CARBS: 25G · FIBER: 6G · SUGARS: 6G · ADDED SUGARS: 0G · PROTEIN: 2G

Green Pea Fritters

PREP TIME	COOK TIME	SERVING SIZE	SERVES
15 MINUTES	25 MINUTES	2 FRITTERS	6

Ingredients

2 teaspoons extra-virgin olive oil

1 yellow onion, diced

3 cloves garlic, minced

2 cups frozen peas

¾ cup almond flour

1 teaspoon baking soda

1 teaspoon Vegitude Power Spice Blend*

½ teaspoon salt

Get ready to "pea-lease" your taste buds with my savory Green Pea Fritters. They make a great protein-packed snack that's fiber-rich and budget friendly. Many people looking for variety in their plant-based proteins often overlook the humble pea, which is rich in plant compounds that may have anti-cancer effects. "Peas" be sure you don't count these out!

Directions

1. Preheat oven to 350°F. Line a sheet pan with parchment paper.

2. Heat olive oil in a skillet over medium heat. Add the onion and garlic to the skillet and sauté 5 minutes.

3. Meanwhile, run the frozen peas under warm water to thaw. Transfer to a food processor.

4. Add the cooked onion and garlic to the peas in the food processor and process until a thick paste has formed.

5. Transfer the pea mixture to a mixing bowl and stir in almond flour, baking soda, spice blend, and salt. Wet your hands and form the mixture into patties. Transfer to the lined sheet pan.

6. Bake 15–20 minutes, flipping fritters halfway through, until lightly browned.

*Substitute spice blend with ¼ teaspoon granulated garlic, ¼ teaspoon granulated onion, ¼ teaspoon ground turmeric, ⅛ teaspoon dried parsley, pinch of black pepper.

CALORIES: 145 · FAT: 9G · CARBS: 11G · FIBER: 5G · SUGARS: 4G · ADDED SUGARS: 0G · PROTEIN: 6G

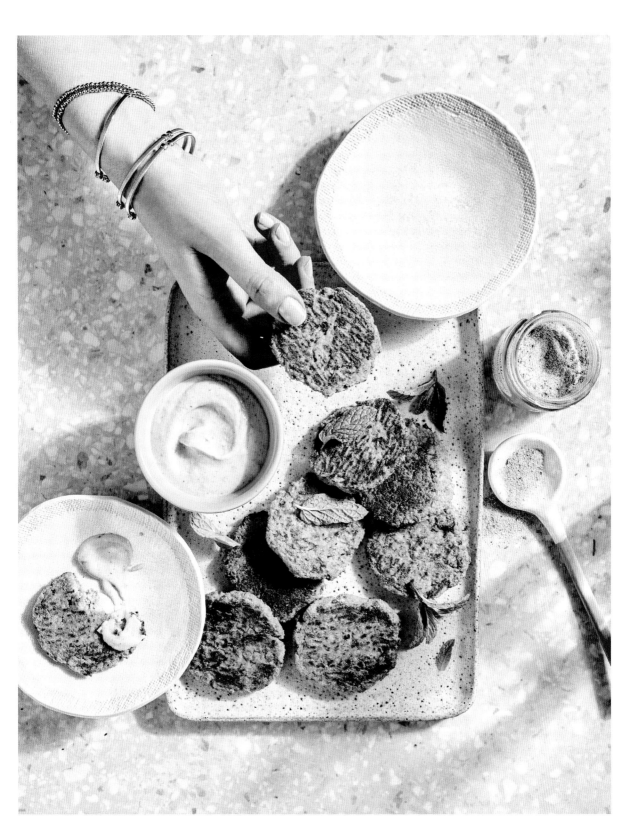

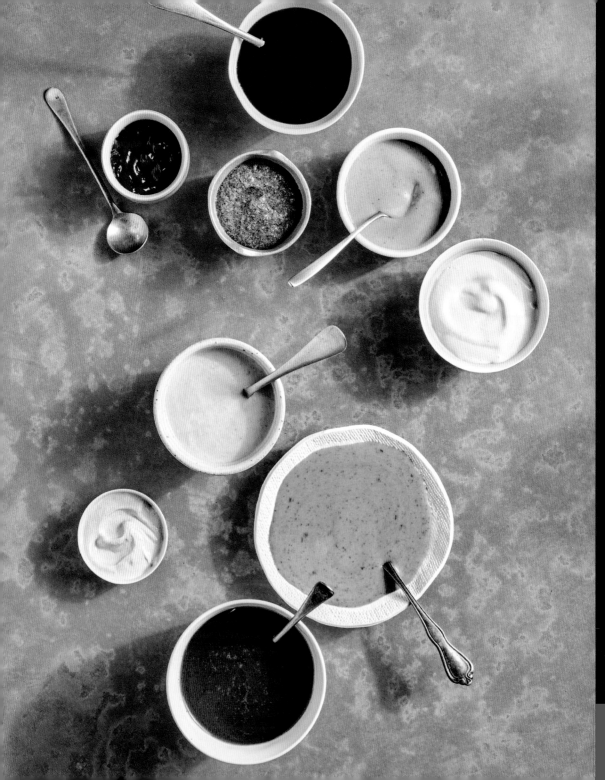

Sauces & Dressings

As they say, the secret is in the sauce. These dips and dressings are made with healthy fats, loaded with spices, and free from unnecessary additives. They're the perfect way to add some pizzazz to your salads, crudités, and everything in between. I suggest having at least one of these dressings on hand throughout the week since this makes adding a dollop of goodness to your meals that much easier. Take your taste buds on a wild ride!

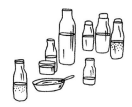

Basic Vinaigrette

PREP TIME	SERVING SIZE	SERVES
5 MINUTES	1 TABLESPOON	8

Ingredients

¼ **cup** balsamic vinegar

¼ **cup** extra-virgin olive oil

2 **teaspoons** Dijon mustard

2 **teaspoons** honey

½ **teaspoon** Italian seasoning

Salt and pepper, to taste

Whipping up a great vinaigrette should be as easy as snapping your fingers! You won't even miss the ultra-refined oils and funky fillers you find typically in store-bought dressings when you try this recipe. It's wholesome, clean, and downright delicious!

Directions

1. In a mixing bowl, whisk together all ingredients until smooth and combined. Store refrigerated for up to 10 days.

TIP: This basic recipe can be adjusted as you please using your choice of vinegar in place of the balsamic, your choice of oil in place of the olive oil, and your choice of dried herbs in place of the Italian seasoning.

CALORIES: 80 · FAT: 7G · CARBS: 5G · FIBER: 0G · SUGARS: 2G · ADDED SUGARS: 1G · PROTEIN: 0G

Miso Dressing

PREP TIME	SERVING SIZE	SERVES
5 MINUTES	2 TABLESPOONS	4

Ingredients

3 tablespoons white miso paste

2 tablespoons water

1 tablespoon sesame oil

1 tablespoon rice vinegar

1 tablespoon coconut aminos or tamari

1 teaspoon honey

This simple "probiotic-rich" dressing is a great way to support your gut health! A flavor-packed addition that goes great on salads or vegetable bowls and will have you coming back for seconds. Say goodbye to unused miso paste and hello to a new staple in your kitchen!

Directions

1. In a mixing bowl, whisk together all ingredients, until smooth and combined. Store refrigerated for up to 4 days.

CALORIES: 65 · FAT: 4G · CARBS: 6G · FIBER: 1G · SUGARS: 3G · ADDED SUGARS: 1G · PROTEIN: 2G

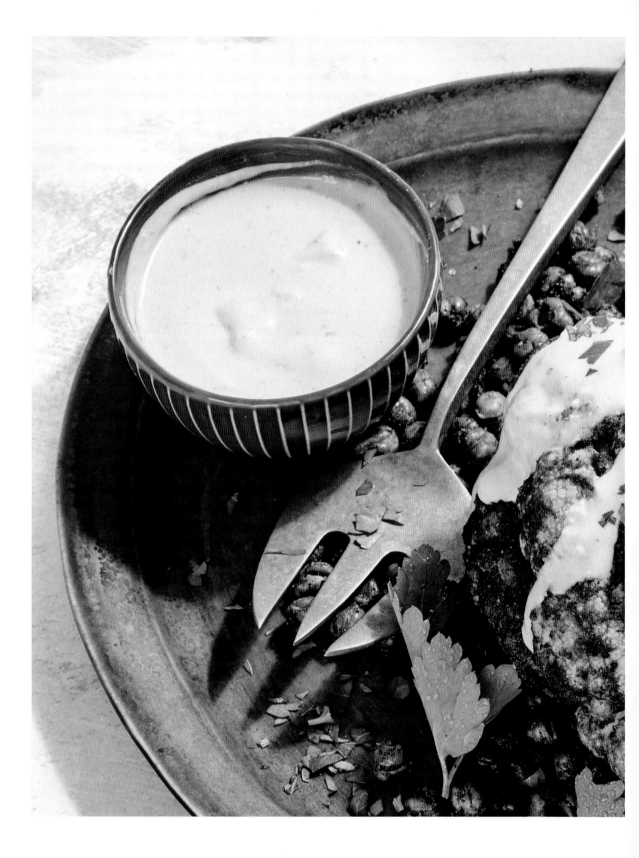

Tahini Sauce Two Ways

PREP TIME	SERVING SIZE	SERVES
5 MINUTES	2 TABLESPOONS	8

Ingredients

½ **cup** tahini paste

½ **cup** water

Juice of lemon

Salt, to taste

GOLDEN TAHINI SAUCE

2 teaspoons Vegitude Power Spice Blend*

GREEN TAHINI SAUCE

½ **cup** parsley, minced

Tahini is a "rock star" as a sauce or salad dressing! It's a win-win as sesame seeds are one of my favorite nutritional superheroes—they add richness, depth, and are packed with protective lignans, which means breast cancer-risk reduction and a total game-changer for cardiac health. Make this on autopilot! Customize it any way you want to fit your taste and power up the nutritional value—add Vegitude Power Blend for a pop of yellow, or fresh parsley for a burst of green.

Directions

1. Place all ingredients in a blender. Blend 20 seconds, until smooth.

2. Add additional ingredients for the version of the sauce that you'd like to make.

3. Store refrigerated for up to 4 days.

TIP: If the blended sauce is too thick, add additional water 1 tablespoon at a time until it has reached your desired consistency.

*Substitute spice blend with ½ teaspoon granulated garlic, ½ teaspoon granulated onion, ½ teaspoon ground turmeric, ¼ teaspoon dried parsley, pinch of black pepper.

CALORIES: 115 · FAT: 9G · CARBS: 3G · FIBER: 2G · SUGARS: 0G · ADDED SUGARS: 0G · PROTEIN: 5G

Vegan Alfredo Sauce

PREP TIME	SERVING SIZE	SERVES
15 MINUTES	¼ CUP	8

Ingredients

1½ cups raw cashews

1 cup hot water

2 cloves garlic

2 tablespoons nutritional yeast

1 teaspoon Vegitude Power Spice Blend*

Juice of ½ lemon

Salt and pepper, to taste

Alfredo, schmalfredo! Who needs heavy cream and butter when you can make an equally luscious and creamy version of this classic sauce that's ALSO packed with nutritional power! Perfectly versatile, this sauce can jazz up your favorite pasta dish, be used as a dressing for your salad, or even mixed with marinara sauce for an irresistible vodka sauce. Try this and you'll never go back to the store-bought stuff again!

Directions

1. Place cashews in a bowl and cover with hot water. Let soak for 10 minutes.

2. Transfer the soaked cashews and water to a blender or food processor.

3. Add the remaining ingredients to the blender and pulse until entirely smooth.

4. Season with salt and pepper to taste before serving.

TIP: If the blended sauce is too thick, add additional water 1 tablespoon at a time until it has reached your desired consistency.

*Substitute spice blend with ¼ teaspoon granulated garlic, ¼ teaspoon granulated onion, ¼ teaspoon ground turmeric, ⅛ teaspoon dried parsley, pinch of black pepper.

CALORIES: 130 · FAT: 9G · CARBS: 7G · FIBER: 1G · SUGARS: 2G · ADDED SUGARS: 0G · PROTEIN: 5G

Spicy Nut Sauce

PREP TIME	SERVING SIZE	SERVES
5 MINUTES	2 TABLESPOONS	4

Ingredients

2 tablespoons nut or seed butter

2 tablespoons coconut aminos or tamari

1 tablespoon sriracha sauce

2 teaspoons minced fresh ginger

2 teaspoons rice vinegar

1 teaspoon honey

1 teaspoon sesame oil

Made with natural nut or seed butter, ginger, and a kick of sriracha, it's the perfect dipping sauce for veggies, or drizzle over a stir-fry or tofu bowl for an extra punch of flavor. It's so good you'll want to lick the bowl clean!

Directions

1. In a mixing bowl, stir together all ingredients until smooth and combined. Store refrigerated for up to 4 days.

TIP: If the blended sauce is too thick, add additional water 1 tablespoon at a time until it has reached your desired consistency.

CALORIES: 70 · FAT: 5G · CARBS: 4G · FIBER: 1G · SUGARS: 3G · ADDED SUGARS: 1G · PROTEIN: 3G

Smoky Ketchup

PREP TIME	SERVING SIZE	SERVES
5 MINUTES	2 TABLESPOONS	4

Ingredients

3 ½ **tablespoons** tomato paste

2 ½ **tablespoons** water

1 **tablespoon** white vinegar

2 **teaspoons** honey

2 **teaspoons** smoked paprika

¼ **teaspoon** onion powder

Salt, to taste

Ketchup on a whole new level with something smoky and delicious! Say farewell to store-bought ketchup, loaded with added refined sugars and preservatives, and say hello to a healthier and tastier alternative that you can easily make at home. Use in moderation to truly savor the flavor.

Directions

1. In a mixing bowl, stir together all ingredients until smooth and combined. Store refrigerated for up to 5 days.

CALORIES: 25 · FAT: 0G · CARBS: 6G · FIBER: 1G · SUGARS: 4G · ADDED SUGARS: 3G · PROTEIN: 1G

Creamy Avocado Lime Dressing

PREP TIME	SERVING SIZE	SERVES
5 MINUTES	2 TABLESPOONS	8

Ingredients

1 avocado

½ cup plant-based plain yogurt

Juice of 2 limes

4 tablespoons fresh cilantro

2 teaspoons honey

2 teaspoons Tex Mex Power Spice Blend*

Salt, to taste

Level up taco nights with this creamy Tex Mex dressing built on avocado, lime, and cilantro! It's great for drizzling over taco salads, burrito bowls, or in place of sour cream on my Bell Pepper Nachos (recipe page 271).

Directions

1. Place all ingredients in a personal blender and process until mostly smooth.

2. Season with salt to taste before serving.

*Substitute spice blend with 1 teaspoon chili powder, ½ teaspoon paprika, ½ teaspoon ground cumin, ¼ teaspoon granulated onion, ¼ teaspoon granulated garlic, ¼ teaspoon dried oregano, ⅛ teaspoon crushed red pepper flakes and ⅛ teaspoon black pepper, pinch of Ceylon cinnamon and pinch of ground cloves.

CALORIES: 45 · FAT: 3G · CARBS: 3G · FIBER: 2G · SUGARS: 2G · ADDED SUGARS: 1G · PROTEIN: 1G

Plant-Based Caesar Dressing

PREP TIME	SERVING SIZE	SERVES
5 MINUTES	2 TABLESPOONS	8

Ingredients

1 cup plant-based plain yogurt

2 tablespoons capers, drained and rinsed

2 tablespoons nutritional yeast

2 cloves garlic

2 teaspoons Dijon mustard

2 teaspoons lemon juice

½ teaspoon pepper

Typically made with anchovy and Parmesan cheese, my creamy dressing is a great plant-based alternative that adds a zesty kick to your standard Caesar.

Directions

1. Place all ingredients in a personal blender and process until mostly smooth.

2. If the mixture is a little thick, thin out with water a few teaspoons at a time, until your desired consistency.

3. For the best flavor, cover and refrigerate 30 minutes before serving.

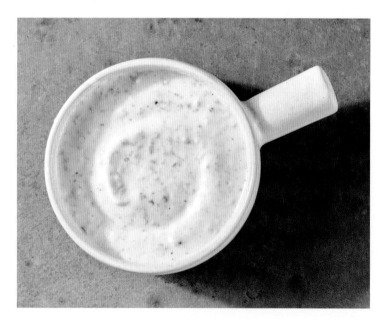

CALORIES: 20 · FAT: 1G · CARBS: 2G · FIBER: 1G · SUGARS: 1G · ADDED SUGARS: 1G · PROTEIN: 2G

Vegan Pesto Sauce

PREP TIME	SERVING SIZE	SERVES
10 MINUTES	¼ CUP	8

Ingredients

2 packed cups fresh basil

3 tablespoons water

2 tablespoons extra-virgin olive oil

2 tablespoons nutritional yeast

1 tablespoon toasted pine nuts

Juice of ½ lemon

2 cloves garlic

Salt and pepper, to taste

Green is the new black in the sauce world and this pesto is no different! It's everything you love about classic pesto with its cheesy, savory flavors but with a plant-based twist that's sure to satisfy.

Directions

1. Add all ingredients to a food processor or personal blender and pulse until mostly smooth.

2. Season with salt and pepper to taste before serving.

TIP: To toast pine nuts, place them in a dry skillet over medium heat and, moving them around the skillet constantly to prevent burning, toast until golden brown and fragrant.

CALORIES: 90 · FAT: 8G · CARBS: 2G · FIBER: 1G · SUGARS: 0G · ADDED SUGARS: 0G · PROTEIN: 2G

Sesame Dressing

PREP TIME	SERVING SIZE	SERVES
5 MINUTES	1 TABLESPOON	16

Ingredients

Juice of 2 limes

¼ **cup** avocado oil

¼ **cup** coconut aminos or tamari

2 tablespoons sesame oil

1½ tablespoons pure maple syrup

Salt, to taste

Sesame-sational news! Fragrant sesame oil meets tangy lime juice and a touch of sweet maple syrup for a flavor-packed dressing that will make any salad shine. I had to include this recipe for all my patients who love the Quinoa and Edamame Salad (recipe page 225) that can't get enough of that sesame goodness.

Directions

1. In a mixing bowl, whisk together all ingredients until smooth and combined.

2. Season with salt to taste. Store refrigerated for up to 5 days.

TIP: For even more flavor, add a few pinches of zest from the lime as well.

CALORIES: 58 · FAT: 5G · CARBS: 3G · FIBER: 0G · SUGARS: 2G · ADDED SUGARS: 1G · PROTEIN: 0G

Caramel Sauce

PREP TIME	COOK TIME	SERVING SIZE	SERVES
5 MINUTES	2 MINUTES	1 TABLESPOON	16

Ingredients

10 pitted dates

¾ cup unsweetened plant milk

½ teaspoon Cinnapeel Spicer Power Spice Blend*

Pinch of salt

½ teaspoon vanilla extract, optional

Made from sweet, succulent dates, it's the perfect addition to everything from oatmeal and breakfast cookies to parfaits, sliced apples, and berries. With its natural sweetness and feel-good flavor, you can indulge in this simple sauce knowing that a little goes a long way toward sweet success!

Directions

1. Soak the dates in hot water for 5 minutes. Drain the water.

2. Place the drained dates and all other ingredients in a blender and blend until smooth. Serve warm or chilled.

TIP: If the blended sauce is too thick, add additional plant milk 1 tablespoon at a time until it has reached your desired consistency.

*Substitute spice blend with ¼ teaspoon Ceylon cinnamon, ¼ teaspoon granulated orange peel, pinch of ground ginger.

CALORIES: 20 · FAT: 0G · CARBS: 5G · FIBER: 1G · SUGARS: 3G · ADDED SUGARS: 0G · PROTEIN: 0.5G

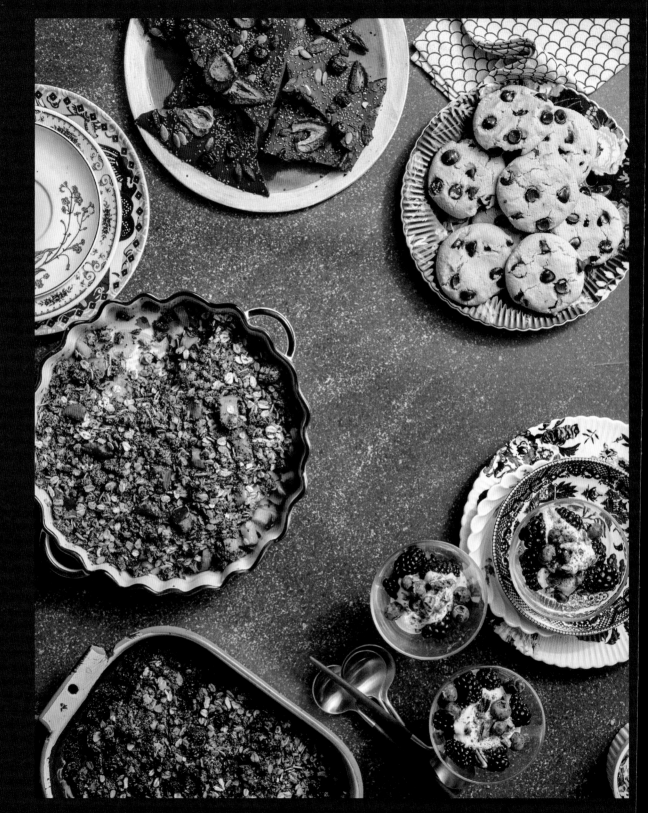

Desserts

I don't encourage having super sweet desserts, as that can intensify sugar cravings. But completely ignoring a sweet tooth may just make you feel deprived and enhance your urges. Enter these Beller Method desserts. They're mildly sweet by design to wean you from intense sugar cravings and contain ingredients that may help modulate your blood sugars rather than spike them. Reach for one of these extra delicious treats on occasion when you need a little extra, and don't feel guilty when you do indulge— just be mindful of portions and enjoy them in moderation. My mantra: It's what you do most of the time, not sometimes, that makes a difference when it comes to your long-term health.

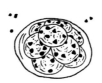

Spiced Blueberry Crumble

PREP TIME	COOK TIME	SERVES
15 MINUTES	45 MINUTES	12

Ingredients

Avocado oil spray

2 ½ **cups** blueberries

1 ½ **tablespoons** arrowroot powder

1 **tablespoon** lemon juice

1 **teaspoon** vanilla extract

3 **tablespoons** pure maple syrup, divided

1 **cup** rolled oats (sprouted preferred)

¼ **cup** ground flaxseed

¼ **cup** chia seeds

¼ **cup** almond flour

1 **teaspoon** Cinnapeel Spicer Power Spice Blend*

2 **tablespoons** avocado or walnut oil

I'm "berry" excited to share one of my favorite desserts (but don't tell the others)! My Spiced Blueberry Crumble will satisfy that sweet tooth while keeping you in that good-for-you mindset. It keeps well and can be eaten chilled or warmed the next day—if I send dinner guests home with desserts, I always make sure to hold onto a slice or two for myself!

Directions

1. Preheat oven to 350°F. Lightly spray a pie plate or 9-inch baking dish with avocado oil spray.

2. In a mixing bowl, toss the blueberries in arrowroot powder, lemon juice, vanilla extract, and ½ of the maple syrup. Transfer to the prepared pie plate.

3. In a separate mixing bowl, toss the oats, flaxseed, chia seeds, almond flour, and spice blend.

4. Whisk the 2 tablespoons of oil with the remaining maple syrup and fold into the oat mixture until oats are evenly coated. Spoon over the fruit in the pie plate. Cover with parchment paper and foil.

5. Bake 45–60 minutes, until the fruit is bubbly hot and oat topping is golden brown. Let cool 10 minutes before serving.

*Substitute spice blend with ¾ teaspoon Ceylon cinnamon, ½ teaspoon granulated orange peel, pinch of ground ginger.

CALORIES: 140 · FAT: 7G · CARBS: 18G · FIBER: 5G · SUGARS: 6G · ADDED SUGARS: 3G · PROTEIN: 4G

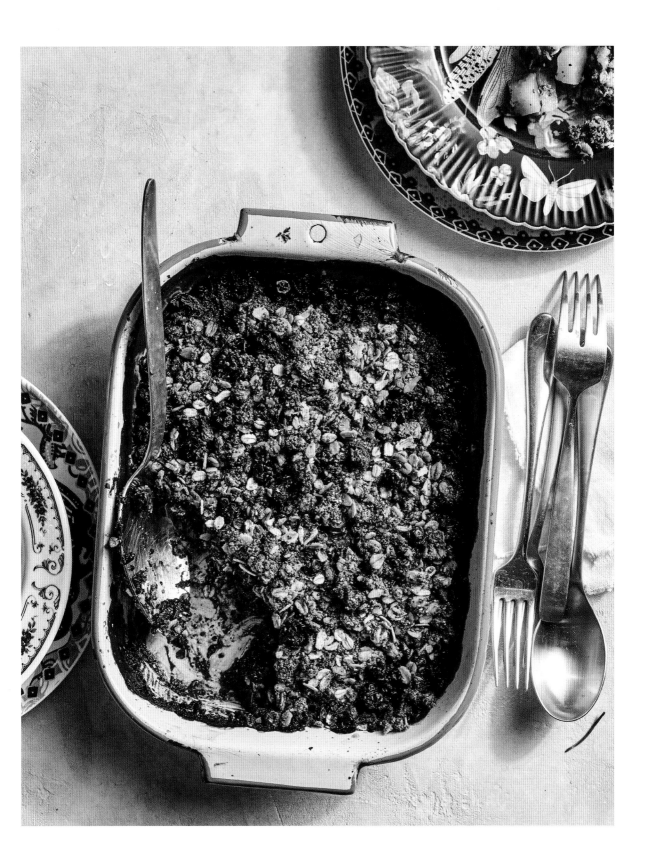

Quinoa Chocolate Crunch Rounds

PREP TIME	COOK TIME	SERVES
10 MINUTES	10 MINUTES	12

Ingredients

1 cup uncooked quinoa

1 cup dark chocolate chips

1 teaspoon avocado oil

My favorite twist on an old favorite—think Nestlé Crunch bar with crunchy quinoa and dark chocolate. The dark chocolate delivers powerful antioxidants while fiber and protein help keep our blood sugars a little more balanced than most chocolate treats. I love and suggest enjoying it as a nice "power treat" with a nice power tonic on the side.

Directions

1. Line a muffin tin with 12 paper liners.

2. Preheat a large skillet over medium-high heat until nearly smoking hot.

3. Add ½ of the quinoa to the skillet and, stirring constantly, toast 3–4 minutes, until you hear the quinoa pop. Quinoa should smell fragrant and toasted and lightly brown.

4. Transfer the toasted quinoa to a mixing bowl and repeat the last step to toast the remaining ½ cup of quinoa. Transfer to the mixing bowl.

5. Reduce heat to low and add the chocolate and avocado oil to the skillet. Stirring constantly, heat just until melted.

6. Remove the chocolate from the heat and stir in the toasted quinoa.

7. Pour the chocolate and quinoa mixture evenly among the 12 lined muffin cups.

8. Freeze for 1 hour before removing from the paper liners to serve. Once cooled in the freezer, the chocolate rounds can be stored in either the fridge or the freezer, though I like them best straight out of the freezer.

CALORIES: 165 · FAT: 7G · CARBS: 22G · FIBER: 2G · SUGARS: 10G · ADDED SUGARS: 9G · PROTEIN: 3G

Crunchy Coconut Clusters

PREP TIME	COOK TIME	SERVES
10 MINUTES	20 MINUTES	20

Ingredients

3 cups unsweetened coconut flakes

½ cup shelled pumpkin seeds

¼ cup pure maple syrup

3 tablespoons avocado oil

2 tablespoons date syrup

1 teaspoon Morning Boost Power Spice Blend*

A satisfyingly crunchy treat for all you coconut lovers out there. Even if you're not usually a fan of coconut, you'll be hooked—my family loves the added touch of date syrup, and they're always a hit at family dinners. Quick and easy to make too—whip up a batch in minutes!

Directions

1. Preheat oven to 325°F. Line a sheet pan with parchment paper.

2. In a mixing bowl, stir together all ingredients.

3. Pour out onto the prepared sheet pan and flatten out with a spatula to form a tight layer.

4. Bake 15–20 minutes, until coconut is golden brown.

5. Let cool for 15 minutes before breaking apart to make bite-sized clusters.

*Substitute spice blend with ¾ teaspoon Ceylon cinnamon, ⅛ teaspoon ground ginger, ⅛ teaspoon nutmeg, pinch of allspice, pinch of ground cloves.

CALORIES: 135 · FAT: 11G · CARBS: 8G · FIBER: 3G · SUGARS: 5G · ADDED SUGARS: 4G · PROTEIN: 2G

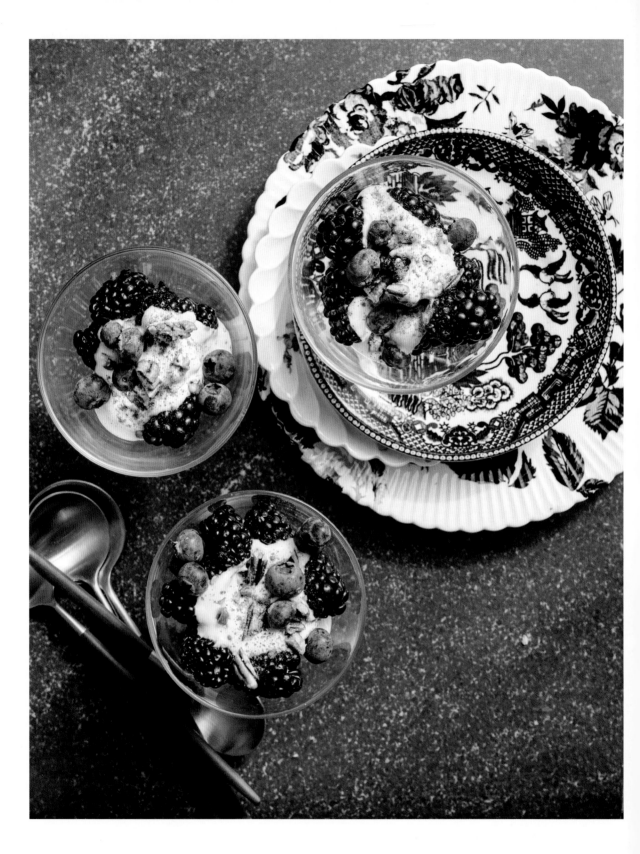

Berry Parfaits, Your Way!

PREP TIME
10 MINUTES

SERVES
1

Ingredients

½ **cup** any berries
(raspberries, blueberries,
blackberries, strawberries)

2 tablespoons plain plant-
based yogurt

1 tablespoon chopped nuts
(almonds, pistachios, pecans
or walnuts)

1 tablespoon Caramel Sauce
(recipe page 305), optional

This fruity delight will leave you feeling light and
wholesome. Customize it to your heart's content with a
beautiful presentation that will make you feel like you're
indulging in something truly special. Fresh and easy-to-
make—a parfait dessert with nutritional perks!

Directions

1. Place berries in a
   serving bowl.

2. Top with yogurt and
   sprinkle with chopped
   nuts of your choice.

3. Drizzle with a small
   amount of caramel
   sauce, if desired.

CALORIES: 80 · FAT: 5G · CARBS: 14G · FIBER: 5G · SUGARS: 3G · ADDED SUGARS: 0G · PROTEIN:3G

Basic Chocolate Chip Cookies

PREP TIME	COOK TIME	SERVES
10 MINUTES	20 MINUTES	12

Ingredients

1½ **cups** almond flour

1½ **teaspoons** baking powder

3 **tablespoons** avocado or walnut oil

3 **tablespoons** pure maple syrup

2 **tablespoons** unsweetened plant milk

1 **teaspoon** vanilla extract

⅓ **cup** dark chocolate chips

My nutritious take on a classic treat, these chocolate chip cookies are sweetened with a touch of 100% pure maple syrup. The almond flour contains cancer protective antioxidants and adds heart-healthy fats and a bit of protein to leave you feeling satisfied.

Directions

1. Preheat oven to 350°F. Line a sheet pan with parchment paper.

2. In a mixing bowl, stir together almond flour and baking powder.

3. Stir in the oil, maple syrup, plant milk, and vanilla extract, until a dough has formed. Fold in chocolate chips.

4. Drop heaping tablespoons of the dough onto the parchment paper-lined sheet pan. Cover with another piece of parchment paper and use your hand to flatten each into a cookie shape. Discard top sheet of parchment.

5. Bake 15–20 minutes for soft cookies, or 20–25 minutes for crunchier cookies. Let cool 5 minutes before serving.

CALORIES: 160 · FAT: 12G · CARBS: 10G · FIBER: 3G · SUGARS: 7G · ADDED SUGARS: 6G · PROTEIN: 5G

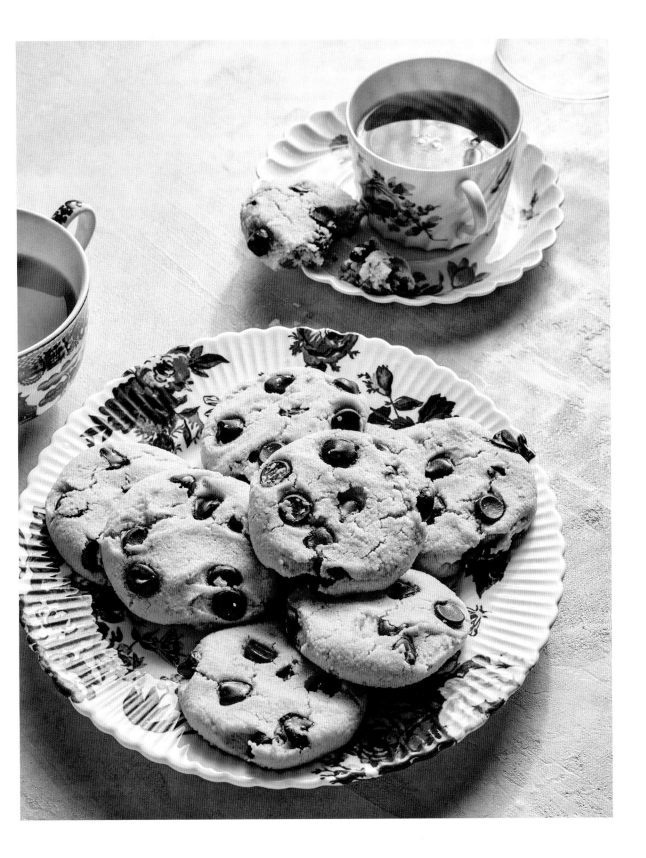

Chocolate Fix Cookies

PREP TIME	COOK TIME	SERVES
10 MINUTES	15 MINUTES	10

Ingredients

¾ **cup** almond flour

⅓ **cup** unsweetened cacao powder

¼ **cup** unsweetened plant milk

3 ½ **tablespoons** coconut sugar

2 teaspoons Golden Breakfast Power Spice Blend*

¾ **teaspoon** baking powder

Dark chocolate chips, chia seeds, or chopped almonds, optional, to top

Indulge in a guilt-free treat with these delicious chocolate cookies! Made with nutrient-rich almond flour, antioxidant-packed cacao powder, and a touch of coconut sugar, these cookies are a satisfying and simple dessert.

Directions

1. Preheat oven to 350°F. Line a sheet pan with parchment paper.

2. In a mixing bowl, fold together all ingredients to create a dough.

3. Drop heaping tablespoons of the dough onto the parchment paper-lined sheet pan. Cover with another piece of parchment paper and use your hand to flatten each into a cookie shape. Discard top sheet of parchment.

4. Top cookies with a few dark chocolate chips, chia seeds, or chopped almonds, if desired.

5. Bake 15 minutes. Let cool 5 minutes before serving.

*Substitute spice blend with 1 teaspoon Ceylon cinnamon, 1 teaspoon cacao powder, ½ teaspoon ground turmeric, dash of ground ginger.

CALORIES: 80 · FAT: 4G · CARBS: 8G · FIBER: 2G · SUGARS: 4G · ADDED SUGARS: 3G · PROTEIN: 3G

Spiced Snickerdoodle Cookies

PREP TIME	**COOK TIME**	**SERVES**
10 MINUTES	15 MINUTES	18

Ingredients

3 cups almond flour

2 teaspoons Cinnapeel Spicer Power Spice Blend*

½ teaspoon baking powder

½ teaspoon salt

½ cup avocado oil

½ cup pure maple syrup

1 tablespoon vanilla extract

1 tablespoon coconut sugar, optional

Satisfy your sweet tooth with these filling snickerdoodle cookies made from almond flour, avocado oil, pure maple syrup, and my Cinnapeel Spicer Power Spice Blend with Ceylon cinnamon—a blend that has you knowing you added more good to your dessert.

Directions

1. Preheat oven to 350°F. Line a sheet pan with parchment paper.

2. In a mixing bowl, stir together almond flour, spice blend, baking powder, and salt.

3. In a separate mixing bowl, stir together avocado oil, maple syrup, and vanilla extract.

4. Fold the wet ingredients into the dry ingredients until all is combined and a dough has formed.

5. Drop heaping tablespoons of the dough onto the parchment paper-lined sheet pan. Cover with another piece of parchment paper and use your hand to flatten each into a cookie shape. Discard top sheet of parchment. If desired, sprinkle additional Cinnapeel Spicer and a small amount of coconut sugar over top of the cookies for more color and flavor.

6. Bake 15 minutes, just until lightly browned. Let cool 5 minutes before serving.

*Substitute spice blend with 1½ teaspoon Ceylon cinnamon, 1 teaspoon granulated orange peel, dash of ground ginger.

CALORIES: 180 · FAT: 14G · CARBS: 10G · FIBER: 14G · SUGARS: 8G · ADDED SUGARS: 6G · PROTEIN: 6G

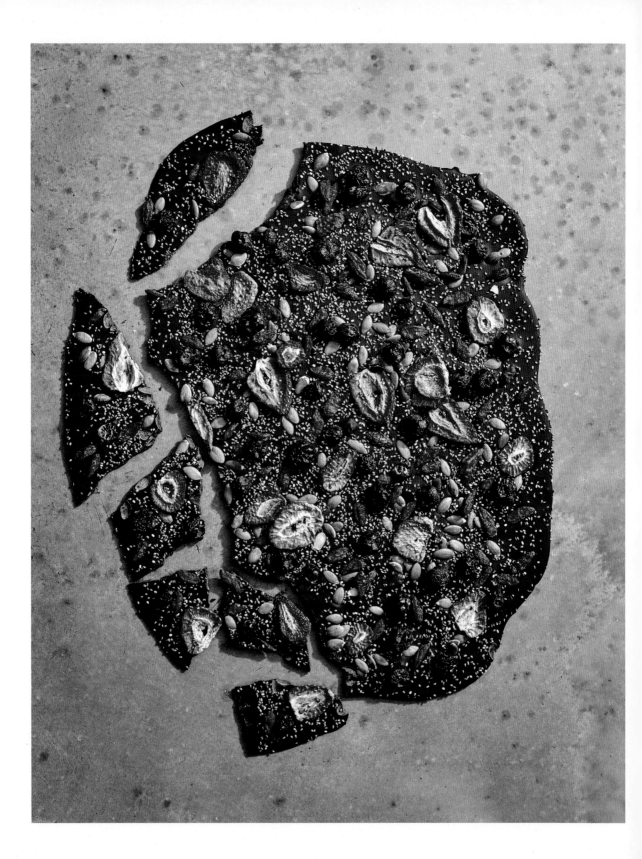

Power Chocolate Bark

PREP TIME	COOK TIME	SERVES
10 MINUTES	3 MINUTES	16

Ingredients

10 ounces dark chocolate chips

⅓ cup freeze dried berries

1 tablespoon goji berries

1 tablespoon shelled pumpkin seeds

1 teaspoon chia seeds

A mix of fiber-rich seeds, antioxidant-packed fruit, and dark chocolate loaded with protective polyphenols makes this a true power bark! With endless possibilities for toppings and mix-ins (think goji berries, pumpkin seeds, and more!), you can customize this bark to your heart's content. It's the perfect treat and sure to become your new go-to indulgence!

Directions

1. Line a sheet pan with parchment paper.

2. Place chocolate in a microwave-safe bowl and microwave in 15-second intervals, stirring in between, until fully melted.

3. Pour the melted chocolate onto the parchment paper and spread until less than ¼-inch thick.

4. Working quickly, top the chocolate with the freeze dried berries, goji berries, pumpkin seeds, and chia seeds. For the best results, use a clean spatula to lightly press the toppings down into the bark.

5. Let cool at least 2 hours before breaking or cutting into pieces to serve.

CALORIES: 100 · FAT: 6G · CARBS: 11G · FIBER: 2G · SUGARS: 9G · ADDED SUGARS: 8G · PROTEIN: 1G

Sesame Cookies

PREP TIME	COOK TIME	SERVES
15 MINUTES	15 MINUTES	18

Ingredients

1½ cups almond flour

½ cup tahini paste

2 tablespoons pure maple syrup

1 teaspoon vanilla extract

1 teaspoon Morning Boost Power Spice Blend*

¼ cup raw sesame seeds

Made with wholesome ingredients like tahini paste and sesame seeds, these nutritional powerhouses offer a delicious and filling treat. But beware: the biggest challenge lies in not devouring the batter before these hearty cookies even make it into the oven!

Directions

1. Preheat oven to 350°F. Line a sheet pan with parchment paper.

2. In a mixing bowl, fold together almond flour, tahini, maple syrup, vanilla extract, and spice blend. If the mixture is too dry to form a dough, add a small amount of plant milk until it can easily be rolled into balls.

3. Place the sesame seeds on a plate. Roll the dough into 18 balls and roll them in the sesame seeds to lightly coat before transferring to the prepared sheet pan.

4. Cover with a second piece of parchment paper and use your hand to flatten each into a cookie shape. Discard top sheet of parchment paper.

5. Bake for 10–15 minutes, until seeds are golden brown. Let cool 10 minutes before serving.

*Substitute ¾ teaspoon Ceylon cinnamon, ⅛ teaspoon ground ginger, ⅛ teaspoon nutmeg, pinch of allspice, pinch of ground cloves.

CALORIES: 90 · FAT: 7G · CARBS: 2G · FIBER: 2G · SUGARS: 2G · ADDED SUGARS: 1G · PROTEIN: 3G

Sweet Potato Brownies

PREP TIME	COOK TIME	SERVES
20 MINUTES	25 MINUTES	16

Ingredients

¾ **cup** baked and cooled sweet potato, scooped from peel

½ **cup** water

¼ **cup** pure maple syrup

1 **tablespoon** balsamic vinegar

2 **teaspoons** pure vanilla extract

1 **cup** oat or spelt flour

⅓ **cup** coconut sugar

⅓ **cup** dark chocolate chips

¼ **cup** unsweetened cocoa powder

1 **teaspoon** Cinnapeel Spicer Power Spice Blend*

1 **teaspoon** baking powder

¾ **teaspoon** baking soda

Pinch salt

A "spud-tacularly" pleasant twist on classic brownies! Not only are they a better-for-you treat, but they also hold a special place in my heart as my niece Karin and daughter Alexia loved making and recipe-testing these with me. Because I keep baked sweet potatoes on hand for breakfast, whipping up these delicious brownies becomes a breeze whenever someone is in need of a delightful treat.

Directions

1. Preheat oven to 350°F. Line an 8-inch square baking dish with parchment paper.

2. Place the sweet potato, water, maple syrup, balsamic vinegar, and vanilla extract in a blender and blend until smooth.

3. In a large mixing bowl, combine flour, coconut sugar, chocolate chips, cocoa powder, spice blend, baking powder, baking soda, and salt.

4. Mix the sweet potato mixture into the flour mixture, until all is well combined. Transfer to the prepared baking dish and smooth out the top.

5. Bake 21–25 minutes. Let cool at least 15 minutes before slicing to serve.

*Substitute spice blend with ¾ teaspoon Ceylon cinnamon, ½ teaspoon granulated orange peel, pinch of ground ginger.

CALORIES: 95 · FAT: 2G · CARBS: 18G · FIBER: 2G · SUGARS: 10G · ADDED SUGARS: 5G · PROTEIN: 2G

Quick Date Oatmeal Cookies

PREP TIME	COOK TIME	SERVES
10 MINUTES	15 MINUTES	16

Ingredients

1½ cups pitted dates

1½ cups rolled oats (sprouted preferred)

½ cup tahini paste or any seed butter

2 tablespoons pure maple syrup or honey, optional

With just 3–4 ingredients, this recipe will be stamped in your mind, making it your go-to when someone asks for a healthy dessert cookie. It's quick, easy, and incredibly satisfying— you can even customize the sweetness to suit your taste buds.

Directions

1. Preheat oven to 350°F. Line a sheet pan with parchment paper.

2. Soak dates for 5 minutes in hot water and drain.

3. Place all ingredients in a food processor and process until a thick dough has formed.

4. Roll the dough into 16 balls and place on the lined sheet pan.

5. Cover with a second piece of parchment paper and use your hand to flatten each into a cookie shape. Discard top sheet of parchment paper.

6. Bake for 10–15 minutes, until lightly browned. Let cool 10 minutes before serving.

CALORIES: 75 · FAT: 2G · CARBS: 12G · FIBER: 2G · SUGARS: 6G · ADDED SUGARS: 0G · PROTEIN: 2G

Chocolate Almond Butter Cake Cups

PREP TIME	COOK TIME	SERVES
15 MINUTES	25 MINUTES	12

Ingredients

2 tablespoons flaxseed to make 2 "flax eggs"

1½ cups black beans (cooked, drained, rinsed)

½ cup cacao powder

⅓ cup pure date or maple syrup

3 tablespoons avocado oil or applesauce

1 tablespoon baking powder

1 teaspoon Golden Breakfast Blend*

2 teaspoons vanilla extract

¼ cup dark chocolate chips

⅓ cup almond or sunflower seed butter, divided

Don't "bean" shy—these are not your ordinary brownies. Black beans are packed with fiber and protein—slip them in and you'll be full in no time. These treats are a smart choice for a wholesome, satisfying indulgence that will nourish your body and please the soul. Prepare to be amazed by how these brownies transform nutritious ingredients into a filling and decadent delight!

Directions

1. Preheat oven to 350°F.

2. Make the "flax eggs" by mixing the ground flaxseed with 5 tablespoons of water. Allow the "flax egg" mixture to gel for about 5 minutes.

3. Place muffin liners in a muffin tin.

4. In a blender, add "flax egg" mixture, black beans, cacao powder, syrup, oil (or applesauce), baking powder, spice blend, and vanilla. Blend for 20 seconds until smooth and creamy. Add in the chocolate chips.

5. Divide the mixture among the muffin cups. Place 1 teaspoon of the nut or seed butter in the center of each cup. Use a toothpick or chopstick to swirl the nut butter into the chocolate mixture.

6. Bake for 25 minutes. Let cool for about 15 minutes.

*Substitute spice blend with ½ teaspoon Ceylon cinnamon, ½ teaspoon cacao powder, ¼ teaspoon ground turmeric, pinch of ground ginger.

CALORIES: 145 · FAT: 6.5G · CARBS: 19.5G · FIBER: 3.5G · SUGARS: 9G · ADDED SUGARS: 0G · PROTEIN: 4.5G

References

DISCOVER THE POWER OF SPICING

1. Ahmadi A, Shadboorestan A. Oxidative stress and cancer; the role of hesperidin, a citrus natural bioflavonoid, as a cancer chemoprotective agent. Nutr Cancer. 2016;68(1):29-39. doi:10.1080/01635581.2015.1078822

2. Alsamr=i H, Athamneh K, Pintus G, Eid AH, Iratni R. Pharmacological and Antioxidant Activities of Rhus coriaria L. (Sumac). Antioxidants (Basel). Jan 8 2021;10(1)doi:10.3390/antiox10010073

3. American Institute for Cancer Research. The Spices of Cancer Prevention. AICR Science Now: American Institute for Cancer Research; 2013.

4. Azimi P, Ghiasvand R, Feizi A, Hariri M, Abbasi B. Effects of Cinnamon, Cardamom, Saffron, and Ginger Consumption on Markers of Glycemic Control, Lipid Profile, Oxidative Stress, and Inflammation in Type 2 Diabetes Patients. Rev Diabet Stud. Fall-Winter 2014;11(3-4):258-66. doi:10.1900/RDS.2014.11.258

5. Azimi P, Ghiasvand R, Feizi A, et al. Effect of cinnamon, cardamom, saffron and ginger consumption on blood pressure and a marker of endothelial function in patients with type 2 diabetes mellitus: A randomized controlled clinical trial. Blood Press. Jun 2016;25(3):133-40. doi:10.3109/08037051.2015.1111020

6. Azzeh FS. Synergistic effect of green tea, cinnamon and ginger combination on enhancing postprandial blood glucose. Pak J Biol Sci. Jan 15 2013;16(2):74-9. doi:10.3923/pjbs.2013.74.79

7. Bachmeier BE, Killian PH, Melchart D. The Role of Curcumin in Prevention and Management of Metastatic Disease. Int J Mol Sci. Jun 9 2018;19(6) doi:10.3390/ijms19061716

8. Bag A, Chattopadhyay RR. Evaluation of Synergistic Antibacterial and Antioxidant Efficacy of Essential Oils of Spices and Herbs in Combination. PLoS One. 2015;10(7):e0131321. doi:10.1371/journal.pone.0131321

9. Bahri S, Jameleddine S, Shlyonsky V. Relevance of carnosic acid to the treatment of several health disorders: Molecular targets and mechanisms. Biomed Pharmacother. Dec 2016;84:569-582. doi:10.1016/j.biopha.2016.09.067

10. Butt MS, Naz A, Sultan MT, Qayyum MM. Anti-oncogenic perspectives of spices/herbs: A comprehensive review. Excli j. 2013;12:1043-65.

11. Carlsen MH, Halvorsen BL, Holte K, et al. The total antioxidant content of more than 3100 foods, beverages, spices, herbs and supplements used worldwide. Nutr J. Jan 22 2010;9:3. doi:10.1186/1475-2891-9-3

12. Crowell PL. Monoterpenes in breast cancer chemoprevention. Breast Cancer Res Treat. Nov-Dec 1997;46(2-3):191-7. doi:10.1023/a:1005939806591

13. Desai G, Schelske-Santos M, Nazario CM, et al. Onion and Garlic Intake and Breast Cancer, a Case-Control Study in Puerto Rico. Nutrition and Cancer. 2020/07/03 2020;72(5):791-800. doi:10.1080/01635581.2019.1651349

14. Dudhatra GB, Mody SK, Awale MM, et al. A comprehensive review on pharmacotherapeutics of herbal bioenhancers. ScientificWorldJournal. 2012;2012:637953. doi:10.1100/2012/637953

15. Fuller S, Stephens JM. Diosgenin, 4-hydroxyisoleucine, and fiber from fenugreek: mechanisms of actions and potential effects on metabolic syndrome. Adv Nutr. Mar 2015;6(2):189-97. doi:10.3945/an.114.007807

16. Gonzalez-Vallinas M, Molina S, Vicente G, et al. Modulation of estrogen and epidermal growth factor receptors by rosemary extract in breast cancer cells. Electrophoresis. Jun 2014;35(11):1719-27. doi:10.1002/elps.201400011

17. Gonzalez-Vallinas M, Reglero G, Ramirez de Molina A. Rosemary (Rosmarinus officinalis L.) Extract as a Potential Complementary Agent in Anticancer Therapy. Nutr Cancer. 2015;67(8):1221-9. doi:10.1080/01635581.2015.1082110

18. Gottumukkala RV, Nadimpalli N, Sukala K, Subbaraju GV. Determination of Catechin and Epicatechin Content in Chocolates by High-Performance Liquid Chromatography. Int Sch Res Notices. 2014;2014:628196. doi:10.1155/2014/628196

19. Gutierrez J, Barry-Ryan C, Bourke P. The antimicrobial efficacy of plant essential oil combinations and interactions with food ingredients. Int J Food Microbiol. May 10 2008;124(1):91-7. doi:10.1016/j.ijfoodmicro.2008.02.028

20. Holt RR, Lazarus SA, Sullards MC, et al. Procyanidin dimer B2 [epicatechin-(4beta-8)-epicatechin] in human plasma after the consumption of a flavanol-rich cocoa. Am J Clin Nutr. Oct 2002;76(4):798-804. doi:10.1093/ajcn/76.4.798

21. Kim HG, Lee JH, Lee SJ, et al. The increased cellular uptake and biliary excretion of curcumin by quercetin: a possible role of albumin binding interaction. Drug Metab Dispos. Aug 2012;40(8):1452-5. doi:10.1124/dmd.111.044123

22. Kim MY, Trudel LJ, Wogan GN. Apoptosis induced by capsaicin and resveratrol in colon carcinoma cells requires nitric oxide production and caspase activation. Anticancer Res. Oct 2009;29(10):3733-40.

23. Li C, Schluesener H. Health-promoting effects of the citrus flavanone hesperidin. Crit Rev Food Sci Nutr. Feb 11 2017;57(3):613-631. doi:10.1080/10408398.2014.906382

24. Liu D, Chen Z. The effect of curcumin on breast cancer cells. J Breast Cancer. Jun 2013;16(2):133-7. doi:10.4048/jbc.2013.16.2.133

25. Lu QY, Summanen PH, Lee RP, et al. Prebiotic Potential and Chemical Composition of Seven Culinary Spice Extracts. J Food Sci. Aug 2017;82(8):1807-1813. doi:10.1111/1750-3841.13792

26. Majdalawieh AF, Carr RI. In vitro investigation of the potential immunomodulatory and anti-cancer activities of black pepper (Piper nigrum) and cardamom (Elettaria cardamomum). J Med Food. Apr 2010;13(2):371-81. doi:10.1089/jmf.2009.1131

27. Martin MA, Goya L, Ramos S. Potential for preventive effects of cocoa and cocoa polyphenols in cancer. Food Chem Toxicol. Jun 2013;56:336-51. doi:10.1016/j.fct.2013.02.020

28. Mirmosayyeb O, Tanhaei A, Sohrabi HR, et al. Possible Role of Common Spices as a Preventive and Therapeutic Agent for Alzheimer's Disease. Int J Prev Med. 2017;8:5. doi:10.4103/2008-7802.199640

29. Moore J, Yousef M, Tsiani E. Anticancer Effects of Rosemary (Rosmarinus officinalis L.) Extract and Rosemary Extract Polyphenols. Nutrients. Nov 17 2016;8(11)doi:10.3390/nu8110731

30. Morre DJ, Morre DM. Synergistic Capsicum-tea mixtures with anticancer activity. J Pharm Pharmacol. Jul 2003;55(7):987-94. doi:10.1211/0022357021521

31. Mukthamba P, Srinivasan K. Protective effect of dietary fenugreek (Trigonella foenum-graecum) seeds and garlic (Allium sativum) on induced oxidation of low-density lipoprotein in rats. J Basic Clin Physiol Pharmacol. Jan 2016;27(1):39-47. doi:10.1515/jbcpp-2015-0037

32. Mutmainah, Susilowati R, Rahmawati N, Nugroho AE. Gastroprotective effects of combination of hot water extracts of turmeric (Curcuma domestica L.), cardamom pods (Ammomum compactum S.) and sembung leaf (Blumea balsamifera DC.) against aspirin-induced gastric ulcer model in rats. Asian Pac J Trop Biomed. May 2014;4(Suppl 1):S500-4. doi:10.12980/APJTB.4.2014C972

33. Nabavi SM, Habtemariam S, Daglia M, Nabavi SF. Apigenin and Breast Cancers: From Chemistry

to Medicine. Anticancer Agents Med Chem. 2015;15(6):728-35. doi:10.2174/18715206156666150304120643

34. Oleaga C, Garcia M, Sole A, Ciudad CJ, Izquierdo-Pulido M, Noe V. CYP1A1 is overexpressed upon incubation of breast cancer cells with a polyphenolic cocoa extract. Eur J Nutr. Jun 2012;51(4):465-76. doi:10.1007/s00394-011-0231-2

35. Otunola GA, Oloyede OB, Oladiji AT, Afolayan AJ. Selected spices and their combination modulate hypercholesterolemia-induced oxidative stress in experimental rats. Biol Res. Mar 26 2014;47(1):5. doi:10.1186/0717-6287-47-5

36. Park JH, Lee M, Park E. Antioxidant activity of orange flesh and peel extracted with various solvents. Prev Nutr Food Sci. Dec 2014;19(4):291-8. doi:10.3746/pnf.2014.19.4.291

37. Patel K. Rosmarinic Acid. Examine. Accessed May 17, 2023. https://examine.com/supplements/rosmarinic-acid/

38. Percival SS, Vanden Heuvel JP, Nieves CJ, Montero C, Migliaccio AJ, Meadors J. Bioavailability of herbs and spices in humans as determined by ex vivo inflammatory suppression and DNA strand breaks. J Am Coll Nutr. Aug 2012;31(4):288-94. doi:10.1080/07315724.2012.10720438

39. Shoba G, Joy D, Joseph T, Majeed M, Rajendran R, Srinivas PS. Influence of piperine on the pharmacokinetics of curcumin in animals and human volunteers. Planta Med. May 1998;64(4):353-6. doi:10.1055/s-2006-957450

40. Sun J. D-Limonene: safety and clinical applications. Altern Med Rev. Sep 2007;12(3):259-64.

41. Vukovic NL, Vukic MD, Obradovic AD, Matic MM, Galovicova L, Kacaniova M. GC, GC/MS Analysis, and Biological Effects of Essential Oils from Thymus mastchina and Elettaria cardamomum. Plants (Basel). Nov 23 2022;11(23)doi:10.3390/plants11233213

42. Zahid Ashraf M, Hussain ME, Fahim M. Antiatherosclerotic effects of dietary supplementations of garlic and turmeric: Restoration of endothelial function in rats. Life Sci. Jul 8 2005;77(8):837-57. doi:10.1016/j.lfs.2004.11.039

CONSIDER THE WEIGHT CONNECTION

1. BreastCancer.org. Being Overweight. BreastCancer.org. Accessed May 17, 2023. https://www.breastcancer.org/risk/risk-factors/being-overweight

2. Centers for Disease Control and Prevention. Obesity and Cancer. cdc.gov. Accessed May 17, 2023. https://www.cdc.gov/cancer/obesity/index.htm

3. Chan DSM, Vieira AR, Aune D, et al. Body mass index and survival in women with breast cancer-systematic literature review and meta-analysis of 82 follow-up studies. Ann Oncol. Oct 2014;25(10):1901-1914. doi:10.1093/annonc/mdu042

4. Eliassen AH, Colditz GA, Rosner B, Willett WC, Hankinson SE. Adult weight change and risk of postmenopausal breast cancer. JAMA. Jul 12 2006;296(2):193-201. doi:10.1001/jama.296.2.193

5. Fourkala E-O, Burnell M, Cox C, et al. Association of skirt size and postmenopausal breast cancer risk in older women: a cohort study within the UK Collaborative Trial of Ovarian Cancer Screening (UKCTOCS). BMJ Open. 2014;4(9):e005400. doi:10.1136/bmjopen-2014-005400

6. Harvie M, Howell A, Vierkant RA, et al. Association of Gain and Loss of Weight before and after Menopause with Risk of Postmenopausal Breast Cancer in the Iowa Women's Health Study. Cancer Epidemiology, Biomarkers & Prevention. 2005;14(3):656-661. doi:10.1158/1055-9965.Epi-04-0001

7. Jiralerspong S, Goodwin PJ. Obesity and Breast Cancer Prognosis: Evidence, Challenges, and Opportunities. J Clin Oncol. Dec 10 2016;34(35):4203-4216. doi:10.1200/JCO.2016.68.4480

8. Keum N, Greenwood DC, Lee DH, et al. Adult weight gain and adiposity-related cancers: a dose-response meta-analysis of prospective observational studies. J Natl Cancer Inst. Feb 2015;107(2)doi:10.1093/jnci/djv088

9. Susan G. Komen. Breast Cancer Risk: Body Weight and Weight Gain. komen.org. Updated April 3, 2023. Accessed May 17, 2023. https://www.komen.org/breast-cancer/risk-factor/weight/#:~:text=Body%20weight%20and%20breast%20cancer%20risk%20after%20menopause,weight%20throughout%20life%20%5B26%5D

10. Teras LR, Goodman M, Patel AV, Diver WR, Flanders WD, Feigelson HS. Weight loss and postmenopausal breast cancer in a prospective cohort of overweight and obese US women. Cancer Causes Control. Apr 2011;22(4):573-9. doi:10.1007/s10552-011-9730-y

11. Underferth D. How does obesity cause cancer? MD Anderson Cancer Center. Accessed May 17, 2023. https://www.mdanderson.org/publications/focused-on-health/how-does-obesity-cause-cancer.h27Z1591413.html

12. World Health Organization. Obesity. who.int. Accessed May 17, 2023. https://www.who.int/health-topics/obesity#tab=tab_1

FIBER UP & DIVERSIFY

1. Aune D, Chan DS, Greenwood DC, et al. Dietary fiber and breast cancer risk: a systematic review and meta-analysis of prospective studies. Ann Oncol. Jun 2012;23(6):1394-402. doi:10.1093/annonc/mdr589

2. Farvid MS, Eliassen AH, Cho E, Liao X, Chen WY, Willett WC. Dietary Fiber Intake in Young Adults and Breast Cancer Risk. Pediatrics. 2016;137(3) doi:10.1542/peds.2015-1226

3. Farvid MS, Spence ND, Holmes MD, Barnett JB. Fiber consumption and breast cancer incidence: A systematic review and meta-analysis of prospective studies. Cancer. Jul 1 2020;126(13):3061-3075. doi:10.1002/cncr.32816

4. Goldin BR, Adlercreutz H, Gorbach SL, et al. Estrogen excretion patterns and plasma levels in vegetarian and omnivorous women. N Engl J Med. Dec 16 1982;307(25):1542-7. doi:10.1056/nejm198212163072502

5. Holmes MD, Liu S, Hankinson SE, Colditz GA, Hunter DJ, Willett WC. Dietary Carbohydrates, Fiber, and Breast Cancer Risk. American Journal of Epidemiology. 2004;159(8):732-739. doi:10.1093/aje/kwh112

6. Suzuki R, Rylander-Rudqvist T, Ye W, Saji S, Adlercreutz H, Wolk A. Dietary fiber intake and risk of postmenopausal breast cancer defined by estrogen and progesterone receptor status—a prospective cohort study among Swedish women. Int J Cancer. Jan 15 2008;122(2):403-12. doi:10.1002/ijc.23060

7. Xu K, Sun Q, Shi Z, et al. A Dose-Response Meta-Analysis of Dietary Fiber Intake and Breast Cancer Risk. Asia Pac J Public Health. May 2022;34(4):331-337. doi:10.1177/10105395211072997

STRIKE A SUGAR BALANCE

1. Christopoulos PF, Msaouel P, Koutsilieris M. The role of the insulin-like growth factor-1 system in breast cancer. Mol Cancer. Feb 15 2015;14:43. doi:10.1186/s12943-015-0291-7

2. Friedrich N, Thuesen B, Jørgensen T, et al. The association between IGF-I and insulin resistance: a general population study in Danish adults. Diabetes Care. Apr 2012;35(4):768-73. doi:10.2337/dc11-1833

3. Liljeberg H, Granfeldt Y, Björck I. Metabolic responses to starch in bread containing intact kernels versus milled flour. Eur J Clin Nutr. Aug 1992;46(8):561-75.

4. Musa-Veloso K, Noori D, Venditti C, et al. A Systematic Review and Meta-Analysis of

Randomized Controlled Trials on the Effects of Oats and Oat Processing on Postprandial Blood Glucose and Insulin Responses. The Journal of Nutrition. 2020;151(2):341-351. doi:10.1093/jn/nxaa349

5. Ng SW, Slining MM, Popkin BM. Use of caloric and noncaloric sweeteners in US consumer packaged foods, 2005-2009. J Acad Nutr Diet. Nov 2012;112(11):1828-34.e1-6. doi:10.1016/j.jand.2012.07.009

VEG OUT

1. Aune D, Chan DS, Vieira AR, et al. Dietary compared with blood concentrations of carotenoids and breast cancer risk: a systematic review and meta-analysis of prospective studies. Am J Clin Nutr. Aug 2012;96(2):356-73. doi:10.3945/ajcn.112.034165

2. Ba DM, Ssentongo P, Beelman RB, Muscat J, Gao X, Richie JP. Higher Mushroom Consumption Is Associated with Lower Risk of Cancer: A Systematic Review and Meta-Analysis of Observational Studies. Adv Nutr. Oct 1 2021;12(5):1691-1704. doi:10.1093/advances/nmab015

3. BreastCancer.org. Foods Containing Phytochemicals. breastcancer.org. Updated July 27, 2022. Accessed May 17, 2023. https://www.breastcancer.org/managing-life/diet-nutrition/breast-cancer-risk-reduction/foods/phytochemicals

4. Busch S. Cooked Vs. Raw for Beta-Carotene. Week&. Updated December 7, 2018. Accessed May 17, 2023. https://www.weekand.com/healthy-living/article/cooked-vs-raw-betacarotene-18007161.php

5. Carlson JL, Erickson JM, Lloyd BB, Slavin JL. Health Effects and Sources of Prebiotic Dietary Fiber. Curr Dev Nutr. Mar 2018;2(3):nzy005. doi:10.1093/cdn/nzy005

6. Davani-Davari D, Negahdaripour M, Karimzadeh I, et al. Prebiotics: Definition, Types, Sources, Mechanisms, and Clinical Applications. Foods. Mar 9 2019;8(3)doi:10.3390/foods8030092

7. Eliassen AH, Hendrickson SJ, Brinton LA, et al. Circulating carotenoids and risk of breast cancer: pooled analysis of eight prospective studies. J Natl Cancer Inst. Dec 19 2012;104(24):1905-16. doi:10.1093/jnci/djs461

8. Eliassen AH, Liao X, Rosner B, Tamimi RM, Tworoger SS, Hankinson SE. Plasma carotenoids and risk of breast cancer over 20 y of follow-up. Am J Clin Nutr. Jun 2015;101(6):1197-205. doi:10.3945/ajcn.114.105080

9. Farvid MS, Chen WY, Rosner BA, Tamimi RM, Willett WC, Eliassen AH. Fruit and vegetable consumption and breast cancer incidence: Repeated measures over 30 years of follow-up. Int J Cancer. Apr 1 2019;144(7):1496-1510. doi:10.1002/ijc.31653

10. Grube BJ, Eng ET, Kao YC, Kwon A, Chen S. White button mushroom phytochemicals inhibit aromatase activity and breast cancer cell proliferation. J Nutr. Dec 2001;131(12):3288-93. doi:10.1093/jn/131.12.3288

11. Higdon J. β-Carotene, β-Carotene, β-Cryptoxanthin, Lycopene, Lutein, and Zeaxanthin. Oregon State University. Updated August 2016. Accessed May 17, 2023. https://lpi.oregonstate.edu/mic/dietary-factors/phytochemicals/carotenoids

12. Higdon J. Cruciferous Vegetables. Oregon State University. Updated December 2016. Accessed May 17, 2023. https://lpi.oregonstate.edu/mic/food-beverages/cruciferous-vegetables

13. Kabat GC, Kim M, Adams-Campbell LL, et al. Longitudinal study of serum carotenoid, retinol, and tocopherol concentrations in relation to breast cancer risk among postmenopausal women. Am J Clin Nutr. Jul 2009;90(1):162-9. doi:10.3945/ajcn.2009.27568

14. Kothari D, Lee WD, Kim SK. Allium Flavonols: Health Benefits, Molecular Targets, and Bioavailability. Antioxidants (Basel). Sep 19 2020;9(9)doi:10.3390/antiox9090888

15. Liu X, Lv K. Cruciferous vegetables intake is inversely associated with risk of breast cancer: a meta-analysis. Breast. Jun 2013;22(3):309-13. doi:10.1016/j.breast.2012.07.013

16. Sengupta A, Ghosh S, Bhattacharjee S. Allium Vegetables in Cancer Prevention: An Overview. Asian Pacific journal of cancer prevention : APJCP. 07/01 2004;5:237-45.

17. Stelmach-Mardas M, Rodacki T, Dobrowolska-Iwanek J, et al. Link between Food Energy Density and Body Weight Changes in Obese Adults. Nutrients. Apr 20 2016;8(4):229. doi:10.3390/nu8040229

18. Nutrition and Health Info Sheet: Phytochemicals. Department of Nutrition, University of California, Davis; 2016. https://nutrition.ucdavis.edu/sites/g/files/dgvnsk426/files/content/infosheets/factsheets/fact-pro-phytochemical.pdf

19. Zhang M, Huang J, Xie X, Holman CD. Dietary intakes of mushrooms and green tea combine to reduce the risk of breast cancer in Chinese women. Int J Cancer. Mar 15 2009;124(6):1404-8. doi:10.1002/ijc.24047

GO PRO WITH PREMIUM PROTEINS

1. Allen NE, Appleby PN, Davey GK, Kaaks R, Rinaldi S, Key TJ. The associations of diet with serum insulin-like growth factor I and its main binding proteins in 292 women meat-eaters, vegetarians, and vegans. Cancer Epidemiol Biomarkers Prev. Nov 2002;11(11):1441-8.

2. American Institute for Cancer Research. Soy: Intake Does Not Increase Risk for Breast Cancer Survivors. Updated April 8, 2021. Accessed May 17, 2023. https://www.aicr.org/cancer-prevention/food-facts/soy/

3. Consumer Concerns About Hormones in Food. Cornell Center for the Environment; 2000. https://ecommons.cornell.edu/bitstream/handle/1813/14514/fs37.hormones.pdf

4. David LA, Maurice CF, Carmody RN, et al. Diet rapidly and reproducibly alters the human gut microbiome. Nature. Jan 23 2014;505(7484):559-63. doi:10.1038/nature12820

5. Ervin SM, Li H, Lim L, et al. Gut microbial β-glucuronidases reactivate estrogens as components of the estrobolome that reactivate estrogens. J Biol Chem. Dec 6 2019;294(49):18586-18599. doi:10.1074/jbc.RA119.010950

6. Fabian CJ, Kimler BF, Hursting SD. Omega-3 fatty acids for breast cancer prevention and survivorship. Breast Cancer Res. May 4 2015;17(1):62. doi:10.1186/s13058-015-0571-6

7. Farvid MS, Cho E, Chen WY, Eliassen AH, Willett WC. Dietary protein sources in early adulthood and breast cancer incidence: prospective cohort study. BMJ : British Medical Journal. 2014;348:g3437. doi:10.1136/bmj.g3437

8. Farvid MS, Cho E, Chen WY, Eliassen AH, Willett WC. Dietary protein sources in early adulthood and breast cancer incidence: prospective cohort study. BMJ : British Medical Journal. 2014;348:g3437. doi:10.1136/bmj.g3437

9. Funk K. Breasts: The Owner's Manual. Thomas Nelson; 2018.

10. Goyens PL, Spilker ME, Zock PL, Katan MB, Mensink RP. Conversion of α-linolenic acid in humans is influenced by the absolute amounts of -linolenic acid and linoleic acid in the diet and not by their ratio. The American Journal of Clinical Nutrition. 2006;84(1):44-53. doi:10.1093/ajcn/84.1.44

11. Harmon BE, Morimoto Y, Beckford F, Franke AA, Stanczyk FZ, Maskarinec G. Oestrogen levels in serum and urine of premenopausal women eating low and high amounts of meat. Public Health Nutrition. 2014;17(9):2087-2093. doi:10.1017/S1368980013002553

12. He Y, Tao Q, Zhou F, et al. The relationship between dairy products intake and breast cancer incidence: a meta-analysis of observational studies. BMC Cancer. 2021/10/15 2021;21(1):1109. doi:10.1186/s12885-021-08854-w

13. HealthDay. Plant-Based Diet May Help Keep Breast Cancer Away. Brigham and Women's Hospital. Updated June 16, 2022. Accessed May 17, 2023. https://healthlibrary.brighamandwomens.org/Conditions/Cancer/NewsRecent/6,1657470151

14. Higdon J. Essential Fatty Acids. Oregon State University. Updated May 2019. Accessed May 17, 2023. https://lpi.oregonstate.edu/mic/other-nutrients/essential-fatty-acids#authors-reviewers

15. HIgdon J. Soy Isoflavones. Oregon State University. Updated August 2016. Accessed May 17, 2023. https://lpi.oregonstate.edu/mic/dietary-factors/phytochemicals/soy-isoflavones#estrogenic-anti-estrogenic-activities

16. Hruby A, Jacques PF. Dietary Protein and Changes in Biomarkers of Inflammation and Oxidative Stress in the Framingham Heart Study Offspring Cohort. Curr Dev Nutr. May 2019;3(5):nzz019. doi:10.1093/cdn/nzz019

17. Keum N, Lee DH, Marchand N, et al. Egg intake and cancers of the breast, ovary and prostate: a dose-response meta-analysis of prospective observational studies. Br J Nutr. Oct 14 2015;114(7):1099-107. doi:10.1017/s0007114515002135

18. Kimbung S, Chang C-y, Bendahl P-O, et al. Impact of 27-hydroxylase (CYP27A1) and 27-hydroxycholesterol in breast cancer. Endocrine-Related Cancer. 01 Jul. 2017 2017;24(7):339-349. doi:10.1530/ERC-16-0533

19. Ko K-P, Kim S-W, Ma SH, et al. Dietary intake and breast cancer among carriers and noncarriers of BRCA mutations in the Korean Hereditary Breast Cancer Study. The American Journal of Clinical Nutrition. 2013;98(6):1493-1501. doi:10.3945/ajcn.112.057760

20. Kristensen MD, Bendsen NT, Christensen SM, Astrup A, Raben A. Meals based on vegetable protein sources (beans and peas) are more satiating than meals based on animal protein sources (veal and pork)—a randomized cross-over meal test study. Food Nutr Res. 2016;60:32634. doi:10.3402/fnr.v60.32634

21. Lane K, Derbyshire E, Li W, Brennan C. Bioavailability and potential uses of vegetarian sources of omega-3 fatty acids: a review of the literature. Crit Rev Food Sci Nutr. 2014;54(5):572-9. doi:10.1080/10408398.2011.596292

22. Li C, Yang L, Zhang D, Jiang W. Systematic review and meta-analysis suggest that dietary cholesterol intake increases risk of breast cancer. Nutr Res. Jul 2016;36(7):627-35. doi:10.1016/j.nutres.2016.04.009

23. Link LB, Canchola AJ, Bernstein L, et al. Dietary patterns and breast cancer risk in the California Teachers Study cohort. Am J Clin Nutr. Dec 2013;98(6):1524-32. doi:10.3945/ajcn.113.061184

24. Ma L, Cho W, Nelson ER. Our evolving understanding of how 27-hydroxycholesterol influences cancer. Biochem Pharmacol. Feb 2022;196:114621. doi:10.1016/j.bcp.2021.114621

25. Maruyama K, Oshima T, Ohyama K. Exposure to exogenous estrogen through intake of commercial milk produced from pregnant cows. Pediatr Int. Feb 2010;52(1):33-8. doi:10.1111/j.1442-200X.2009.02890.x

26. Murphy N, Knuppel A, Papadimitriou N, et al. Insulin-like growth factor-1, insulin-like growth factor-binding protein-3, and breast cancer risk: observational and Mendelian randomization analyses with ∼430 000 women. Annals of Oncology. 2020;31(5):641-649. doi:10.1016/j.annonc.2020.01.066

27. Nechuta SJ, Caan BJ, Chen WY, et al. Soy food intake after diagnosis of breast cancer and survival: an in-depth analysis of combined evidence from cohort studies of US and Chinese women. Am J Clin Nutr. Jul 2012;96(1):123-32. doi:10.3945/ajcn.112.035972

28. Nelson M. Major New Analysis: Fiber May Prevent Breast Cancer. American Institute for Cancer Research. Accessed May 17, 2023. https://www.aicr.org/resources/blog/major-new-analysis-fiber-may-prevent-breast-cancer/#:~:text=The%20study%20found%20that%20for,lower%20risk%2C%20and%20so%20on

29. Paruthiyil S, Parmar H, Kerekatte V, Cunha GR, Firestone GL, Leitman DC. Estrogen receptor beta inhibits human breast cancer cell proliferation and tumor formation by causing a G2 cell cycle arrest. Cancer Res. Jan 1 2004;64(1):423-8. doi:10.1158/0008-5472.can-03-2446

30. Pastorino B. New study associates intake of dairy milk with greater risk of breast cancer. Loma Linda University Health. Accessed May 17, 2023. https://news.llu.edu/research/new-study-associates-intake-of-dairy-milk-with-greater-risk-of-breast-cancer

31. Richman EL, Kenfield SA, Stampfer MJ, Giovannucci EL, Chan JM. Egg, red meat, and poultry intake and risk of lethal prostate cancer in the prostate-specific antigen-era: incidence and survival. Cancer Prev Res (Phila). Dec 2011;4(12):2110-21. doi:10.1158/1940-6207.Capr-11-0354

32. Rigi S, Mousavi SM, Benisi-Kohansal S, Azadbakht L, Esmaillzadeh A. The association between plant-based dietary patterns and risk of breast cancer: a case−control study. Scientific Reports. 2021/02/09 2021;11(1):3391. doi:10.1038/s41598-021-82659-6

33. Romo Ventura E, Konigorski S, Rohrmann S, et al. Association of dietary intake of milk and dairy products with blood concentrations of insulin-like growth factor 1 (IGF-1) in Bavarian adults. Eur J Nutr. Jun 2020;59(4):1413-1420. doi:10.1007/s00394-019-01994-7

34. Si R, Qu K, Jiang Z, Yang X, Gao P. Egg consumption and breast cancer risk: a meta-analysis. Breast Cancer. May 2014;21(3):251-61. doi:10.1007/s12282-014-0519-1

35. Simon S. Soy and Cancer Risk: Our Expert's Advice. American Cancer Society. Updated April 29, 2019. Accessed May 17, 2023. https://www.cancer.org/cancer/latest-news/soy-and-cancer-risk-our-experts-advice.html

36. Sui Y, Wu J, Chen J. The Role of Gut Microbial β-Glucuronidase in Estrogen Reactivation and Breast Cancer. Front Cell Dev Biol. 2021;9:631552. doi:10.3389/fcell.2021.631552

37. Tantamango-Bartley Y, Jaceldo-Siegl K, Fan J, Fraser G. Vegetarian diets and the incidence of cancer in a low-risk population. Cancer Epidemiol Biomarkers Prev. Feb 2013;22(2):286-94. doi:10.1158/1055-9965.Epi-12-1060

38. Taylor EF, Burley VJ, Greenwood DC, Cade JE. Meat consumption and risk of breast cancer in the UK Women's Cohort Study. Br J Cancer. Apr 10 2007;96(7):1139-46. doi:10.1038/sj.bjc.6603689

39. Watling CZ, Schmidt JA, Dunneram Y, et al. Risk of cancer in regular and low meat-eaters, fish-eaters, and vegetarians: a prospective analysis of UK Biobank participants. BMC Medicine. 2022/02/24 2022;20(1):73. doi:10.1186/s12916-022-02256-w

40. Zheng JS, Hu XJ, Zhao YM, Yang J, Li D. Intake of fish and marine n-3 polyunsaturated fatty acids and risk of breast cancer: meta-analysis of data from 21 independent prospective cohort studies. Bmj. Jun 27 2013;346:f3706. doi:10.1136/bmj.f3706

GET AN OIL CHANGE

1. Blackburn GL, Wang KA. Dietary fat reduction and breast cancer outcome: results from the Women's Intervention Nutrition Study (WINS)2, 3. The American Journal of Clinical Nutrition. 2007/09/01 2007;86(3):878S-881S. doi:https://doi.org/10.1093/ajcn.86.3.878S

2. BreastCancer.org. Diet High in Saturated Fat Linked to Higher Risk of HER2-Negative, Hormone-Receptor-Positive Breast Cancer. breastcancer.org. Updated May 28, 2014. Accessed May 18, 2023. https://www.breastcancer.org/research-news/high-fat-diet-linked-to-breast-cancer

3. BreastCancer.org. Location of Fat May Affect Type of Breast Cancer Risk. breastcancer.org. Updated September 20, 2017. Accessed May 18, 2023. https://www.breastcancer.org/research-news/location-of-fat-may-affect-type-of-bc-risk

4. Brennan SF, Woodside JV, Lunny PM, Cardwell CR, Cantwell MM. Dietary fat and breast cancer mortality: A systematic review and meta-analysis. Crit Rev Food Sci Nutr. Jul 3 2017;57(10):1999-2008. doi:10.1080/10408398.2012.724481

5. Chlebowski RT, Aragaki AK, Anderson GL, et al. Dietary Modification and Breast Cancer Mortality: Long-Term Follow-Up of the Women's Health Initiative Randomized Trial. Journal of Clinical Oncology. 2020;38(13):1419-1428. doi:10.1200/jco.19.00435

6. Chlebowski RT, Blackburn GL, Hoy MK, et al. Survival analyses from the Women's Intervention Nutrition Study (WINS) evaluating dietary fat reduction and breast cancer outcome. Journal of Clinical Oncology. 2008;26(15_suppl):522-522. doi:10.1200/jco.2008.26.15_suppl.522

7. Fabian CJ, Kimler BF, Hursting SD. Omega-3 fatty acids for breast cancer prevention and survivorship. Breast Cancer Res. May 4 2015;17(1):62. doi:10.1186/s13058-015-0571-6

8. Garcia-Estevez L, Moreno-Bueno G. Updating the role of obesity and cholesterol in breast cancer. Breast Cancer Research. 2019/03/01 2019;21(1):35. doi:10.1186/s13058-019-1124-1

9. Harvard T.H. Chan School of Public Health. Types of Fat. Harvard T.H. Chan School of Public Health. Accessed May 18, 2023. https://www.hsph.harvard.edu/nutritionsource/what-should-you-eat/fats-and-cholesterol/types-of-fat/

10. Leibniz-Institut für Lebensmittel-Systembiologie an der TU München. Why stored linseed oil tastes bitter — and what you could do about it. ScienceDaily. Accessed May 18, 2023. www.sciencedaily.com/releases/2022/04/220421141625.htm

11. Riccardi G, Giacco R, Rivellese AA. Dietary fat, insulin sensitivity and the metabolic syndrome. Clin Nutr. Aug 2004;23(4):447-56. doi:10.1016/j.clnu.2004.02.006

12. Sieri S, Chiodini P, Agnoli C, et al. Dietary Fat Intake and Development of Specific Breast Cancer Subtypes. JNCI: Journal of the National Cancer Institute. 2014;106(5)doi:10.1093/jnci/dju068

13. Thalheimer JC. Coconut Oil. Today's Dietitian. Accessed May 18, 2023. https://www.todaysdietitian.com/newarchives/1016p32.shtml

14. The Harvard Gazette. Diets high in animal fat may impact breast cancer risk: Researchers turn attention to younger women. Harvard University. Accessed May 18, 2023. https://news.harvard.edu/gazette/story/2003/07/diets-high-in-animal-fat-may-impact-breast-cancer-risk/#:~:text=%E2%80%9COverall%2C%20we%20observed%20that%20there,medicine%20at%20Harvard%20Medical%20School

15. UCSF Osher Center for Integrative Health. Animal Protein and Cancer Risk. University of California San Francisco. Accessed May 18, 2023. https://osher.ucsf.edu/patient-care/integrative-medicine-resources/cancer-and-nutrition/faq/animal-protein-cancer-risk

16. Willett WC. Ask the doctor: Coconut oil and health. Harvard Health Publishing. Accessed May 18, 2023. https://www.health.harvard.edu/staying-healthy/coconut-oil

17. Wolk A, Bergström R, Hunter D, et al. A Prospective Study of Association of Monounsaturated Fat and Other Types of Fat With Risk of Breast Cancer. Archives of Internal Medicine. 1998;158(1):41-45. doi:10.1001/archinte.158.1.41

POWER UP YOUR PANTRY!

1. Bimonte S, Cascella M, Barbieri A, Arra C, Cuomo A. Current shreds of evidence on the anticancer role of EGCG in triple negative breast cancer: an update of the current state of knowledge. Infect Agent Cancer. 2020;15:2. doi:10.1186/s13027-020-0270-5

2. Bramen L. Nigella Seeds: What the Heck Do I Do with Those? Smithsonian Magazine. Accessed May 18, 2023. https://www.smithsonianmag.com/arts-culture/nigella-seeds-what-the-heck-do-i-do-with-those-29298883/#:~:text=The%20seeds%20have%20a%20slightly,of%20a%20toasted%20everything%20bagel

3. Butt MS, Sultan MT. Ginger and its Health Claims: Molecular Aspects. Critical Reviews in Food Science and Nutrition. 2011/04/14 2011;51(5):383-393. doi:10.1080/10408391003624848

4. Chang HC, Peng CH, Yeh DM, Kao ES, Wang CJ. Hibiscus sabdariffa extract inhibits obesity and fat accumulation, and improves liver steatosis in humans. Food Funct. Apr 2014;5(4):734-9. doi:10.1039/c3fo60495k

5. Chiu CT, Chen JH, Chou FP, Lin HH. Hibiscus sabdariffa Leaf Extract Inhibits Human Prostate Cancer Cell Invasion via Down-Regulation of Akt/NF-kB/MMP-9 Pathway. Nutrients. Jun 24 2015;7(7):5065-87. doi:10.3390/nu7075065

6. Das G, Tantengco OAG, Tundis R, et al. Glucosinolates and Omega-3 Fatty Acids from Mustard Seeds: Phytochemistry and Pharmacology. Plants (Basel). Sep 1 2022;11(17)doi:10.3390/plants11172290

7. Di Noia J. Defining Powerhouse Fruits and Vegetables: A Nutrient Density Approach. Preventing Chronic Disease. 2014;11:E95. doi:10.5888/pcd11.130390

8. Gioia FD. The ABCs of Microgreens. Pennsylvania State University. Updated May 8, 2020. Accessed May 18, 2023. https://extension.psu.edu/the-abcs-of-microgreens

9. Greger M. Amla vs. Cancer Cell Growth. NutritionFacts.org. Accessed May 18, 2023. https://nutritionfacts.org/video/amla-versus-cancer-cell-growth/

10. HealthEssentials. 7 Benefits of Hibiscus Tea. Cleveland Clinic. Accessed May 18, 2023. https://health.clevelandclinic.org/benefits-of-hibiscus/

11. Higdon J. Cruciferous Vegetables. Oregon State University. Updated December 2016. Accessed May 17, 2023. https://lpi.oregonstate.edu/mic/food-beverages/cruciferous-vegetables

12. Higdon J. Indole-3-Carbinol. Oregon State University. Updated January 2017. Accessed May 18, 2023. https://lpi.oregonstate.edu/mic/dietary-factors/phytochemicals/indole-3-carbinol#authors-reviewers

13. Hong KJ, Lee CH, Kim SW. Aspergillus oryzae GB-107 fermentation improves nutritional quality of food soybeans and feed soybean meals. J Med Food. Winter 2004;7(4):430-5. doi:10.1089/jmf.2004.7.430

14. Hu ML, Rayner CK, Wu KL, et al. Effect of ginger on gastric motility and symptoms of functional dyspepsia. World J Gastroenterol. Jan 7 2011;17(1):105-10. doi:10.3748/wjg.v17.i1.105

15. Icahn School of Medicine at Mount Sinai. Psyllium. MountSinai.org. Accessed May 18, 2023. https://www.mountsinai.org/health-library/supplement/psyllium#:~:text=The%20soluble%20fiber%20found%20in,levels%20in%20people%20with%20diabetes

16. Khan N, Mukhtar H. Tea and health: studies in humans. Curr Pharm Des. 2013;19(34):6141-7. doi:10.2174/1381612811319340008

17. Kreydiyyeh SI, Usta J. Diuretic effect and mechanism of action of parsley. J Ethnopharmacol. Mar 2002;79(3):353-7. doi:10.1016/s0378-8741(01)00408-1

18. Kuran D, Pogorzelska A, Wiktorska K. Breast Cancer Prevention-Is there a Future for Sulforaphane and Its Analogs? Nutrients. May 27 2020;12(6)doi:10.3390/nu12061559

19. Lee KW, Kim YJ, Lee HJ, Lee CY. Cocoa has more phenolic phytochemicals and a higher antioxidant capacity than teas and red wine. J Agric Food Chem. Dec 3 2003;51(25):7292-5. doi:10.1021/jf0344385

20. Lin BW, Gong CC, Song HF, Cui YY. Effects of anthocyanins on the prevention and treatment of cancer. Br J Pharmacol. Jun 2017;174(11):1226-1243. doi:10.1111/bph.13627

21. Lin HH, Huang HP, Huang CC, Chen JH, Wang CJ. Hibiscus polyphenol-rich extract induces apoptosis in human gastric carcinoma cells via p53 phosphorylation and p38 MAPK/FasL cascade pathway. Mol Carcinog. Jun 2005;43(2):86-99. doi:10.1002/mc.20103

22. Liu D, Chen Z. The effect of curcumin on breast cancer cells. J Breast Cancer. Jun 2013;16(2):133-7. doi:10.4048/jbc.2013.16.2.133

23. Long X, Fan M, Bigsby RM, Nephew KP. Apigenin inhibits antiestrogen-resistant breast cancer cell growth through estrogen receptor-alpha-dependent and estrogen receptor-alpha-independent mechanisms. Mol Cancer Ther. Jul 2008;7(7):2096-108. doi:10.1158/1535-7163.Mct-07-2350

24. Malacrida A, Maggioni D, Cassetti A, Nicolini G, Cavaletti G, Miloso M. Antitumoral Effect of Hibiscus sabdariffa on Human Squamous Cell Carcinoma and Multiple Myeloma Cells. Nutr Cancer. Oct 2016;68(7):1161-70. doi:10.1080/01635581.2016.1208830

25. Mao QQ, Xu XY, Cao SY, et al. Bioactive Compounds and Bioactivities of Ginger (Zingiber officinale Roscoe). Foods. May 30 2019;8(6)doi:10.3390/foods8060185

26. Martin MA, Goya L, Ramos S. Potential for preventive effects of cocoa and cocoa polyphenols in cancer. Food and Chemical Toxicology. 2013/06/01/ 2013;56:336-351. doi:https://doi.org/10.1016/j.fct.2013.02.020

27. Milder IE, Arts IC, van de Putte B, Venema DP, Hollman PC. Lignan contents of Dutch plant foods: a database including lariciresinol, pinoresinol, secoisolariciresinol and matairesinol. Br J Nutr. Mar 2005;93(3):393-402. doi:10.1079/bjn20051371

28. Ngamkitidechakul C, Jaijoy K, Hansakul P, Soonthornchareonnon N, Sireeratawong S. Antitumour effects of Phyllanthus emblica L.: induction of cancer cell apoptosis and inhibition of in vivo tumour promotion and in vitro invasion of human cancer cells. Phytother Res. Sep 2010;24(9):1405-13. doi:10.1002/ptr.3127

29. O'Neill T. High Fiber Diet. Michigan Bowel Control Program. Updated June 2022. Accessed May 18, 2023. https://www.med.umich.edu/1libr/MBCP/HighFiberDietAdults.pdf

30. Park SY, Kim YH, Kim Y, Lee SJ. Aromatic-turmerone attenuates invasion and expression of MMP-9 and COX-2 through inhibition of NF-βB activation in TPA-induced breast cancer cells. J Cell Biochem. Dec 2012;113(12):3653-62. doi:10.1002/jcb.24238

31. Pathak DR, Stein AD, He JP, et al. Cabbage and Sauerkraut Consumption in Adolescence and Adulthood and Breast Cancer Risk among US-Resident Polish Migrant Women. Int J Environ Res Public Health. Oct 14 2021;18(20)doi:10.3390/ijerph182010795

32. Patton D. Sauerkraut consumption may fight off breast cancer. FoodNavigator Europe. Updated July 19, 2008. Accessed May 18, 2023. https://www.foodnavigator.com/Article/2005/11/04/Sauerkraut-consumption-may-fight-off-breast-cancer#

33. Rodriguez-Leyva D, Pierce GN. The cardiac and haemostatic effects of dietary hempseed. Nutr Metab (Lond). Apr 21 2010;7:32. doi:10.1186/1743-7075-7-32

34. Santiago LA, Hiramatsu M, Mori A. Japanese soybean paste miso scavenges free radicals and inhibits lipid peroxidation. J Nutr Sci Vitaminol (Tokyo). Jun 1992;38(3):297-304. doi:10.3177/jnsv.38.297

35. Scherbakov AM, Andreeva OE. Apigenin Inhibits Growth of Breast Cancer Cells: The Role of ERβ and HER2/neu. Acta Naturae. Jul-Sep 2015;7(3):133-9.

36. Schor J. Health Effects of Tart Cherries. Natural Medicine Journal. Accessed May 18, 2023. https://www.naturalmedicinejournal.com/journal/health-effects-tart-cherries#:~:text=Anthocyanin%20Content&text=Tart%20cherries%20contain%20more%20anthocyanins,higher%20than%20in%20sweet%20cherries.&text=Tart%20cherries%20yield%20about%2090,1%20and%202%20than%20raspberries

37. Soares APdC, Faria NCd, Graciano GF, et al. Ginger infusion increases diet-induced thermogenesis in healthy individuals: A randomized crossover trial. Food Bioscience. 2022/12/01/ 2022;50:102005. doi:https://doi.org/10.1016/j.fbio.2022.102005

38. Tasdemir SS, Sanlier N. An insight into the anticancer effects of fermented foods: A review. Journal of Functional Foods. 2020/12/01/ 2020;75:104281. doi:https://doi.org/10.1016/j.jff.2020.104281

39. The Japan Times. Miso a day keeps breast cancer away. japantimes.co.jp. Updated June 19, 2003. Accessed May 18, 2023. https://www.japantimes.co.jp/news/2003/06/19/national/miso-a-day-keeps-breast-cancer-away/

40. Thompson LU. Experimental studies on lignans and cancer. Baillieres Clin Endocrinol Metab. Dec 1998;12(4):691-705. doi:10.1016/s0950-351x(98)80011-6

41. Thompson LU, Chen JM, Li T, Strasser-Weippl K, Goss PE. Dietary Flaxseed Alters Tumor Biological Markers in Postmenopausal Breast Cancer. Clinical Cancer Research. 2005;11(10):3828-3835. doi:10.1158/1078-0432.Ccr-04-2326

42. Tříska J, Balík J, Houška M, et al. Factors Influencing Sulforaphane Content in Broccoli Sprouts and Subsequent Sulforaphane Extraction. Foods. Aug 19 2021;10(8)doi:10.3390/foods10081927

43. University of Illinois College of Agricultural, Consumer and Environmental Sciences (ACES). Cancer-fighting properties of horseradish revealed. ScienceDaily. Accessed May 18, 2023. https://www.sciencedaily.com/releases/2016/05/160517122054.htm

44. Watanabe H. Beneficial biological effects of miso with reference to radiation injury, cancer and hypertension. J Toxicol Pathol. Jun 2013;26(2):91-103. doi:10.1293/tox.26.91

45. Weiss DJ, Anderton CR. Determination of catechins in matcha green tea by micellar electrokinetic chromatography. J Chromatogr A. Sep 5 2003;1011(1-2):173-80. doi:10.1016/s0021-9673(03)01133-6

46. Wojdyło A, Nowicka P, Tkacz K, Turkiewicz IP. Sprouts vs. Microgreens as Novel Functional Foods: Variation of Nutritional and Phytochemical Profiles and Their In Vitro Bioactive Properties. Molecules. Oct 12 2020;25(20)doi:10.3390/molecules25204648

47. Yamamoto S, Sobue T, Kobayashi M, Sasaki S, Tsugane S. Soy, isoflavones, and breast cancer risk in Japan. J Natl Cancer Inst. Jun 18 2003;95(12):906-13. doi:10.1093/jnci/95.12.906

48. Yang YJ, Nam S-J, Kong G, Kim MK. A case–control study on seaweed consumption and the risk of breast cancer. British Journal of Nutrition. 2010;103(9):1345-1353. doi:10.1017/S0007114509993242

49. Zeng Y, Pu X, Yang J, et al. Preventive and Therapeutic Role of Functional Ingredients of Barley Grass for Chronic Diseases in Human

Beings. Oxid Med Cell Longev. 2018;2018:3232080. doi:10.1155/2018/3232080

50. Zhao T, Sun Q, Marques M, Witcher M. Anticancer Properties of Phyllanthus emblica (Indian Gooseberry). Oxid Med Cell Longev. 2015;2015:950890. doi:10.1155/2015/950890

RECONSIDER THAT DRINK

1. Al-Sader H, Abdul-Jabar H, Allawi Z, Haba Y. Alcohol and breast cancer: the mechanisms explained. J Clin Med Res. Aug 2009;1(3):125-31. doi:10.4021/jocmr2009.07.1246

2. American Cancer Society. Alcohol Use and Cancer. cancer.org. Updated June 9, 2020. Accessed May 18, 2023. https://www.cancer.org/cancer/risk-prevention/diet-physical-activity/alcohol-use-and-cancer.html

3. American Institute for Cancer Research. Alcohol: Drinking Increases Cancer Risk. aicr.org. Updated March 31, 2021. Accessed May 18, 2023. https://www.aicr.org/cancer-prevention/food-facts/alcohol/

4. Anderson BO, Berdzuli N, Ilbawi A, et al. Health and cancer risks associated with low levels of alcohol consumption. The Lancet Public Health. 2023;8(1):e6-e7. doi:10.1016/S2468-2667(22)00317-6

5. Badrick E, Bobak M, Britton A, Kirschbaum C, Marmot M, Kumari M. The relationship between alcohol consumption and cortisol secretion in an aging cohort. J Clin Endocrinol Metab. Mar 2008;93(3):750-7. doi:10.1210/jc.2007-0737

6. Bagnardi V, Rota M, Botteri E, et al. Alcohol consumption and site-specific cancer risk: a comprehensive dose-response meta-analysis. Br J Cancer. Feb 3 2015;112(3):580-93. doi:10.1038/bjc.2014.579

7. Cancer Research UK. Does alcohol cause cancer? cancerresearchuk.org. Updated March 31, 2021. Accessed May 18, 2023. https://www.cancerresearchuk.org/about-cancer/causes-of-cancer/alcohol-and-cancer/does-alcohol-cause-cancer

8. Cedars-Sinai Staff. Red Wine: Is It Good for You or Not? Cedars-Sinai. Updated Apr 16, 2017. Accessed May 18, 2023. https://www.cedars-sinai.org/blog/health-benefits-of-red-wine.html

9. Chen WY, Rosner B, Hankinson SE, Colditz GA, Willett WC. Moderate alcohol consumption during adult life, drinking patterns, and breast cancer risk. Jama. Nov 2 2011;306(17):1884-90. doi:10.1001/jama.2011.1590

10. Engen PA, Green SJ, Voigt RM, Forsyth CB, Keshavarzian A. The Gastrointestinal Microbiome: Alcohol Effects on the Composition of Intestinal Microbiota. Alcohol Res. 2015;37(2):223-36.

11. Hamajima N, Hirose K, Tajima K, et al. Alcohol, tobacco and breast cancer—collaborative reanalysis of individual data from 53 epidemiological studies, including 58,515 women with breast cancer and 95,067 women without the disease. Br J Cancer. Nov 18 2002;87(11):1234-45. doi:10.1038/sj.bjc.6600596

12. Harvard Health Blog. Diet rich in resveratrol offers no health boost. Harvard Health Publishing. Updated May 15, 2014. Accessed May 18, 2023. https://www.health.harvard.edu/blog/diet-rich-resveratrol-offers-health-boost-201405157153

13. Higdon J. Resveratrol. Oregon State University. Updated May 2015. Accessed May 18, 2023. https://lpi.oregonstate.edu/mic/dietary-factors/phytochemicals/resveratrol#authors-reviewers

14. Mayo Clinic Staff. Breast cancer. Mayo Clinic. Accessed May 18, 2023. https://www.mayoclinic.org/diseases-conditions/breast-cancer/symptoms-causes/syc-20352470

15. National Cancer Institute. Alcohol and Cancer Risk. National Institutes of Health. Updated July 14, 2021. Accessed May 18, 2023. https://www.cancer.gov/about-cancer/causes-prevention/risk/alcohol/alcohol-fact-sheet

16. NTP (National Toxicology Program). Alcoholic Beverage Consumption. Report on Carcinogens. 5th ed. U.S. Department of Health and Human Services, Public Health Service; 2021.

17. Nutrition Action. The effect of alcohol on breast cancer. Center for Science in the Public Interest. Accessed May 18, 2023. https://www.cspinet.org/daily/what-to-eat/the-effect-of-alcohol-on-breast-cancer/

18. Susan G. Komen. Alcohol. komen.org. Accessed May 18, 2023. https://www.komen.org/breast-cancer/risk-factor/alcohol-consumption/

Index

Universal Conversion Chart

OVEN TEMPERATURE EQUIVALENTS

250°F = 120°C

275°F = 135°C

300°F = 150°C

325°F = 160°C

350°F = 180°C

375°F = 190°C

400°F = 200°C

425°F = 220°C

450°F = 240°C

500°F = 260°C

UNIVERSAL MEASUREMENT EQUIVALENTS
(Measurements should always be level unless directed otherwise

⅛ teaspoon = 0.5 ml

¼ teaspoon = 1 ml

½ teaspoon = 2 ml

1 teaspoon = 5 ml

1 tablespoon = 3 teaspoons = ½ fluid ounce = 15 ml

2 tablespoons = ⅛ cup = 1 fluid ounce = 30 ml

4 tablespoons = ¼ cup = 2 fluid ounces = 60 ml

5⅓ tablespoons = ⅓ cup = 3 fluid ounces = 80 ml

8 tablespoons = ½ cup = 4 fluid ounces = 120 ml

10⅔ tablespoons = ⅔ cup = 5 fluid ounces = 160 ml

12 tablespoons = ¾ cup = 6 fluid ounces = 180 ml

16 tablespoons = 1 cup = 8 fluid ounces = 240 ml

Simplify Your Life with My Power Spice Blends!

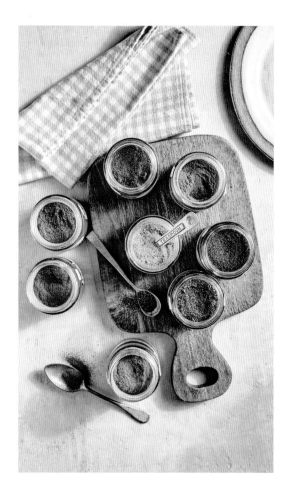

As you can see from my recipes in this book, I love and recommend spices. Not only do spices take healthy dishes from bland to in-demand, but my years of research revealed that spices also add "daily power" in the form of nutritional value. I carefully crafted spice blends that have extra synergistic powers. When used together, certain spice combos synergistically boost each other's powerful nutritional effects. Think of these as the ultimate power couples... or threesomes... or more!

The goal for creating my best-selling line of Power Spice Blends is to forever change the way you think about your pantry. You will shift your mindset from flavor enhancers to a must-have pharmacy in your very own power pantry. Plus, I want to make it easy for you too!

Give my Power Spice Blends a try! I hope you'll find them as fun and flavorful as I do.

Go to bellernutrition.com and order now! In addition, stay in touch @bellernutrition to learn more about the latest releases, recipes, nutrition programs, special offers, and more!

Happy Spicing!

Want to Further Refine Your Transformation with Me?

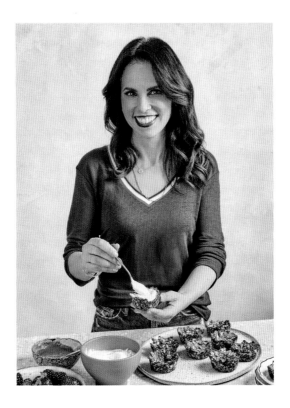

Join my next online Beller Nutrition Masterclass, a simple, all-in-one action plan that will help you reduce cancer risk, lose excess weight, and forever change how you think about the food you choose to put in your body. Designed for busy women to help them feel their amazing best.

It is a hands-on program where my team of experts and I work with you directly to help you achieve your goals.

Learn more at bellernutrition.com

To your health!

Acknowledgments

This book would not be possible without an amazing array of support, love, and dedication from some very special people in my life that I want to acknowledge and thank for their tireless efforts in making this book a reality.

To all the amazing dietitians who are part of the team at Beller Nutrition:

Leanna Teng: There isn't a pedestal high enough to hold up your awesomeness. Year in and year out, you are there and always come through for me. A humongous thank you as an incredible dietitian extraordinaire. Your dedication to this project, attention to detail, and ongoing support throughout the years are something I will cherish forever. Your knowledge and expertise through every process of fact-checking, researching, and writing were invaluable. I appreciate all the weekends and late nights that you put in. This book would not have happened without you, literally.

Laura Cannon: Thank you for always supporting my vision and seeing things through. You are my sounding board for everything BNI – the book, masterclass, private counseling, and so much more. You are a big part of the reason we thrive!

Kayee Liu: Thank you for assisting with the nutritional analyses and recipe descriptions. Your work is appreciated and invaluable in getting the job done.

Julie Shimko: Thank you for your hard work, research, fact-checking and dedication to this book.

To the creative people and those that support me and make this book so special:

Freddy Nager: Thank you for your words of encouragement to pursue *SpiceRack*. We both know the truth behind the title of the book and it would never have happened without you.

Sarah Conant: Your creativity and artwork made all the difference in the world for the design of this book. The overall style would not have come together without you. I am amazed by your vision and artistic talents. Thank you for also designing the book cover and all of your contributions.

Teri Lyn Fisher: You are an incredibly artistic and innovative food photographer, and you never cease to amaze me. You always make the food look so good that I could almost eat the pages. You elevate the quality of all my work. You are a genius, plain and simple.

Marian Cooper Cairns and Natalie Pavich Drobny: food stylists extraordinaire. Your creative and inventive presentation style and attention to detail made such a great impact in the look and feel of the book.

Emily Dorio: Your behind the camera talent captured the real me in the moment. Thank you for your talented contribution to this book.

Chef Ben Harel: Thank you for being there when I needed help with recipe development. You made the food recipes not only simple, but incredibly inviting and delicious, elevating them to the highest quality. Your hard work and expertise is admirable and I will always appreciate your advice.

Mona Dolgov, President of You Live Right Publishers: Thanks for believing in me and making my dream of having this book come true. You inspired and empowered me to make it happen as you are so passionate about giving your heart and soul. I can't thank you enough for all of your brilliant ideas, healthy-delicious recipes, and for spearheading the entire creative process of this book right to the finish line (and beyond!). You guided me and helped me through every step of the way. I have no other words than thank you.

Many thanks to the following people at the You Live Right Publishers team for all of their contributions and support: graphic designer Leslie Feagley for her detailed work in pulling the book together, Christian Stella for helping in recipe development and writing and nutritional analyses, and Abe Ogden, who helped keep us on track.

My patients and masterclass participants: Thank you for allowing me to share my passion and knowledge with you. It is my greatest hope to empower each and every one of you to forever change the way you think about the power of food.

My friends and colleagues: Your ongoing support means the world to me. I appreciate the enthusiasm and feedback and encouragement. I'm so grateful to each and every one of you.

And...to my loving family:

My brothers, my sisters-in-law, nieces, and nephews—you share my journey, provide invaluable insight and feedback, and your words of support and encouragement keep me going. I'm blessed to have a loving family.

My mother (my go-to best friend for all), Shula. Thank you for always encouraging me to aim high. To my father, Joe. You are the spark plug and biggest inspiration for my life's work and mission. I carry you with me always and I miss you so much.

My four kids, Alexia, Jonah, Keira, and Evan: Being your mom has made me the luckiest woman in the world. Thank you for your love, laughter, and ongoing support for my work.

My best friend and husband, Mark. Thank you for ALWAYS being on my side and loving me. You enrich my life and are such an amazing father to our four kids. I LOVE YOU!

youliveright.com

The health advice presented in this book is intended only as an informative resource guide to help you make informed decisions. It is not meant to replace the advice of a physician or to serve as a guide to self-treatment. Always seek competent medical care for any health condition or if there is any question about the appropriateness of a procedure or health recommendation. The information is not intended to diagnose, prevent, treat or cure any disease.

The author and publisher will in no event be held liable for any loss or other damages, including but not limited to special, incidental, consequential, or any other damages.

Nutritional information is given as a reference and may vary due to differences in sizes, brands, and types of ingredients. Nutritional calculations were done using multiple resources, including the USDA database, and nutritional information provided by the most popular manufacturers of a given food. Nutritional information was rounded to the nearest 0.5 gram.

The author's reference to any brands does not imply endorsement or sponsorship. Product names are the trademarks of their respected owners.

Executive and Managing Editor: Mona Dolgov

Food Photography: Teri Lyn Fisher

Cover and Lifestyle Photography: Emily Dorio, Teri Lyn Fisher

Cover and Book Design: Sarah Conant

ISBN: 978-1-7366756-5-6

Library of Congress Control Number: 2023910790

First Edition

10 9 8 7 6 5 4 3 2 1

YOU
LIVE
RIGHT
PUBLISHERS